2012
YEAR BOOK OF
PLASTIC AND
AESTHETIC SURGERY™

The 2012 Year Book Series

Year Book of Anesthesiology and Pain Management™: Drs Chestnut, Abram, Black, Gravlee, Lien, Mathru, and Roizen

Year Book of Cardiology®: Drs Gersh, Cheitlin, Elliott, Gold, Graham, and Thourani

Year Book of Critical Care Medicine®: Drs Dellinger, Parrillo, Balk, Dorman, Dries, and Zanotti-Cavazzoni

Year Book of Dermatology and Dermatologic Surgery™: Dr Del Rosso

Year Book of Diagnostic Radiology®: Drs Osborn, Abbara, Elster, Manaster, Oestreich, Offiah, Rosado de Christenson, Stephens, and Walker

Year Book of Emergency Medicine®: Drs Hamilton, Bruno, Handly, Mullin, Quintana, and Ramoska

Year Book of Endocrinology®: Drs Schott, Apovian, Clarke, Eugster, Ludlam, Meikle, Schinner, Schteingart, and Toth

Year Book of Gastroenterology™: Drs Talley, DeVault, Harnois, Murray, Pearson, Philcox, Picco, and Smith

Year Book of Hand and Upper Limb Surgery®: Drs Yao and Steinmann

Year Book of Medicine®: Drs Barker, Garrick, Gersh, Khardori, LeRoith, Panush, Talley, and Thigpen

Year Book of Neonatal and Perinatal Medicine®: Drs Fanaroff, Benitz, Donn, Neu, Papile, Polin, and Van Marter

Year Book of Neurology and Neurosurgery®: Drs Klimo and Rabinstein

Year Book of Obstetrics, Gynecology, and Women's Health®: Drs Dungan and Shulman

Year Book of Oncology®: Drs Arceci, Bauer, Chiorean, Gordon, Lawton, Murphy, Thigpen, and Tsao

Year Book of Ophthalmology®: Drs Rapuano, Cohen, Flanders, Fudemberg, Hammersmith, Milman, Myers, Nagra, Nelson, Penne, Pyfer, Sergott, Shields, Talekar, and Vander

Year Book of Orthopedics®: Drs Morrey, Beauchamp, Huddleston, Swiontkowski, and Trigg

Year Book of Otolaryngology-Head and Neck Surgery®: Drs Sindwani, Balough, Franco, Gapany, and Mitchell

Year Book of Pathology and Laboratory Medicine®: Drs Raab, Parwani, Bejarano, and Bissell

Year Book of Pediatrics®: Dr Stockman

Year Book of Plastic and Aesthetic Surgery™: Drs Miller, Gosman, Gurtner, Gutowski, Ruberg, Salisbury, and Smith

Year Book of Psychiatry and Applied Mental Health®: Drs Talbott, Ballenger, Buckley, Frances, Krupnick, and Mack

Year Book of Pulmonary Disease®: Drs Barker, Jones, Maurer, Raza, Tanoue, and Willsie

Year Book of Sports Medicine®: Drs Shephard, Cantu, Feldman, Jankowski, Khan, Lebrun, Nieman, Pierrynowski, and Rowland

Year Book of Surgery®: Drs Copeland, Behrns, Daly, Eberlein, Fahey, Huber, Klodell, Mozingo, and Pruett

Year Book of Urology®: Drs Andriole and Coplen

Year Book of Vascular Surgery®: Drs Moneta, Gillespie, Starnes, and Watkins

2012

The Year Book of PLASTIC AND AESTHETIC SURGERY™

Editor-in-Chief
Stephen H. Miller, MD, MPH
Voluntary Clinical Professor of Surgery and Family Medicine, University of California San Diego, San Diego, California

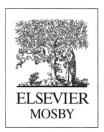

ELSEVIER
MOSBY

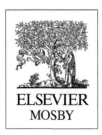

ELSEVIER
MOSBY

Vice President, Continuity: Kimberly Murphy
Editor: Joanne Husovski
Production Manager, Electronic Year Books: Donna M. Skelton
Electronic Article Manager: Mike Sheets
Illustrations and Permissions Coordinator: Dawn Vohsen

2012 EDITION
Copyright 2012, Mosby, Inc. All rights reserved.

Printed and bound by CPI Group (UK) Ltd, Croydon, CR0 4YY

Transferred to Digital Print 2011

Editorial Office:
Elsevier
1600 John F. Kennedy Blvd.
Suite 1800
Philadelphia, PA 19103-2899

International Standard Serial Number: 1535-1513
International Standard Book Number: 978-0-323-08891-6

Table of Contents

Journals Represented

Journals represented in this YEAR BOOK are listed below.

Aesthetic Plastic Surgery
Aesthetic Surgery Journal
Allergy
American Journal of Otolaryngology
American Journal of Sports Medicine
Annals of Otology Rhinology & Laryngology
Annals of Plastic Surgery
Annals of Surgical Oncology
Annals of Thoracic Surgery
Archives of Dermatology
Archives of Facial Plastic Surgery
Archives of Otolaryngology Head & Neck Surgery
Breast Journal
British Journal of Surgery
Burns
Cleft Palate Craniofacial Journal
Dermatologic Surgery
Dermatology
European Journal of Plastic Surgery
Injury
Journal of Burn Care & Research
Journal of Bone & Joint Surgery
Journal of Clinical Oncology
Journal of Hand Surgery
Journal of Hand Surgery (America)
Journal of Oral and Maxillofacial Surgery
Journal of Orthopaedic Research
Journal of Pediatric Surgery
Journal of Plastic Reconstructive & Aesthetic Surgery
Journal of Reconstructive Microsurgery
Journal of Surgical Research
Journal of the American Academy of Dermatology
Journal of the American Medical Association
Journal of the European Academy of Dermatology and Venereology
Journal of the National Cancer Institute
Journal of Trauma
Laryngoscope
Microsurgery
Oral Oncology
Orthopedics
Otolaryngology-Head and Neck Surgery
Otology & Neurotology
Plastic and Reconstructive Surgery

Surgical Oncology
Wound Repair and Regeneration

STANDARD ABBREVIATIONS

The following terms are abbreviated in this edition: acquired immunodeficiency syndrome (AIDS), cardiopulmonary resuscitation (CPR), central nervous system (CNS), cerebrospinal fluid (CSF), computed tomography (CT), deoxyribonucleic acid (DNA), electrocardiography (ECG), health maintenance organization (HMO), human immunodeficiency virus (HIV), intensive care unit (ICU), intramuscular (IM), intravenous (IV), magnetic resonance (MR) imaging (MRI), ribonucleic acid (RNA), ultrasound (US), and ultraviolet (UV).

NOTE

The YEAR BOOK OF PLASTIC AND AESTHETIC SURGERY is a literature survey service providing abstracts of articles published in the professional literature. Every effort is made to assure the accuracy of the information presented in these pages. Neither the editors nor the publisher of the YEAR BOOK OF PLASTIC AND AESTHETIC SURGERY can be responsible for errors in the original materials. The editors' comments are their own opinions. Mention of specific products within this publication does not constitute endorsement.

To facilitate the use of the YEAR BOOK OF PLASTIC AND AESTHETIC SURGERY as a reference tool, all illustrations and tables included in this publication are now identified as they appear in the original article. This change is meant to help the reader recognize that any illustration or table appearing in the YEAR BOOK OF PLASTIC AND AESTHETIC SURGERY may be only one of many in the original article. For this reason, figure and table numbers will often appear to be out of sequence within the YEAR BOOK OF PLASTIC AND AESTHETIC SURGERY.

Introduction

This is the fourth year in which the YEAR BOOK OF PLASTIC AND AESTHETIC SURGERY has been published in electronic on-line and hard-copy formats. It seems evident that the future for dual formats for the YEAR BOOK will be constrained by economics as hard-copy circulation of all of the YEAR BOOK has declined dramatically in the last few years.

Once again, we have had several changes in the associate editorial staff. We welcome Dr Amanda Gosman of the University of California San Diego School of Medicine; she is replacing Dr Arun Gosain. Her responsibility will primarily be in the selection of articles for the congenital section of the YEAR BOOK. We also welcome Dr Jeremy Warner, an associate of Dr Karol Gutkowski. Dr Warner's primary responsibility will be to select articles related to surgery of the nose.

I am grateful for the continuing contributions and support of several of our long-standing associate editors: Drs Geoffrey Gurtner, Karol Gutkowski, Robert Ruberg, Roger Salisbury, and David Smith, Jr. These people have done yeoman's work in combing the plastic surgical literature as well as the literature of related disciplines to select worthwhile articles to review and present to our readership.

I also acknowledge the contributions of several of my plastic surgical colleagues from the University of California San Diego: Drs Marek Dobke, Ralph Holmes, and Mayer Tennenhaus.

Thanks to Joanne Husovski, Senior Clinics Editor with Elsevier, who took over the job of aiding and assisting us. Her gentle reminders were most helpful in encouraging many of the associate editors to meet and in several instances exceed their goals for selections.

One of the highlights this year is that the associate editors have felt free to submit selections in several different areas beyond those to which they had been assigned. Not infrequently, this has resulted in having more than one editor review and critique the same selection, potentially providing the reader with differing viewpoints on the same article.

I call the reader's attention to several noteworthy articles: (1) Venous thromboembolism following microsurgical breast reconstruction: An objective analysis in 225 consecutive patients using low-molecular-weight heparin prophylaxis; (2) Aesthetic and oncologic outcome after microsurgical reconstruction of complex scalp and forehead defects after malignant tumor resection: An algorithm for treatment; (3) Secondary surgery in paediatric facial paralysis reanimation; (4) A 12-year anthropometric evaluation of the nose in bilateral cleft lip-cleft palate patients following nasoalveolar molding and cutting bilateral cleft lip and nose reconstruction; (5) Prevention of acute hematoma after face-lifts; (6) Painless abdominoplasty: The efficacy of combined intercostal and pararectus blocks in reducing postoperative pain and recovery time; (7) Evidence-based recommendations for the use of negative pressure wound therapy in traumatic wounds and reconstructive surgery: Steps towards an international consensus; (8) Breast prostheses and connective tissue disease (CTD): Myth or reality; and (9) Reporting clinical outcomes of breast reconstruction: A systematic review.

Stephen H. Miller, MD, MPH

1 Congenital

Auricular Deformities

Biomechanical Evaluation of Surgical Correction of Prominent Ear
Miyamoto J, Nagasao T, Tamaki T, et al (Keio Univ, Tokyo, Japan)
Plast Reconstr Surg 123:889-896, 2009

Background.—Mustardé sutures and conchal setback are widely used for surgical correction of prominent ear, and numerous cartilage-manipulation techniques accompanying these two methods are also available. However, it is unknown how each technique works biomechanically. The effects of otoplasty were evaluated by finite element analysis.

Methods.—Data of eight prominent ears were obtained with a noncontact three-dimensional digitizer, and three-dimensional auricular cartilage models were produced. These models were modified to cartilage-manipulation models: scaphal-incision, abrasion, conchal-incision, and conchal-excision models. The loads corresponding to Mustardé sutures were then applied to the no-manipulation, scaphal-incision, and abrasion models. Loads corresponding to conchal setback were applied to the no-manipulation, conchal-incision, and conchal-excision models. Stresses and deformed shapes were evaluated using finite element method.

Results.—When Mustardé sutures and conchal setback were compared in the no-manipulation models, maximal stresses occurred around loads in Mustardé sutures and at the root of the helix in conchal setback. The entire ear laid down in conchal setback, whereas in Mustardé sutures, strong bending occurred at the upper third. In Mustardé sutures, maximal stresses decreased to 82 percent with scaphal incision and 95 percent with abrasion. However, the setback effect was also reduced in these two models. In conchal setback, high stresses were markedly decreased with conchal incision or excision. There was no significant difference between incision and excision.

Conclusions.—For successful otoplasty, precise understanding of biomechanical reactions is essential. This study provides improved insight into otoplasty for many surgeons.

▶ The authors of this study have developed an interesting digitized biomechanical model of the prominent ear for evaluating the cartilage stress, tension, and shape deformity associated with different otoplasty techniques. The study looks at 2 common techniques for surgical correction of the prominent ear: restoration of the antihelical fold (Mustardé sutures) and conchal setback. These 2 no-manipulation cartilage technique models are evaluated for the degree and location of maximal stress and also for the resultant change in the shape of the ear on anterior and lateral view when the mechanical load of Mustardé sutures or conchal setback are applied. The authors also evaluate models of different cartilage manipulation techniques, including incision, excision, and abrasion, which were used in conjunction with antihelical fold restoration and/or conchal setback. Cartilage manipulation techniques were analyzed for how effectively they release the tension in the cartilage when mechanical loads are applied, which is important in the prevention of recurrence of a prominent ear deformity.

In comparison of the no-manipulation Mustardé suture versus conchal setback models, the authors found that there were different shape deformities. In the conchal setback model, the ears were wide on lateral view. In the Mustardé suture model, the antihelix was more conspicuous on frontal view because of the strong setback of the superior helix. The Mustardé suture load was applied to the no-manipulation cartilage model, scaphal-incision model, and abrasion models. The abrasion model reduced the cartilage thickness by 50%. Both cartilage manipulation models significantly reduced the maximal stresses compared with the no-manipulation model, and the incision model stress was a significant reduction from the abrasion model. In the scaphal-incision model, the position of the helix did not change position when the load was applied and the cut edges around the suture loads became irregular. In the abrasion model, the setback effect of the helix was reduced in comparison with the no-manipulation model. Both of these cartilage manipulation technique models demonstrated reduction in the tension or maximal stress on the cartilage but also resulted in less-effective helical setback when the load of Mustardé sutures was applied.

In the conchal setback group, the conchal-incision and conchal-excision models had significantly reduced maximal stress compared with the no-manipulation model. All of these techniques demonstrated widening of the ear on lateral view, and there were no significant differences between the degrees of stress reduction for the manipulation techniques.

This study uses a unique biomechanical cartilage model to investigate the effects of load bearing on different cartilage configurations. The authors' analysis provides insight into the balance between effective surgical correction and reducing the tension in the cartilage that may lead to recurrence. As demonstrated in the Mustardé suture models, these are often opposing forces, and manipulation techniques that may reduce the risk of recurrence of the prominent ear also result in a less-effective setback, thus highlighting the importance of understanding these biomechanical forces to achieve the desired lasting effect. Reported shape changes are also an important consideration. Cartilage manipulation with incision or excision in conjunction with conchal setback did effectively reduce the tension in the cartilage; however, widening of the ear on lateral view was demonstrated on all the conchal setback models.

This study is limited in that it represents a theoretical digitized model that does not take into account the influence of the overlying soft tissue and skin. The cartilage response to load application was evaluated in isolation for each technique, and most otoplasty procedures may incorporate more than 1 of these techniques in addition to skin excision. This model did not evaluate the additive effects of conchal setback and Mustardé sutures. However, I think that the results are very representative of the clinical findings of the isolated surgical techniques, and this study helps to clarify the biomechanical effects that should be considered when generating a balanced individual surgical treatment plan for the correction of the prominent ear. Moreover, the cartilage biomechanical model has many potential applications such as in the evaluation of rhinoplasty techniques and tip suturing.

A. Gosman, MD

Bilateral microtia reconstruction
Liu X, Zhang Q, Quan Y, et al (Plastic Surgery Hosp, Peking, China)
J Plast Reconstr Aesth Surg 63:1275-1278, 2010

Background.—Ear reconstruction for congenital microtia is a challenge for the plastic and reconstructive surgeon. Ten percent of microtia cases are bilateral. However, the published literature contains relatively little information about auricular reconstruction in bilateral microtia. Some authorities prefer to reconstruct each side at different stages. In this article, we introduce an operative method to reconstruct both sides simultaneously. This is completely feasible, and saves time and cost. Furthermore, this method allows comparison between sides during surgery, and facilitates carving of bilateral ear frameworks of equal size and shape.

Methods.—From March 2007 to June 2008, 21 cases of congenital bilateral microtia were treated by post-auricular skin flap expansion, autogenous rib cartilage framework implantation, post-auricular fascial flap lifting, followed by split-thickness free skin grafting to reconstruct bilateral external ears during the same stage.

Results.—With a follow-up duration of 6 months to 1 year, two cases in a total of 21 showed different levels of absorption and cartilage deformation. The rest (19 cases) of the bilateral reconstructed ears showed good symmetry in size, shape and location. The bilateral reconstructed ears looked symmetrical and similar in outline, with well-defined structures.

Conclusion.—Simultaneous bilateral congenital microtia reconstruction is feasible and effective. The authors recommend it as the treatment of choice for bilateral microtia reconstruction.

▶ Plastic surgeons continually strive to achieve reconstructive goals with as few surgeries as possible, and this article is an excellent example of that effort. The authors use the same 3-stage technique that they use for unilateral microtia reconstruction at their institution.[1] However, in this 21-patient series, they performed ear reconstructions on both sides at the same time. In stage I, bilateral tissue expanders are inserted and expanded. In stage II, bilateral rib cartilage grafts are harvested, carved, positioned, and covered with the expanded mastoid skin, post-auricular fascial flap, and split-thickness skin graft. In stage III, both sides undergo removal of the vestigial cartilage remnant, formation of a tragus, and deepening of the conchal bowl. The major upside is the decreased patient burden of undergoing 3 rather than 6 surgeries. And the major downside is the increased patient burden of dealing with twice the discomfort for stages I and II. During stage I, bilateral tissue expanders limit head positioning, require greater cooperation of the child, and may increase the potential for complications if cooperation is not optimal. In stage II, bilateral rib cartilage donor sites increase postoperative pain and limited head positioning continues to be required to minimize the ischemic effect of pressure on the expanded skin now draped over the new framework. Only in stage III is the added burden inconsequential. The Brent's 4-stage technique could similarly be used to reconstruct bilateral microtia in 4 surgeries, again with twice the discomfort for stages I and III. Stages II and IV are already routinely performed bilaterally. However, in my experience, minimizing discomfort is very important to maintain the enthusiasm of the child for subsequent procedures. The authors are to be applauded for their efforts, and I wonder if they have considered sequencing their stages to increase patient comfort. Tissue expansion on one side could be followed in the second surgery with a cartilage framework on the same side and insertion of a tissue expander in the contralateral side. During the 1 or 2 weeks before expansion begins, the patient can lie on that side. After the third surgery, the child can easily lie on the side undergoing stage III, thus protecting the side undergoing stage II and reducing the risk of complications. Discomfort would be reduced at the burden of 1 additional surgical procedure.

R. E. Holmes, MD

Reference

1. Jiang H, Pan B, Lin L, Cai Z, Zhuang H. Ten-year experience in microtia reconstruction using tissue expander and autogenous cartilage. *Int J Pediatr Otorhinolaryngol.* 2008;72:1251-1259.

Donor site reconstitution for ear reconstruction
Fattah A, Sebire NJ, Bulstrode NW (Great Ormond St Hosp for Children NHS Trust, London, UK)
J Plast Reconstr Aesth Surg 63:1459-1465, 2010

Background.—Current techniques of autologous ear reconstruction involve the soft tissue coverage of a carved costal cartilage framework. However, assessment of the morbidity associated with this donor site has been little documented. This study describes a method to reconstruct the defect and analyses the outcomes with or without donor site reconstruction.

Methods.—The donor site was reconstituted by wrapping morcelised cartilage in a vicryl mesh. Twenty-one patients with reconstitution and nine without were recruited to the study. Scar quality and length, dimensions of donor defect and visible deformity were recorded according to a modified Vancouver scar scale. Patients were also assessed by the SF36 questionnaire, a well-validated health survey. In a subset of our study group, we assessed the fate of the donor site reconstitution by direct visualisation *in situ* and histological analysis.

Results.—Fifteen donor sites of patients without donor site reconstitution were compared to 23 reconstructed donor sites. In those without, all had a palpable defect with nearly half exhibiting visible chest deformity. In contrast, those that had rib reconstitution did not demonstrate significant chest wall deformity. Intraoperative examination demonstrated formation of a neo-rib, histologically proven to comprise hyaline cartilage admixed with fibrous tissue. Analysis of SF36 results showed a higher satisfaction in the reconstituted group, but in both groups, the donor site was of little overall morbidity.

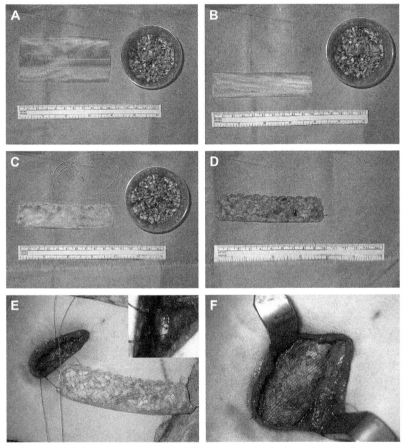

FIGURE 1.—Method of rib reconstitution. A. Vicryl mesh and morcelised cartilage. B. Mesh is folded in half lengthwise. C. Two sides are sutured. D. The mesh is packed with cartilage and closed to create a 'sausage'. E. 'Sausage' is inset by 'parachuting' it down onto the cut end of the ninth rib. It is then sutured medially to the 5th rib. Inset: two vicryl sutures through the synchondrosis of the rib. F. 'Sausage' *in situ* prior to repair of rectus sheath and wound closure. Note the intact rectus abdominis medially in the wound. (Reprinted from Fattah A, Sebire NJ, Bulstrode NW. Donor site reconstitution for ear reconstruction. *J Plast Reconstr Aesthet Surg.* 2010;63:1459-1465, with permission from British Association of Plastic, Reconstructive and Aesthetic Surgeons.)

Conclusions.—Although there is little difference between the groups in terms of subjectively perceived benefit, rib reconstitution is objectively associated with better costal margin contour and less chest wall deformity (Fig 1).

▶ This is an interesting and apparently successful approach to dealing with the obvious donor site deformity that results from harvesting rib cartilage for ear reconstruction. The concept of creating a minor deformity in a less noticed area to correct a major readily visible deformity is a basic tenet of plastic surgery. Yet if one, with little risk, can minimize even that minor deformity, should the technique not be considered? The authors' use of the discarded pieces of costal cartilage made into a sausage using vicryl mesh, as the external sausage casing, seems to limit the contour deformities usually seen after rib cartilage harvest[1] as well as clicking at the site. In future studies, it would be desirable for the authors to document the increased operative time and cost necessary for this technique as compared with not performing reconstruction of the donor sites. In future studies, preoperative short form (SF)-36 evaluations can be compared with postoperative SF-36, which was not possible in this retrospective review. It might also be worthwhile to the postoperative evaluations performed by others rather than the surgeon who developed the technique.

S. H. Miller, MD, MPH

Reference

1. Uppal RS, Sabbagh W, Chana J, et al. Donor site morbidity after autologous cartilage harvest in ear reconstruction and approaches to reducing donor-site contour deformity. *Plast Reconstr Surg.* 2008;121:1949e55.

A New Postoperative Otoplasty Dressing Technique Using Cyanoacrylate Tissue Adhesives

Vetter M, Foehn M, Wedler V (Kantonsspital Frauenfeld, Switzerland)
Aesth Plast Surg 34:212-213, 2010

There are many techniques for cosmetic surgery of the ears and also many different procedures for postoperative treatment. The postoperative dressing is described as important for a successful outcome. We present our method of postoperative dressing in the form of liquid bonding. Cyanoacrylate tissue adhesives as liquid bonding agents are used for fixation of the pinna at the mastoid area. After 10–14 days the bonding can be easily removed. No huge dressings, tapes, or plasters are necessary. The patients are satisfied with the light dressing; they do not feel ashamed to appear in public. We have found this dressing technique to be simple and economical, especially because of the use of the bonding for skin closure before. It can be used after otoplasty with an anterior or a posterior approach.

▶ Theoretically, this technique for bandaging an ear after otoplasty is appealing, but does it really prevent postoperative hematomas in children and adults? Is the postoperative shape and position maintained with this type of dressing, especially in young children? The authors did not provide us with the number of patients on whom this has been used and, other than to state that most of their patients are adults, did not give us any indication of how many children have had this type of dressing. Nonetheless, considering the drawbacks of using bulky ear dressings with elasticized bandages, this technique is worthy of further study.

S. H. Miller, MD, MPH

Cleft Lip and Palate

A 12-Year Anthropometric Evaluation of the Nose in Bilateral Cleft Lip—Cleft Palate Patients following Nasoalveolar Molding and Cutting Bilateral Cleft Lip and Nose Reconstruction

Garfinkle JS, King TW, Grayson BH et al (Oregon Health and Science Univ, Portland; Univ of Wisconsin School of Medicine and Public Health, Madison; New York Univ Med Ctr)
Plast Reconstr Surg 127:1659-1667, 2011

Background.—Patients with bilateral cleft lip—cleft palate have nasal deformities including reduced nasal tip projection, widened ala base, and a deficient or absent columella. The authors compare the nasal morphology of patients treated with presurgical nasoalveolar molding followed by primary lip/nasal reconstruction with age-matched noncleft controls.

Methods.—A longitudinal, retrospective review of 77 nonsyndromic patients with bilateral cleft lip—cleft palate was performed. Nasal tip protrusion, alar base width, alar width, columella length, and columella width were measured at five time points spanning 12.5 years. A one-sample *t* test was used for statistical comparison to an age-matched non cleft population published by Farkas.

Results.—All five measurements demonstrated parallel, proportional growth in the treatment group relative to the noncleft group. The nasal tip protrusion, alar base width, alar width, columella length, and columella width were not statistically different from those of the noncleft, age-matched control group at age 12.5 years. The nasal tip protrusion also showed no difference in length at 7 and 12.5 years. The alar width and alar base width were significantly wider at the first four time points.

Conclusions.—This is the first study to describe nasal morphology following nasoalveolar molding and primary surgical repair in patients with bilateral cleft lip—cleft palate through the age of 12.5 years. In this investigation, the authors have shown that patients with bilateral cleft lip—cleft palate treated at their institution with nasoalveolar molding and primary nasal reconstruction, performed at the time of their lip repair, attained nearly normal nasal morphology through 12.5 years of age.

▶ This article reports the most extensive long-term follow-up (12.5 years) comparison of the nasal morphology in patients with bilateral cleft lip and palate treated with nasoalveolar molding (NAM), followed by cutting primary cleft lip and nasal repair with age-matched noncleft controls. Anthropometric analysis was performed on nasal casts of patients at 5 different time points and compared with the age-matched noncleft controls published by Farkas. At the age of 12.5 years, the difference in the 5 anthropometric measurements in the 2 groups was not significant, and the authors state that the treatment group appears to be on a parallel growth curve with the controls (Fig 5 in the original article).

The anthropometric trend of alar base width and alar width has specific clinical significance. For the first 4 time points, these anthropometric parameters were of significantly greater width in the treatment group versus the control group. However, at the last time point (12.5 years), this difference was no longer statistically significant for either parameter. According to the authors, these data imply that they might need to further decrease the alar base width and alar width at the time of primary reconstruction.

The clinical results and anthropometric data in this study are impressive and strongly support the effectiveness of NAM and Cutting primary nasal reconstruction (Fig 1 in the original article). The patients in the study have not had any additional surgical procedures on the nose other than the primary reconstruction. One of the shortcomings of the study is the decreasing sample size at each subsequent time point. The sample size at the last time point (12.5 years) is only 9 patients, which may contribute to the lack of statistically significant differences detected in this oldest group.

A. Gosman, MD

A Microcosting Approach for Isolated, Unilateral Cleft Lip Care in the First Year of Life

Abbott MM, Meara JG (Children's Hosp Boston, MA; Massachusetts Eye and Ear Infirmary, Boston)
Plast Reconstr Surg 127:333-339, 2011

Background.—The concept of value-based health care underlies many new improvement initiatives in U.S. health care. To determine value, accurate measures of both outcomes and costs are essential, which may then be compared for the same provider or system over time or between providers, to foster improvement. Although outcomes measurement has received a great deal of attention since the quality movement began in the United States, costing methodologies are lacking.

Methods.—A basic microcosting methodology was used to obtain direct medical costs, including physician compensation, for individuals with isolated, unilateral cleft lip deformity receiving their full course of care from one surgeon. The authors analyzed costs associated with the timeline of care during the first year of life.

Results.—The median cost for the first year of life was $13,013 (range, $10,426 to $16,115; $n = 12$). Ninety-one percent of costs were associated with the cleft lip repair, which occurred at a median age of 3.7 months.

The majority of these costs stemmed from time in the operating room and the inpatient stay, which accounted for 68 and 19 percent of first-year costs, respectively.

Conclusions.—Using a microcosting approach, the authors identified specific cost drivers and outlined a distinct timeline of care for patients with isolated cleft lip in the first year of life. This approach may serve as a template for the cost side of the value equation, for which accurate methodologies are needed. When combined with key outcomes measures, it will be possible to measure and improve value at the patient and provider levels.

▶ This is a timely article that uses costing methodologies to identify components of care that drive costs for patients who undergo unilateral cleft lip repair during the first year of life. In the current climate of health care reform, providers are required to become involved in the fiscal responsibility of their practice. In the evolving system of value-based health care, providers and health care systems will be evaluated based on patient-centered outcomes and the cost of care over the duration of a patient's treatment. It is important that physicians and surgeons participate in the cost conversion side of this value equation to ensure that the quality of care does not suffer and that all aspects of care are included in the calculations.

The goal of this study is to define specific costs that can be linked to outcomes to determine where value may be improved for a patient. Microcosting measures discrete resources used by patients over a continuum of care, and the authors contend that this is the best method for determining drivers of cost and potential areas for value improvement. Microcosting methodology is applied in this study to the least complex subtype of cleft—the isolated cleft lip. A detailed analysis of hospital and physician costs is performed, and the authors calculated what percentage of the total cost was attributed to each component of the care provided. Time was identified as the main driver of cost for the operating room costs (facility and staff costs greater than equipment and medication), physician reimbursement (anesthesia greater than surgeon), and inpatient stay.

This study is an important contribution toward the development of useful methodologies for evaluating the cost of plastic surgery procedures. The shortcomings of this analysis are that the costs measured are not complete and that the cycle of care analyzed is only 1 year. Furthermore, to truly evaluate the value of the care provided by this single-surgeon sample, the cost data will have to be correlated with outcome measures. However, the development of accurate costing methodology is an important step toward the assessment of value-based health care in plastic surgery.

A. Gosman, MD

A New Yardstick for Rating Dental Arch Relationship in Patients With Complete Bilateral Cleft Lip and Palate

Ozawa TO, Shaw WC, Katsaros C, et al (Univ of São Paulo, Bauru, Brazil; Univ of Manchester, UK; Univ of Bern, Switzerland; et al)
Cleft Palate Craniofac J 48:167-172, 2011

Objective.—To develop yardsticks for assessment of dental arch relationship in young individuals with repaired complete bilateral cleft lip and palate appropriate to different stages of dental development.

Participants.—Eleven cleft team orthodontists from five countries worked on the projects for 4 days. A total of 776 sets of standardized plaster models from 411 patients with operated complete bilateral cleft lip and palate were available for the exercise.

Statistics.—The interexaminer reliability was calculated using weighted kappa statistics.

Results.—The interrater weighted kappa scores were between .74 and .92, which is in the "good" to "very good" categories.

Conclusions.—Three bilateral cleft lip and palate yardsticks for different developmental stages of the dentition were made: one for the deciduous dentition (6-year-olds' yardstick), one for early mixed dentition (9-year-olds' yardstick), and one for early permanent dentition (12-year-olds' yardstick).

▶ This study marks an important accomplishment in the international effort to evaluate outcomes and provide evidence-based treatment for children with cleft lip and palate. The authors are an international team of cleft orthodontists who have collaborated to develop a reliable tool for assessing the dental arch relationships for patients with bilateral cleft lip and palate at 3 different development stages. Although instruments are available for assessing the treatment outcomes in patients with unilateral cleft lip and palate, no such standardized tool exists to the evaluation of bilateral cleft lip and palate. This new yardstick will be important in assessing the dental arch outcomes and comparing different treatment protocols for patients with bilateral cleft lip and palate. Although the bilateral deformity is less common, it has been particularly amenable to newer treatment modalities such as infant nasoalveolar molding and passive columellar lengthening. It will be important to assess the growth and dental arch relationships as an outcome measure in this particular subset of patients and in all patients with bilateral cleft lip and palate to optimize treatment protocols.

A. Gosman, MD

Prevalence at Birth of Cleft Lip With or Without Cleft Palate: Data From the International Perinatal Database of Typical Oral Clefts (IPDTOC)

IPDTOC Working Group (ICBDSR Centre, Rome, Italy; et al)
Cleft Palate Craniofac J 48:66-81, 2011

As part of a collaborative project on the epidemiology of craniofacial anomalies, funded by the National Institutes for Dental and Craniofacial Research and channeled through the Human Genetics Programme of the World Health Organization, the International Perinatal Database of Typical Orofacial Clefts (IPDTOC) was established in 2003. IPDTOC is collecting case-by-case information on cleft lip with or without cleft palate and on cleft palate alone from birth defects registries contributing to at least one of three collaborative organizations: European Surveillance Systems of Congenital Anomalies (EUROCAT) in Europe, National Birth Defects Prevention Network (NBDPN) in the United States, and International Clearinghouse for Birth Defects Surveillance and Research (ICBDSR) worldwide. Analysis of the collected information is performed centrally at the ICBDSR Centre in Rome, Italy, to maximize the comparability of results. The present paper, the first of a series, reports data on the prevalence of cleft lip with or without cleft palate from 54 registries in 30 countries over at least 1 complete year during the period 2000 to 2005. Thus, the denominator comprises more than 7.5 million births. A total of 7704 cases of cleft lip with or without cleft palate (7141 livebirths, 237 stillbirths, 301 terminations of pregnancy, and 25 with pregnancy outcome unknown) were available. The overall prevalence of cleft lip with or without cleft palate was 9.92 per 10,000. The prevalence of cleft lip was 3.28 per 10,000, and that of cleft lip and palate was 6.64 per 10,000. There were 5918 cases (76.8%) that were isolated, 1224 (15.9%) had malformations in other systems, and 562 (7.3%) occurred as part of recognized syndromes. Cases with greater dysmorphological severity of cleft lip with or without cleft palate were more likely to include malformations of other systems.

▶ This is an impressive collaboration of international registries to analyze the prevalence of typical orofacial clefts. The primary aim of the study was to document international variation in the prevalence of cleft lip and palate (CLP), according to a standardized protocol. Registries were analyzed individually and grouped into 11 geographic areas. An evaluation of the 11 geographic areas showed that the registries in Japan, Mexico-South America, Western Europe, and Canada had a statistically higher prevalence than the overall estimate of 9.2 per 10 000 births. Registries in Eastern Europe, South-Mediterranean Europe, and South Africa had a statistically lower prevalence (Fig 1 in the original article). In Europe, 34 registries demonstrated a statistically significant correlation between CLP prevalence and the latitude of the largest city in the catchment area for total and isolated cases, but not for multiple malformed cases or syndromes. The proportion of CLP of the total CLP cases was statistically significantly higher than the total estimate of 66.9% in Mexico-South America and in the United States, whereas in Eastern Europe, the British Isles, and South-Mediterranean Europe, it is slightly lower (Fig 4 in the original article). In 9 geographic areas, the CLP prevalence correlated with the proportion of all cases of CLP out of the total CLP ($P = .0025$), which supports previous reports and the model predicting that the higher the overall CLP prevalence, the greater the genetic liability within that particular gene pool and therefore the more CLP as opposed to cleft lip. The International Perinatal Database of Typical Orofacial Clefts initiative is an excellent example of the importance of international cooperation among cleft registries to collect accurate data. The collaborators discuss the shortcomings of their data collection and caution against extrapolation of data from specific registry areas to an entire country.

A. Gosman, MD

Revision of pharyngeal flaps causing obstructive airway symptoms: An analysis of treatment with three different techniques over 39 years

Por Y-C, Tan Y-C, Chang FC-S, et al (Kandang Kerbau Women's and Children's Hosp, Singapore; Chang Gung Univ, Taiwan)
J Plast Reconstr Aesth Surg 63:930-933, 2010

Background.—Pharyngeal flaps are used to treat velopharyngeal insufficiency. Occasionally the flap exceeds its intended function and results in an obstructive airway. In this article, the results of management of these cases are analysed.

Methods.—This is a 39-year retrospective review of patients who had revision of pharyngeal flaps causing obstructive airway symptoms. Three methods of relieving the airway obstruction were used, and the patients were thus separated into three groups, namely group 1 (release and Z-plasty of the lateral ports), group 2 (division of the pharyngeal flap) and group 3 (division of the pharyngeal flap combined with Furlow palatoplasty). The results obtained were based on four parameters: symptomatic improvement, velopharyngeal sufficiency, the presence of re-attachment of the pharyngeal flap and the necessity for re-operation. These results were then pooled into two groups: 'good result' and 'bad result'. The respiratory disturbance index (RDI) was also obtained and analysed separately. Statistical analysis was performed with the Fisher's exact test and the paired t-test in SPSS v.11.

Results.—A total of 44 patients were included in the study. There were 20, 11 and 13 patients in groups 1, 2 and 3, respectively. The Pearson's chi-square test indicated that group 3 patients had a statistically significant proportion of 'good results' when compared to groups 1 ($p = 0.019$) and 2 ($p = 0.004$). There was a statistically significant reduction in RDI in group 3 ($p = 0.003$). There was no statistically significant difference between the groups 1 and 2.

Conclusions.—Division of a pharyngeal flap for obstructive airway complications should be accompanied by a Furlow palatoplasty to reduce the myriad complications that arise from either a release + Z-plasty or a simple division of the pharyngeal flap.

▶ Generally speaking, in my experience, failures secondary to surgery for velopharyngeal incompetence (VPI) typically are more likely continued VPI rather than airway obstruction. Once faced with the problem of chronic airway obstruction, that which exists beyond the immediate postoperative period and usually results from edema, the surgeon must determine the degree of obstruction and the best remedy. The authors of this study clearly suggest that in their hands, at least those of the senior author, the best results can be achieved by dividing the flap and performing a Furlow palatoplasty. My experience leads me to accept the premise espoused, but clearly this study's retrospective nature, involving pharyngeal flaps performed by many different surgeons, inability to assess the degree of postflap obstruction, the cause of postflap obstruction, and any variability amongst the patients and surgeons performing the secondary surgery make it difficult to assess the comparisons made.

S. H. Miller, MD, MPH

Cranio-Maxillo-Facial

Influence of Bone-Derived Matrices on Generation of Bone in an Ectopic Rat Model

Bahar H, Yaffe A, Boskey A, et al (Tel Aviv Univ, Israel; Hebrew Univ Hadassah School, Jerusalem, Israel; Hosp for Special Surgery, NY)
J Orthop Res 28:664-670, 2010

Most bone regeneration experimental models that test bone-derived matrices take place in conjunction with the native bone. Here, we compared the relative effectiveness of bone matrix components on bone-marrow-directed osteogenesis in an ectopic model. Cortical bone cylinders consisted of diaphysis of DA rat femurs. They were either demineralized (DBM), deproteinized (HABM), or nontreated (MBM). Fresh bone marrow was placed into cylinders and implanted at subcutaneous thoracic sites of 2-month-old DA rats. At designated times the cylinders were surgically removed from the animals. Microradiographs of DBM and histology of DBM and MBM cylinders demonstrated progressive increase in mineralized bone volume and its trabecular configuration. Bone filled the inner volume of DBM and MBM cylinders within 4 weeks, while in HABM cylinders mostly granulation tissue developed. In the DBM cylinders cartilage deposited within 10 days, while in the MBM cylinders bone was directly deposited. As early as day 3 after marrow transplantation, marrow cells interacting with DBM increased significantly the genes that express the cartilage and the bone phenotype. In conclusion, organic components of bone are needed for marrow-directed osteogenesis.

▶ This experimental comparison of the effectiveness of bone matrix components on bone marrow—directed osteogenesis in an ectopic model yields interesting conclusions. The experimental model evaluates osteogenesis in demineralized (demineralized bone matrix [DBM]), deproteinized (hydroxyapatite bone mineral matrix [HABM]), or nontreated (mineralized bone matrix [MBM]) cortical bone cylinders that were filled with fresh bone marrow and implanted subcutaneously in rats. In the nontreated (MBM) cylinders, the interaction with bone marrow cells stimulated osteogenesis and the development of woven trabecular bone without developing cartilage. In the demineralized bone (DBM) cylinders filled with bone marrow cells, cartilage developed first, followed by trabecular bone formation. No bone or cartilage was observed on the inner or outer surface of DBM cylinders that were not filled with bone marrow. In contrast to some reports that ceramic hydroxyapatite (HA) has the capability to support osteogenic differentiation when combined with mesenchymal stem cells (see references 26-29 in original article), the deproteinized (HABM) cylinder composed of mostly mineral components (HA) in this model did not form any bone when filled with bone marrow cells. The authors conclude that the organic bone matrix components, not just a mineral scaffold, are required to effectively interact with bone marrow cells and result in bone formation.

A. Gosman, MD

Distraction Osteogenesis of Costocartilaginous Rib Grafts and Treatment Algorithm for Severely Hypoplastic Mandibles
Wan DC, Taub PJ, Allam KA, et al (Univ of California, Los Angeles; Los Angeles Med Ctr, CA; Mount Sinai Med Ctr, NY)
Plast Reconstr Surg 127:2005-2013, 2011

Background.—In craniofacial microsomia, patients with severely hypoplastic mandibles (Pruzansky type III) require replacement of the ramus and condyle unit. Autogenous costocartilaginous rib graft and distraction osteogenesis are the most important techniques used, but long-term results need to be looked at to determine optimal management.

Methods.—Of the 485 patients with craniofacial microsomia and mandibular abnormality identified by the authors' craniofacial multidisciplinary clinic, 31 patients were identified with Pruzansky type III mandibles who underwent treatment and were available for study. Patients primarily had either costocartilaginous grafts or mandibular distraction after molar extraction. Outcomes assessed rib failure, undergrowth, or overgrowth. Reoperation included regrafting for graft failure, rib distraction for undergrowth, and mandibular setback for overgrowth. Details surrounding complications for each modality including osteotomy site were recorded.

Results.—For primary mandibular reconstruction, 27 patients underwent costocartilaginous rib graft surgery (30 grafts, three bilateral) at 9.9 ± 4.1 years; four patients underwent mandibular distraction at 7.4 ± 2.3 years. Rib graft failure in seven of 30 cases (23 percent) required regrafting. Undergrowth in 17 cases (57 percent) required rib distraction. Overgrowth in three cases (10 percent) required correction at the time of orthognathic correction. For rib graft distraction, osteotomy site locations included native mandible (25 percent), rib-mandible junction (19 percent), and rib graft (56 percent). The rib-mandible junction site had graft-related complications (100 percent) that the other sites did not.

Conclusions.—For the severely hypoplastic mandibles (Pruzansky type III), costocartilaginous grafts are an accepted modality. However, when rib graft growth is insufficient, secondary distraction should be performed within the native mandible or rib graft and not at the rib graft-mandible junction site.

▶ Osteocartilaginous rib grafts for patients with Pruzansky type III craniofacial microsomia have become the accepted standard of care. Based on this study, these authors are now able to provide additional information about the success rate of this procedure and offer useful guidelines for the treatment of cases in which the result has been less than optimal. It is important to note when counseling patients and families that more than three-fourths of the graft cases required additional surgical treatment before an optimal result was achieved. The authors' documentation of 100% complications when distraction is done at the rib-mandible junction site is at first surprising, because this site already has evidence of adequate bone healing of the initial graft. The authors provide an explanation for this phenomenon (cellular mismatch) and advise using an alternative distraction site. The algorithm described by the authors in this article provides a useful, logical approach to this sometimes challenging problem.

R. L. Ruberg, MD

Miscellaneous

Poland Syndrome: Evaluation and Treatment of the Chest Wall in 63 Patients

Seyfer AE, Fox JP, Hamilton CG (F. Edward Hebert School of Medicine, Bethesda, MD; Walter Reed Army Med Ctr; Wright State Univ and Wright-Patterson U.S. Air Force Med Ctr, Dayton, OH; et al)
Plast Reconstr Surg 126:902-911, 2010

Background.—Poland syndrome is a sporadic, congenital unilateral absence of the sternocostal head of the pectoralis major muscle that can occur with other ipsilateral chest wall and limb derangements. The chest wall deficiency is primarily cosmetic, its incidence is unknown, male patients may be affected more than female patients, the right side is affected more than the left, and associated comorbidities may exist. Chest wall repair depends on anatomical type and gender.

Methods.—Sixty-three patients with Poland syndrome were divided into two treatment groups by chest wall anatomy and gender. Surgical repair was based on this division. Seventy-six operations were performed by the senior author (A.E.S.) during a 30-year period, and long-term outcomes are presented. Corrective methods included use of custom-made chest wall prostheses, mammary prostheses, latissimus dorsi muscle transfers, transverse rectus abdominis musculocutaneous flaps, sternal/rib reconstruction, or a combination of methods. Follow-up ranged from 1 to 21 years.

TABLE 5.—Chest Wall Repair of Poland Syndrome Based on Gender and Severity

	Type of Repair
Male patients	
Simple form	Latissimus dorsi transfer* alone
Complex form	Chest wall repair with latissimus transfer*
Female patients	
Simple form	Latissimus transfer with breast prostheses[†]
Complex form	Chest wall repair with latissimus transfer[†] and breast prostheses

*A total of 11 latissimus transfers were performed on male patients.
[†]A total of seven latissimus transfers were performed on female patients.

Results.—Two anatomical forms of the disorder are described, each with unique surgical requirements. The *simple* deformity was effectively repaired with a latissimus dorsi muscle transfer plus, in female patients, a sublatissimus mammary prosthesis. Repair of the *complex* deformity, in addition to the latissimus transfer, selectively included musculoskeletal chest wall realignment. Custom-made chest wall prostheses carried a higher risk of complications.

Conclusions.—Poland syndrome of the chest wall exists in two forms: the more common *simple* variety and a *complex* form (as originally described by Poland). Repair of the chest wall can be effectively tailored to these anatomical types, gender, and patient preference (Table 5).

▶ This article is valuable from a number of perspectives. First of all, it represents a critically evaluated single-surgeon large volume experience (63 patients) in the management of this sometimes challenging problem. Secondly, it provides a carefully outlined approach to surgical correction that is tailored to both the deformity and the gender of the patient. Finally, it provides a summary of useful procedures for assessing various anatomic aspects of the Poland syndrome deformity. The authors note that some of the approaches historically used for the chest wall deformity, namely, custom prostheses, were less than satisfactory, especially from a patient comfort standpoint. An aggressive direct approach to correcting the chest wall appears to have significant benefit, as illustrated by photos in the article. One aspect of the surgical approach to this problem, which was only minimally addressed in the article, was the necessity of creating additional scars for full correction of the complex deformity. When significant bony rearrangement of the thorax is needed in a woman, a midline scar might create aesthetic concerns. The only photographic example of the correction of this type of problem was in a male patient. No other views of the attendant scars are provided. The authors mention the possibility of using endoscopic techniques for muscle harvest but don't indicate whether this was done in any of their cases. Because the objective of this surgery is largely aesthetic improvement, modern endoscopic techniques could certainly be applied to these patients with additional cosmetic benefit.

R. L. Ruberg, MD

2 Neoplastic, Inflammatory and Degenerative Conditions

Benign and Malignant Tumors of the Skin

Mohs micrographic surgery at the Skin and Cancer Foundation Australia, 10 years later (1997 vs 2007)
Lim P, Paver R, Peñas PF (Kuala Lumpur Hosp, Malaysia; Skin and Cancer Foundation Australia, Westmead)
J Am Acad Dermatol 63:832-835, 2010

Background.—Mohs micrographic surgery (MMS) provides a combination of high cure rate and tissue conservation. Epidemiologic factors and changes in techniques may affect the way MMS is performed.

Objective.—We sought to evaluate changes over time in the type of patients and skin cancers that are treated using MMS, and the repairs used to close the defects.

Methods.—We conducted a retrospective study on patients treated with MMS at the Skin and Cancer Foundation Australia, Westmead, in 1997 against those treated in 2007. Patient demographics (age, sex), pathology of tumor, anatomic site of the tumor, preoperative tumor size, postoperative defect size, and repair method were analyzed.

Results.—There was a 260% increase in the number of procedures (596 in 1997 vs 1587 in 2007). The 2007 cohort was a little older (62 vs 64 years), but there were no differences in sex, anatomic site, rate of basal/squamous cell carcinoma, squamous cell carcinoma histologic subtypes, or preoperative tumor size. However, there were fewer superficial basal cell carcinomas, and the postoperative defect size was smaller in 2007 ($P < .0001$). There was also a decrease in the use of grafts and second-intention healing to close the defects and an increase in the number of side-to-side closures ($P < .0001$).

Limitations.—Retrospective study at one institution is a limitation.

Conclusion.—Although tumor size and the percentage of tumors in each anatomic site did not change over 10 years, the size of the defect created after MMS has become smaller. This reduction in defect size may explain why more defects are now repaired by side-to-side closure and flap repairs whereas fewer defects are repaired by skin grafting.

▶ This is an interesting comparison in trends of Mohs micrographic surgery. The 260% increase and increased number of primary closures probably directly reflect the number of dermatologists trained to do this procedure. What is not addressed is the cost-effectiveness. If we are going to stay competitive, true outcomes must be generated, or this part of our practice will be lost.

D. J. Smith, Jr, MD

Facial Paralysis

Computerized Objective Measurement of Facial Motion: Normal Variation and Test-Retest Reliability

Neely JG, Wang KX, Shapland CA, et al (Washington Univ School of Medicine, St Louis, MO; Students and Teachers as Res Scientists (STARS) Program for High School Scholars, St Louis, MO)

Otol Neurotol 31:1488-1492, 2010

Objective.—Objective quantitative measurements of facial motion for the assessment of outcomes in patients with facial paralysis have been elusive. This paper will reintroduce an objective computerized program for measurement of facial motion and present data on symmetry in healthy subjects and test-retest reliability in patients with facial paralysis.

Study Design.—Cross-sectional analysis of archived images.

Setting.—Tertiary referral center.

Patients.—Good quality video-recordings of 38 healthy subjects and 30 facial paralysis subjects with a wide range of paralysis that had been tested twice were selected.

Intervention.—Using image subtraction techniques of digital video recordings, computer-generated strength-duration curves of prescribed facial movements were automatically constructed.

Main Outcome Measures.—The areas under the curve for specific regions of each side of the face were compared as a proportion described as a percentage (left/right in healthy subjects, abnormal/normal side in paralysis) in which 100% would be perfect symmetry.

Results.—Thirty-eight healthy subjects had the following left/right symmetry means (95% confidence interval): brow, 98.95 (93.94–103.95); eye, 99.18 (96.31–102.06); and mouth, 96.87 (93.10–100.63). Thirty patients with varying degrees of facial paralysis, tested twice, were evaluated to determine the degree of agreement between trials as measured by the intraclass correlation coefficient. The results showed the intraclass correlation coefficient (95% confidence interval) for brow was 0.972 (0.943–0.987), eye 0.950 (0.898–0.976), and mouth 0.951 (0.901–0.976).

Conclusion.—These results demonstrate no substantial side bias in healthy subjects and excellent test-retest reliability in patients with facial paralysis. This program may be made available for interested investigators upon request.

▶ One of the most difficult problems for surgeons to assess is the results achieved after performing surgery to alleviate the stigmata of facial paralysis. Still photographs, even in rapid sequence, fail to capture the nuances of facial movements, and using video to demonstrate results is cumbersome and impractical when dealing with many patients. Moreover, results can't be replicated or duplicated frequently by one's own team, much less others. Development of a system that allows computer-assisted analysis of digital video recordings seems to be a promising solution. In this early study, the authors suggest that their technique, Facial Analysis Computerized Evaluation, demonstrates no or little bias in side-to-side measurements of health subjects and good test-retest reliability in 30 patients with facial paralysis. Another group has also reported using similar techniques.[1] It is quite evident that the protocols for the collection of data, including standardization of the techniques for video capture, are essential to generalize these techniques and have other centers begin to use them for further study. At the very least, one would hope that the 2 centers currently using these techniques will collaborate in the near future to develop appropriate protocols to evaluate the effectiveness and efficacy of these techniques.

S. H. Miller, MD, MPH

Reference

1. Meier-Gallati V, Scriba H, Fisch U. Objective scaling of facial nerve function based on area analysis (OSCAR). *Otolaryngol Head Neck Surg.* 1998;118:545-550.

A systematic algorithm for the management of lower lip asymmetry

Lindsay RW, Edwards C, Smitson C, et al (Massachusetts Eye and Ear Infirmary and Harvard Med School, Boston)
Am J Otolaryngol 32:1-7, 2011

Purpose.—An asymmetric smile, caused by loss of function of the lip depressors, can be functionally and cosmetically debilitating. Although some surgeons report excellent results with muscle transfer to the lower lip, many facial reanimation surgeons find that dynamic techniques do not consistently address the lower lip. Our objectives were to retrospectively review our outcomes after treatment of the asymmetric lower lip, and to propose a progressive, stepwise algorithm for the management of lower lip asymmetry in facial paralysis.

Material/Methods.—Retrospective chart review was performed on all patients treated in a multidisciplinary facial nerve center with lower lip asymmetry over an eighteen month period. Treatment ranged from a temporary trial of lidocaine, to chemodenervation with botulinum toxin, to pedicled digastric muscle transfer, and/or resection of the nonparetic depressor labii inferioris (DLI).

Results.—Fifty-seven patients were treated with chemodenervation with botulinum toxin, four with anterior belly of the digastric transfer, and 3 with DLI resection. All patients with DLI resection had undergone chemodenervation to the contralateral lower lip with botulinum toxin and were pleased with the appearance of their smile.

Conclusions.—We have found that lower lip asymmetry is optimally managed by adherence to a standardized protocol that offers patients insight into the likely outcome of chemodenervation or surgery and progresses systematically from the reversible to the irreversible. We present our algorithm for the management of the asymmetric lower lip, which reflects this graduated approach and has resulted in high patient satisfaction (Fig 4).

▶ The concept of weakening/removing or permanently paralyzing unaffected musculature to achieve symmetry in patients with facial paralysis has long been known. The authors provide an algorithm for the management of lower lip asymmetry (Fig 4) with the intention of allowing patients an opportunity

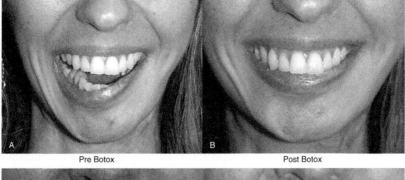

Pre Botox   Post Botox

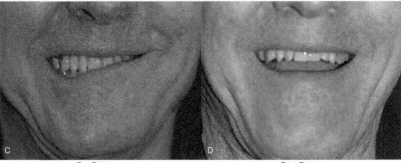

Pre Botox   Post Botox

FIGURE 4.—Chemodenervation with botulinum toxin. (A and B) Note the asymmetry of the lower lip prior to chemodenervation. (C and D) Observe the improved symmetry of the lower lip after chemodenervation. (Reprinted from Lindsay RW, Edwards C, Smitson C, et al. A systematic algorithm for the management of lower lip asymmetry. *Am J Otolaryngol.* 2011;32:1-7, with permission from Elsevier Inc.)

to see the result of temporary paralysis using botulism injections every 4 to 6 weeks for a total of 2 to 3 treatments. Use of botulism toxin builds on the original concept of using a single dose of lidocaine for temporary paralysis proposed by Godwin et al.[1] Having said that, I am unsure of why they propose 2 to 3 treatments with botulism (each lasting 4-6 months) as the standard before going to the more permanent solution of surgical removal of the depressor labii inferioris (DLI). One would assume that living with temporary paralysis of the DLI for a period of 4 to 6 months is more than adequate for patients to decide if they like the results achieved. They do extend the indications for this technique to patients with lip asymmetry remaining even after successful facial reanimation.

S. H. Miller, MD, MPH

Reference

1. Godwin Y, Tomat I, Manktelow R. The use of local anesthetic motor block to demonstrate the potential outcome of depressor labii inferioris resection in patients with facial paralysis. *Plast Reconstr Surg.* 2005;116:957-961.

Secondary surgery in paediatric facial paralysis reanimation
Terzis JK, Olivares FS (Eastern Virginia Med School, Norfolk, VA)
J Plast Reconstr Aesth Surg 63:1794-1806, 2010

Ninety-two children, the entire series of paediatric facial reanimation by a single surgeon over thirty years, are presented. The objective is to analyse the incidence and value of secondary revisions for functional and aesthetic refinements following the two main stages of reanimation. The reconstructive strategy varied according to the denervation time, the aetiology, and whether the paralysis was uni- or bilateral, complete or partial. Irrespective of these variables, 89% of the patients required secondary surgery. Post-operative videos were available in seventy-two cases. Four independent observers graded patients' videos using a scale from poor to excellent.

The effect of diverse secondary procedures was measured computing a mean-percent-gain score. Statistical differences between treatment groups means were tested by the t-test and one-way ANOVA. Two-thirds of the corrective and ancillary techniques utilized granted significantly higher mean-scores post-secondary surgery. A comparison of pre- and post-operative data found valuable improvements in all three facial zones after secondary surgery. In conclusion, inherent to dynamic procedures is the need for secondary revisions. Secondary surgery builds in the potential of reanimation surgery, effectively augmenting functional faculties and aesthesis.

▶ This impressive patient series highlights the importance of secondary revisions for refinement after facial reanimation procedures for the upper, middle, and lower face. The article provides useful information for counseling patients and their families about the number of surgeries that may be required to achieve an optimal result. The authors attempt to assess the value of the different revisionary surgical techniques for each anatomic area in 72 of 92 patients by computing the postoperative percent-gain-score using independent observer evaluations of patient videos before and after initial and revisionary surgery. Although the authors emphasize that procedure selection should be based on each specific clinical situation, they were able to make several interesting conclusions based on their patient population. For example, in midface procedures, patients with poor or fair outcomes after the initial reconstruction had greater secondary improvement after transposition of an additional muscle unit (minitemporalis procedure) than by manipulation of the original muscle graft. Similarly to counter excessive muscular contraction of the muscle graft, revision by augmenting the contralateral commissure with transposition of an additional muscle unit (platysma or digastric) achieved a greater percent gain than manipulation or myectomies of the ipsilateral muscle graft. Secondary revisional surgeries resulted in significantly higher mean scores for most patients in this series. The authors reiterate that the goal of surgery is the coordinated reanimation of the eye-smile-depressor centers of the face, and currently this is not possible with any single procedure. The value of secondary revisional procedures is clearly exemplified in this study and is recommended for functional and aesthetic refinement after the free muscle flap has reached final functional recovery (12-18 months after transfer).

A. Gosman, MD

Head and Neck Reconstruction

Paradigm shifts in the management of osteoradionecrosis of the mandible
Jacobson AS, Buchbinder D, Hu K, et al (Albert Einstein College of Medicine, NY)
Oral Oncol 46:795-801, 2010

Osteoradionecrosis (ORN) of the mandible is a significant complication of radiation therapy for head and neck cancer. In this condition, bone within the radiation field becomes devitalized and exposed through the overlying skin or mucosa, persisting as a non-healing wound for three months or more. In 1926, Ewing first recognized the bone changes associated with radiation therapy and described them as "radiation osteitis". In 1983, Marx proposed the first staging system for ORN that also served as a treatment protocol. This protocol advocated that patients whose disease progressed following conservative therapy (hyperbaric oxygen (HBO), local wound care, debridement) were advanced to a radical resection with a staged reconstruction utilizing a non-vascularized bone graft. Since the introduction of Marx's protocol, there have been advances in surgical techniques (i.e. microvascular surgery), as well as in imaging techniques, which have significantly impacted on the diagnosis and management of ORN. High resolution CT scans and orthopantamograms have become a key component in evaluating and staging ORN, prior to formulating a treatment plan. Patients can now be stratified based on imaging and clinical findings, and treatment can be determined based on the stage of disease, rather than determining the stage of disease based on a patient's response to a standardized treatment protocol. Reconstructions are now routinely performed immediately after resection of the diseased tissue rather than in a staged fashion. Furthermore, the transfer of well-vascularized hard and soft tissue using microvascular surgery have brought the utility of HBO treatment in advanced ORN into question.

▶ This is a very good review article updating the diagnosis and management of osteoradionecrosis of the mandible. For many of us, the complication, osteonecrosis of the mandible, following successful treatment of a carcinoma involving the mandible often caused us to question whether the cure was not worse than the disease. While Marx was a major contributor to the diagnosis and care of this condition, it made little sense to my surgical brain that classification of the severity of the disease should be based retrospectively on the response to treatment. I congratulate the authors and others who have questioned that and now propose a system of preoperative evaluation, using high-resolution CT scans and orthopantamograms, which allow severity ranking and staging, from which treatment protocols and outcomes can be reliably assessed. I too have long been impressed that hyperbaric oxygen is of limited use in treating many different situations despite great enthusiasm for it when first promoted. Logically, a treatment that is applied episodically to pathological circumstances, extant all of the time, is not likely to produce major changes other than in circumstances that are relatively minor. While looking to the new, one must not forget some time-honored lessons from the past: prevention of osteoradionecrosis is more desirable than its treatment. To that end, using newer modalities of radiation, intensity-modulated radiation, with appropriate fractionation and reducing the dosage to susceptible tissues while aiming for cure and meticulous dental hygiene prior to, during, and following radiation treatment are key components of reducing the incidence of osteoradionecrosis. Finally, the concept of bringing in vascularized bone to replace the bone afflicted with osteoradionecrosis should dramatically improve the outcomes for these unfortunate patients.

S. H. Miller, MD, MPH

Nasal Reconstruction
Menick FJ (St Joseph's Hosp and the Univ of Arizona, Tucson)
Plast Reconstr Surg 125:138e, 2010

The face tells the world who we are and materially influences what we can become. The nose is a primary feature. Thin, supple cover and lining are shaped by a middle layer of bone and cartilage support to create its characteristic skin quality, border outline, and three-dimensional contour. The delicacy of its tissues, its central projecting location, and the need to reestablish both a normal appearance and functional breathing make its reconstruction difficult. Nasal repair requires careful analysis of the anatomical and aesthetic deficiencies. Because the wound does not accurately reflect the tissue deficiency, the repair is determined by the "normal." A preliminary operation may be required to ensure clear margins, recreate the defect, reestablish a stable nasal platform on which to build the nose, and prepare tissues for transfer. Major nasal defects require resurfacing with forehead tissue; support with septal, ear, or rib grafts; and replacement of missing lining. This requires a staged approach.

▶ While little new material is offered in this article, it is an excellent summary of the author's well-thought-out, comprehensive, and organized approach to nasal reconstruction. It should prove invaluable to the practicing physician faced with the need to perform major nasal reconstruction and even more so to the plastic surgeon in training. In addition, it should prove helpful to the candidate for certification and to the certified plastic surgeon preparing to take the cognitive portion of American Board of Plastic Surgery Maintenance of Certification program.

S. H. Miller, MD, MPH

Anchor-shaped nasal framework designed for total nasal reconstruction
Li Q, Weng R, Gu B, et al (Shanghai Jiao Tong Univ, PR China)
J Plast Reconstr Aesth Surg 63:954-962, 2010

Background.—Nasal frame grafting has been widely used in nasal reconstruction; however, a stable nasal frame with satisfactory functional and aesthetic results is hard to achieve in total nasal reconstruction. In this study, we devised a technique to create an individually designed anchor-shaped nasal frame composed of an L-strut and two C-battens, and applied it in the total nasal reconstruction procedure to achieve satisfactory functional and aesthetic results.

Method.—In a 9-year period, 17 patients with total nasal defect were treated with autogenous costal grafting utilising forehead flap as the covering. The techniques of the individualised design of the anchor-shaped nasal frame were applied to fit the facial features. All cases were followed for at least 18 months, and outcomes were evaluated separately by the patients and plastic surgeons in terms of aesthetics, stability and function.

Results.—Satisfactory results were achieved in most of the cases after the operation. More than 82.4% of the patients in this series were assessed as satisfactory by both groups in the aesthetics survey; more than 76.5% in the stability survey; and more than 64.7% in the function survey. Complications included flap hyperpigmentation (one case), flap-skin paleness (one case), L-strut distortion (three cases) and stuffiness of the nostrils (one case) as well as minor brow elevation of the donor side (five cases).

Conclusions.—The procedure of applying individually designed anchor-shaped nasal frame with forehead flap technique has obvious advantages for restoration of distinct and delicate subunits, stable nasal structure and good nasal function (Figs 1, 2, and 5).

▶ The authors present an outstanding series of total and subtotal nasal reconstructions. Their handling of the soft tissue defects and their results mirror those presented by Burget and Menick and others. The use of the anchor-shaped framework constructed of rib cartilage is clearly the major contribution of this report (Fig 1). While virtually all authors report the use of an L-shaped strut, the construction of the C-battens from the same rib cartilage using a silicone model and ultimately the union of the 2 provides their patients with excellent results (Fig 2). The 18-month follow-up tends to suggest that these

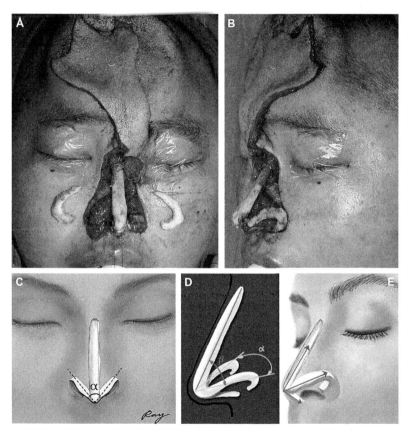

FIGURE 1.—The anchor-shaped nasal frame. A. The design of the L-strut and the C-battens. B. The anchoring of the L-strut and the C-battens. C–D. Illustration of the anchor-shaped nasal frame. E. Illustration of the soft tissue retraction forces, the red arrows indicates the direction of retraction forces. (Reprinted from Li Q, Weng R, Gu B, et al. Anchor-shaped nasal framework designed for total nasal reconstruction. *J Plast Reconstr Aesth Surg.* 2010;63:954-962, with permission from British Association of Plastic, Reconstructive and Aesthetic Surgeons.)

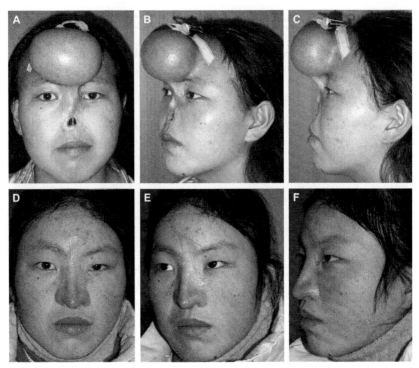

FIGURE 2.—A 25-year-old female with severe nasal defect. A—C. Preoperative view with a well defined and sharp-featured profile. D—F. Postoperative view 13 months after surgery, a pointed nose contour was achieved. (Reprinted from Li Q, Weng R, Gu B, et al. Anchor-shaped nasal framework designed for total nasal reconstruction. *J Plast Reconstr Aesth Surg.* 2010;63:954-962, with permission from British Association of Plastic, Reconstructive and Aesthetic Surgeons.)

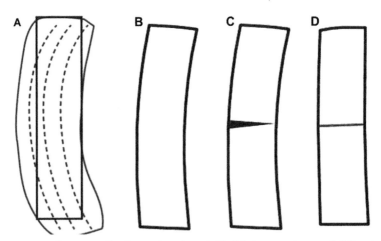

FIGURE 5.—Illustration of bending tension release. A. Physiologic curves shown as dash lines. B. The graft bended after harvested because of the rib bending tension. C. A wedge shaped slice was cut from the convex side. D. The bending tension is released. (Reprinted from Li Q, Weng R, Gu B, et al. Anchor-shaped nasal framework designed for total nasal reconstruction. *J Plast Reconstr Aesth Surg.* 2010;63:954-962, with permission from British Association of Plastic, Reconstructive and Aesthetic Surgeons.)

reconstructions remain stable over time. The adoption of a tension-releasing wedge excision of the convex side of the rib cartilage L-strut appears to be a worthwhile modification (Fig 5) in addition to the actual positioning of the C-battens so as to individualize the reconstruction for the patients' features. This is certainly an article that should be studied carefully by those interested in total and subtotal nasal reconstructions.

S. H. Miller, MD, MPH

Secondary intention healing in lower eyelid reconstruction — a valuable treatment option

Morton J (Whiston Hosp, Prescot, Merseyside, UK)
J Plast Reconstr Aesth Surg 63:1921-1925, 2010

Secondary intention healing — or laissez-faire technique — is the first rung on the reconstructive ladder but may often be overlooked in favour of more elegant reconstructive options. Whilst the nose and medial canthus of eye have long been considered suitable sites for secondary intention healing, most plastic surgeons would hesitate to employ this technique with full-thickness lower eyelid wounds. There are currently no reports in the plastic surgery literature advocating its use, but the technique is gaining credence in the field of oculoplastics as a genuinely useful alternative to formal reconstruction.

Four cases are presented where tumours excised from the lower eyelid were allowed to heal by secondary intention. The largest involved 75% of the lid margin. All were elderly patients in whom formal reconstruction was either declined by the patient or considered unwise by the surgeon.

The cosmetic and functional results were quite remarkable, so much so that this technique demands serious consideration as a valuable treatment option, and quite possibly the treatment of choice in elderly or infirm patients whose tolerance of more complicated procedures may be limited (Figs 2 and 4).

▶ This is an interesting report that is counterintuitive for most plastic surgeons. We have all had experiences with patients who have had healing by laissez-faire. We have always been taught that healing by secondary intention when the wound involves a free margin is problematic because of scar contracture. Yet the authors of this study have shown that in elderly patients with full thickness defects of the lower lid, that may not happen—at least in the 4 patients presented. All healed relatively well without evidence of ectropion. The authors posit that perhaps this was true because the defects included tarsus and thus, the wound could contract more favorably than wounds with tarsal plate present. This hypothesis should be tested. Although the wounds healed well, I am surprised that patients did not have difficulty with bleeding from the open wounds because many, if not most, should be on some type of blood

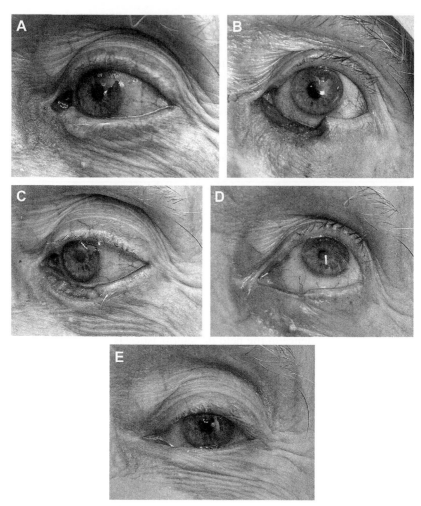

FIGURE 2.—Patient 2, showing medial lid BCC (A), the immediate defect (B), and at 6 days (C), 15 days (D), and 2 months (E). (Reprinted from Morton J. Secondary intention healing in lower eyelid reconstruction — a valuable treatment option. *J Plast Reconstr Aesth Surg.* 2010;63:1921-1925, with permission from British Association of Plastic, Reconstructive and Aesthetic Surgeons.)

thinning regimen. Finally, please note that the length of time required for healing is significant and requires a compliant patient and/or an attentive caretaker.

S. H. Miller, MD, MPH

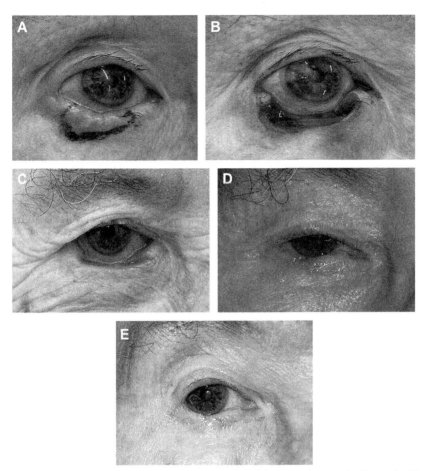

FIGURE 4.—Patient 4, showing the lesion (A), immediate defect (B), and at 1 week (C), 5 weeks (D) and 6 months (E). (Reprinted from Morton J. Secondary intention healing in lower eyelid reconstruction — a valuable treatment option. *J Plast Reconstr Aesth Surg.* 2010;63:1921-1925, with permission from British Association of Plastic, Reconstructive and Aesthetic Surgeons.)

Orbital floor reconstruction: A case for silicone. A 12 year experience

Prowse SJB, Hold PM, Gilmour RF, et al (The Royal Hobart Hosp, Tasmania, Australia)
J Plast Reconstr Aesth Surg 63:1105-1109, 2010

Introduction.—Controversy still exists regarding the choice of implant material for orbital floor reconstructions, in particular the use of silicone. We aimed to evaluate the long-term outcomes of orbital floor reconstructions with silicone versus other non-silicone implants.

Patients and methods.—We conducted a 12 year retrospective review of patients who had orbital floor reconstructions for fractures at the Royal Hobart Hospital, Tasmania, Australia, from 1995 to 2007. Surgical admission notes, CT reports, operation records, outpatient notes, and complications were recorded. Long-term follow-up consisted of a structured telephone interview assessing patient outcomes and satisfaction, including ongoing disability, following orbital floor repair.

Results.—Eighty one patients were identified as having had orbital floor reconstruction with an implant. Mean long-term follow-up was 63 months. Outcomes of Silicone implants ($n = 58$) were compared to non-silicone implant materials ($n = 23$) including titanium mesh, 'Lactasorb', 'Resorb-X', autologous cartilage, and bone graft. Statistically significant advantages in the silicone group were found in the number of patients with palpable implants (24% vs 63%, $p = 0.005$), the number of patients without any complaint (67% vs 32%, $p = 0.004$), and the number of patients requiring subsequent surgery for complications related to their implants (5% vs 23%, $p = 0.046$).

Conclusion.—The appropriate use of silicone implants for orbital floor reconstruction can have good results, contrary to much of the literature, with low complication rates including an acceptably low rate of infection and extrusion, as well as high patient satisfaction. To establish definite guidelines for best surgical practise, particularly amongst synthetic implant materials, prospective study is required.

▶ The conclusion reached in this study run counter to that generally present in the literature. Close evaluation of the study demonstrates some of the failures inherent in reporting a retrospective study without clearly defined protocols and adequate number of patients to truly assess the results. For example, some 19 different surgeons each chose the incision, the implant used, etc. The basis for the analysis of the data revolves around follow-up in person at a mean of 3.5 months and a structured telephone survey asking the patients about potential complications. The timing of the latter was not clearly stated. While the statistics regarding extrusion seem to favor the silicone implant over the other implant group, the latter was a lumped group made up of several different types of implants, including bone. In fact, the gross extrusion rate in each group was almost identical, but the statistics favored the silicone group as the numbers of patients in that group were 3 times greater than in the other implant group. In light of the proposal that silicone is appropriate for orbital floor fractures with and without rim involvement, it behooves the authors to develop a protocol that allows meaningful comparisons.

S. H. Miller, MD, MPH

Versatility of the Posterior Auricular Flap in Partial Ear Reconstruction

Schonauer F, Vuppalapati G, Marlino S, et al (Univ Federico II, Naples, Italy)
Plast Reconstr Surg 126:1213-1221, 2010

Background.—The posterior auricular flap alone has always been popular because of its prompt availability, its rich vascularity, and the ease of closing the donor-site defect primarily.

Methods.—Fifty-seven patients with partial ear defects covered with posterior auricular flaps during the period between 2002 and 2007 were reviewed. In the authors' series, posterior auricular flaps were harvested based on a simple random vascularization and tailored to reach almost any defect of the ear by a simplified and standardized approach.

Results.—The authors propose a simple nomenclature after grouping the flaps according to skin paddle type, pedicle type, pedicle base, flap transfer method, and flap movement; they present a standardized algorithm with which to choose the flap design for a given defect from this group.

Conclusions.—The authors contribute three new flap designs to enhance the versatility of the posterior auricular flap. These are the superiorly and inferiorly based twisted island flaps and the posterior auricular propeller flap (Figs 5 and 7, Table 1).

▶ The posterior auricular flap, in many different iterations, has long been a favorite method to repair skin defects of the surfaces of the ear. This anecdotal report of the experiences, using a posterior auricular flap at a single center in

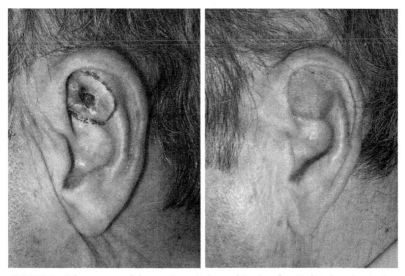

FIGURE 5.—Subcutaneous pedicle posterior auricular revolving door flap. (*Left*) Left ear: basal cell carcinoma of the inferior crus and excision margins. (*Right*) Aesthetic result at 3-month follow-up after subcutaneous pedicle flap transfer. (Reprinted from Schonauer F, Vuppalapati G, Marlino S, et al. Versatility of the posterior auricular flap in partial ear reconstruction. *Plast Reconstr Surg.* 2010;126:1213-1221.)

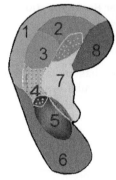

Region		Flap
1	Anterior upper half of helix	Superiorly based transposition flap
2	Scapha	Superiorly based folded de-epithelialized skin pedicle or Revolving door flap
3	Upper antihelix	Inferiorly based twisted de-epithelialized skin pedicle
4	Middle antihelix	Superiorly based twisted de-epithelialized skin pedicle
5	Lower antihelix, antitragus	Inferiorly based folded de-epithelialized skin pedicle
6	Lobule and lower helix	Inferiorly based transposition flap
7	Concha	Revolving door flap
8	Helical root	Propeller flap

FIGURE 7.—Flap algorithm: auricular regions and corresponding flaps. (Reprinted from Schonauer F, Vuppalapati G, Marlino S, et al. Versatility of the posterior auricular flap in partial ear reconstruction. *Plast Reconstr Surg.* 2010;126:1213-1221.)

TABLE 1.—Classification of Posterior Auricular Flaps

Skin Paddle Type	Pedicle Type	Pedicle Base	Method of Transfer	Movement
Island	Deepithelialized skin pedicle	Superior	Folded pedicle Twisted pedicle	Through the cartilage
		Inferior	Folded pedicle Twisted pedicle	
	Subcutaneous pedicle	Central Eccentric	Revolving door Propeller	Around the cartilage
Peninsular	Skin pedicle	Superior Inferior	Transposition	

Italy, contributes to the literature by proposing a nomenclature (Table 1) and a versatile algorithm (Fig 7) to enable a surgeon to select the appropriate flap design that will best address the defect. While the flap is hardy and safe, the posterior auricular skin, coming from an area less exposed to the sun than the skin of the anterior ear, often leads to obvious color mismatch when placed onto the anterior surface of the ear (Fig 5).

S. H. Miller, MD, MPH

Reconstruction of Temporal and Suprabrow Defects
Warren SM, Zide BM (New York Univ School of Medicine)
Ann Plast Surg 64:298-301, 2010

Large temple and suprabrow lesions can pose a reconstructive challenge. When the lesion extends anterior to the hairline, esthetically acceptable local flaps may be difficult to design. We describe a modified scalp flap (ie, part Converse scalping flap and part scalp rotation flap) that can be tailored to reconstruct a variety of difficult temple and suprabrow lesions while simultaneously maintaining eyebrow position.

The modified scalp flap is raised in a subgaleal plane until approximately 2.5 cm above the brow. At this level, dissection proceeds in the subcutaneous plane to protect the frontal branch of the facial nerve and to keep the flap thin. (The key to the modified scalp flap is the dissection plane change that protects the frontal branch of the facial nerve.) The extent of posterior subgaleal dissection is dictated by the amount of anterior rotation necessary. A temporal dog-ear is removed subfollicularly to permit modified flap rotation and preserve the superficial temporal artery.

The modified scalp flap has been used to reconstruct temple and suprabrow lesions in 10 patients ranging in age from 4 months to 22 years. There were no complications. Four typical cases are presented.

Temple and suprabrow lesions can be excised and successfully reconstructed in one stage using a modified scalp flap that is extended from the hair-bearing scalp onto the glabrous skin of the forehead. This novel modified scalp flap prevents eyebrow/hairline distortion and avoids facial nerve injury (Fig 4).

► The authors present their experiences in reconstructing temporal and suprabrow defects using modifications of the Converse scalping flap, a scalp rotation

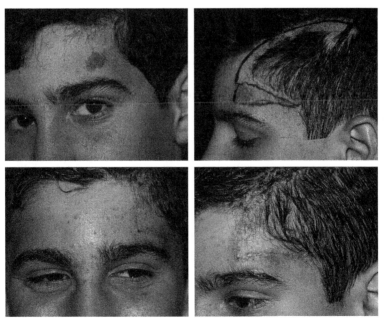

FIGURE 4.—Top left, Preoperative views of a 15-year-old boy with a 2.5 × 2.5 cm sebaceous nevus affecting the left, suprabrow. Top Right, A hatchet-type modified scalp flap was designed with a back-cut at the midhelical point. Bottom Left and Bottom Right, Three months later, the patient had a symmetric eyebrows and fronto-temporal hairlines. (Reprinted from Warren SM, Zide BM. Reconstruction of temporal and suprabrow defects. *Ann Plast Surg.* 2010;64:298-301.)

flap, and where necessary, a cheek flap and skin grafts as in case 4. The major goal of maintaining the position of the eyebrow appears to have been accomplished because of the flexibility of the authors' technique and their attention to detail, specifically, the 2-plane dissection, switching from subgaleal to subcutaneous approximately 1 inch superior to the eyebrow, and the care in removing the dog-ear to prevent injury to the superficial temporal artery. That being said, several of the photos do demonstrate reduction in the distance between the eyebrow and the hairline and some prominent scars and discolorations of the distal end of the flap at least in the photos shown in Fig 4.

S. H. Miller, MD, MPH

Maxillomandibular-Labial Reconstruction: An Autogenous Transplant as an Alternative to Allogenic Face Transplantation
Chepcha DB, Malloy KM, Moyer JS, et al (Univ of Pennsylvania, Philadelphia; Univ of Minnesota, Minneapolis)
Plast Reconstr Surg 126:2007-2011, 2010

Background.—Large-volume maxillomandibular-labial defects are unusual and present reconstructive challenges. Such injuries impair oral sphincter function and cause debilitating and disfiguring soft tissue and bone loss that affect speech and swallowing. Limited local tissue is available, multiple autogenous transplants are needed, and few techniques permit reconstruction of near-total oral sphincter defects. Face transplantation is associated with functional challenges and chronic immunosuppression risks. An alternative technique was used in two patients with traumatic defects of the premaxilla, mandible, and oral sphincter.

Methods.—One patient was age 3 years and the other age 26 years. The technique was accomplished in two steps. First, the intraoral mucosal defect was reconstructed using an independent skin paddle. The design is based on measurements obtained with the patient in "open-mouth" position to accommodate the labial sulcus, labial height, and labial width. A second independent skin paddle was used for the cutaneous defect. The template-based technique maintained the proportions of the oral sphincter and surrounding soft tissues. The remaining native lip and oral sphincter were tacked in place on the external cutaneous skin paddle to avoid contraction, and the maxilla and mandible were projected to correct position. The paddles were allowed to heal for at least 6 weeks, with a small port for suctioning secretions and monitoring mucosal restoration provided.

In the second step, the oral fissure was opened between the maxilla and mandible, carefully placing it midway between the two and in an anatomically proportional site for the individual's face. The part of the flap that the native lip was to replace was resected, then the remnant of native lip inlayed into the oral fissure. It is important to avoid making the oral fissure too wide to control oral secretions. To ensure oral competence, the oral fissure can only exceed the width of the native lip tissue by a small amount.

Twelve months or more after the procedure, patients underwent analysis of their speech and swallowing function, diet, oral competence, functional status, and quality of life.

Results.—Both patients have the midface restored to pretrauma projections. They also both maintain a completely oral diet with no supplementation, tolerate a full range of liquids, have minimal restriction of their solid diet, speak understandably, minimally restrict their public speaking, and have normal function outside the home, with one in school and the other employed full-time.

Conclusions.—The goals of reconstruction were to maintain oral competence, project the maxilla and mandible, position bone grafts to facilitate future implant placement, and ensure good tongue mobility to manage secretions. As much native labial tissue as possible was retained, oral stoma sensation was protected, native tissue mobility was maximized, labial and floor-of-mouth sulci were made to facilitate secretion drainage to the posterior oral cavity, the length and width of the lips were over-reconstructed to measure templates for mucosal and cutaneous reconstructions, a template-based design was used in making skin paddles, and adequate bulk of the oral stoma reconstruction was ensured to generate pressure between the upper and lower lips with jaw closure. Both patients had oral function restored and engage in normal social interactions despite their trauma. This approach is a viable alternative to allogenic face transplantation without the drawbacks of immunosuppression (Figs 1, 2, 3 and 5).

▶ This is an interesting report of 2 cases of staged autologous maxillomandibular-labial reconstruction purporting to provide functional outcomes such as, speaking and eating in public, comparable to those achieved after facial transplantation without the risks of lifetime immunosuppression. The goals of the procedure are primarily related to achieving oral competence, projection of the maxillomandibular components, developing a bony platform for future implants, and allowing tongue mobility. The procedure is described in detail with good

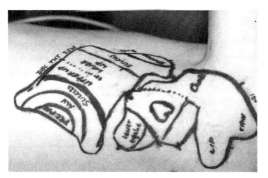

FIGURE 1.—The patient's left lateral thorax, with the patient's head to the right of the figure. (Reprinted from Chepeha DB, Malloy KM, Moyer JS, et al. Maxillomandibular-labial reconstruction: an autogenous transplant as an alternative to allogenic face transplantation. *Plast Reconstr Surg.* 2010;126:2007-2011.)

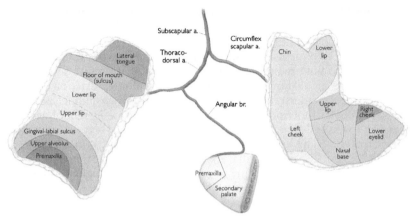

FIGURE 2.—The latissimus dorsi skin paddle for internal reconstruction of the oral mucosa (*left*) and the parascapular skin paddle for external reconstruction are shown (*right*). The bone for the maxillary reconstruction was harvested from the scapular tip and is shown (*center*). Note the mobility of the three components of the reconstruction relative to one another and the length of the vascular pedicle. The components of the transplant have been labeled with the structures they were used to reconstruct and the coloring of the transplant used in this figure is maintained in subsequent figures. (Reprinted from Chepeha DB, Malloy KM, Moyer JS, et al. Maxillomandibular-labial reconstruction: an autogenous transplant as an alternative to allogenic face transplantation. *Plast Reconstr Surg.* 2010;126:2007-2011.)

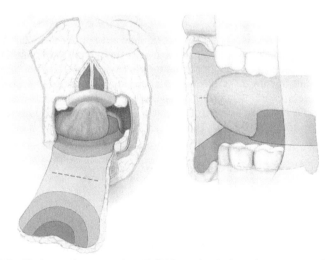

FIGURE 3.—The intraoral reconstruction. (*Left*) The patient is shown in an open-mouth position, with the skin paddle shown after it has been inset to reconstruct the floor of the mouth, the left lateral tongue, and the mandibular alveolus. The most inferior aspect of the skin paddle will be rotated superiorly to reconstruct the palate, labial sulci, and mucosal surface of the upper lip. (*Right*) The view from the posterior lateral is shown after the latissimus dorsi skin paddle has been rotated into place to provide a perspective of the intraoral inset. The native tongue is seen in good contact with the reconstruction of the upper and lower labial mucosal subunits, and adequate tissue is shown for the labial sulci to help the flow of secretions. (Reprinted from Chepeha DB, Malloy KM, Moyer JS, et al. Maxillomandibular-labial reconstruction: an autogenous transplant as an alternative to allogenic face transplantation. *Plast Reconstr Surg.* 2010;126:2007-2011.)

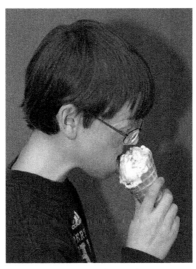

FIGURE 5.—Patient demonstrating tongue protrusion, oral competence, and management of complex food items 7 years after reconstruction. He attends public school, plays sports, and is well socialized. (Reprinted from Chepeha DB, Malloy KM, Moyer JS, et al. Maxillomandibular-labial reconstruction: an autogenous transplant as an alternative to allogenic face transplantation. *Plast Reconstr Surg*. 2010;126:2007-2011.)

line drawings (Figs 1-3), but the authors fail to adequately demonstrate a patient's appearance because they only include a lateral view of one of the patients several years after reconstruction (Fig 5). It seems apparent to this reader that functional comparisons between this technique and facial transplantation in patients with such devastating deformities must include aesthetic outcomes.

S. H. Miller, MD, MPH

Pressure Ulcers

Flap surgery for pressure sores: Should the underlying muscle be transferred or not?
Thiessen FE, Andrades P, Blondeel PN, et al (Gent Univ Hosp, Belgium)
J Plast Reconstr Aesth Surg 64:84-90, 2011

Background.—Musculocutaneous flaps have become the first choice in the surgical repair of pressure sores, but the indication for including muscle in the transferred flaps still remains poorly defined. This study compares outcomes after muscle and non-muscle flap coverage of pressure sores to investigate whether it is still necessary to incorporate muscle tissue as part of the surgical treatment of these ulcers.

Methods.—A retrospective revision of 94 consecutive patients with ischial or sacral pressure sores operated between 1996 and 2002 was performed. Depending on the inclusion of muscle into the flap, the patients were divided in two groups: musculocutaneous flap group and fasciocutaneous flap group. Charts were reviewed for patient characteristics, ulcer features and reconstructive information. Data between groups were compared with emphasis on early (haematoma or seroma, dehiscence, infections, necrosis and secondary procedures) and late (recurrence) postoperative complications.

Results.—A total of 37 wounds were covered with muscle and 57 wounds covered without muscle tissue. The groups were comparable in relation to age, gender, ulcer characteristics and timing for surgery. There were no significant differences in early complications between the study groups. The mean follow-up period was 3.10 ± 1.8 years (range: 0.5 to 6.7). There were no statistical differences in ulcer recurrence between the groups. The type of flap used was not associated with postoperative morbidity or recurrence in the univariate and multivariate analyses.

Conclusions.—The findings of this clinical study indicate that the musculocutaneous flaps are as good as fasciocutaneous flaps in the reconstruction of pressure sores, and they question the long-standing dogma that muscle is needed in the repair of these ulcers.

▶ The treatment of pressure sores remains a significant part of reconstructive plastic surgery practice. Despite this, there is little objective evidence as to the best surgical approach for this difficult problem. Many of us were taught that musculocutaneous flaps were the gold standard for the management of pressure sores. This article calls this teaching into question. In this retrospective analysis, the authors examined a consecutive single-institution series of pressure sores treated with either musculocutaneous or fasciocutaneous flaps in over 100 patients. They found no differences in immediate complication rates or long-term recurrence (which averaged about 30% in both groups). The authors conclude that recent advances in perforator flap technique and understanding of vascular anatomy make fasciocutaneous flaps equally effective for pressure sore management as the previous gold standard muscle flaps. They make the excellent point that muscle is more susceptible to ischemia than skin or fascia, and that in normal anatomy pressure points are never covered by muscle. Thus, it seems likely that it is time to reexamine clinical dogma as it relates to pressure sore management.

G. C. Gurtner, MD

Frequent manual repositioning and incidence of pressure ulcers among bed-bound elderly hip fracture patients
Rich SE, Margolis D, Shardell M, et al (Univ of Maryland School of Medicine, Baltimore; Univ of Pennsylvania School of Medicine, Philadelphia)
Wound Rep Reg 19:10-18, 2011

Frequent manual repositioning is an established part of pressure ulcer prevention, but there is little evidence for its effectiveness. This study examined the association between repositioning and pressure ulcer incidence among bed-bound elderly hip fracture patients, using data from a 2004–2007 cohort study in nine Maryland and Pennsylvania hospitals. Eligible patients (*n*=269) were age a ≥65 years, underwent hip fracture surgery, and were bed-bound at index study visits (during the first 5 days of hospitalization). Information about repositioning on the days of index visits was collected from patient charts; study nurses assessed presence of stage 2+ pressure ulcers 2 days later. The association between frequent manual repositioning and pressure ulcer incidence was estimated, adjusting for pressure ulcer risk factors using generalized estimating equations and weighted estimating equations. Patients were frequently repositioned (at least every 2 hours) on only 53% (187/354) of index visit days. New pressure ulcers developed at 12% of visits following frequent repositioning vs. 10% following less frequent repositioning; the incidence rate of pressure ulcers per person-day did not differ between the two groups (incidence rate ratio 1.1, 95% confidence interval 0.5–2.4). No association was found between frequent repositioning of bed-bound patients and lower pressure ulcer incidence, calling into question the allocation of resources for repositioning.

▶ This is a very well-done and important study examining the conventional wisdom in pressure sore prevention. Clinical teaching and various guidelines advocate turning bedbound patients every 2 hours to prevent decubitus formation. In this prospective observational study, the authors actually sent teams of nurses into 9 hospitals in Maryland and evaluated more than 1000 elderly patients with hip fractures who were at risk for pressure sores. These teams evaluated documentation of patient repositioning every 2 hours and followed up a day later to determine whether a new stage 2 or higher pressure sore was present by direct examination. Surprisingly, there was no difference in pressure sore occurrence between those patients who had been turned every 2 hours and those patients who had not. This piece of data supports a growing body of evidence suggesting that pressure relief and purely physical approaches to pressure sore prevention may never be sufficient to prevent ulceration in high-risk patients. Given the high financial cost of these measures (ie, nursing) and the medicolegal consequences of hospital-developed pressure ulceration, this suggests that new more effective measures are desperately needed to have an impact on this huge problem.

G. C. Gurtner, MD

Treatment of Ischial Pressure Sores Using a Modified Gracilis Myofasciocutaneous Flap

Lin H, Hou C, Chen A, et al (The Second Military Med Univ, Shanghai, P. R. China)
J Reconstr Microsurg 26:153-158, 2010

Despite the availability of a variety of flap reconstruction options, ischial pressure sores continue to be the most difficult pressure sores to treat. This article describes a successful surgical procedure for the coverage of ischial ulcers using a modified gracilis myofasciocutaneous flap. From August 2000 to April 2004, 12 patients with ischial sores were enrolled in the study. All patients underwent early aggressive surgical debridement followed by surgical reconstruction with a modified gracilis myofasciocutaneous flap. The follow-up period ranged from 13 to 86 months, with a mean of 44 months. Overall, 91.7% of the flaps (11 of 12) survived primarily. Partial flap necrosis occurred in one patient. Primary wound healing occurred without complications at both the donor and recipient sites in all cases. In one patient, grade II ischial pressure sores recurred

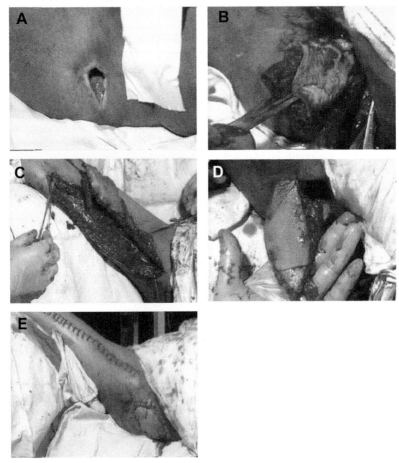

FIGURE 1.—Operative procedure. (A) Preoperative appearance of patient 3. (B) Complete excision of the bursa. (C) Elevation of gracilis myofasciocutaneous flap. (D) Adaptation of the flap to the ischial area through the subcutaneous tunnel formed between the ischial and femoral incision site. (E) Closure of the wound at the end of the operation. (Reprinted from Lin H, Hou C, Chen A, et al. Treatment of ischial pressure sores using a modified gracilis myofasciocutaneous flap. *J Reconstr Microsurg.* 2010;26: 153-158.)

13 months after the operation. There was no recurrence in other 11 patients. A modified gracilis myofasciocutaneous flap provides a good cover for ischial pressure sores. Because it is easy to use and has favorable results, it can be used in the primary treatment for large and deep ischial pressure sores (Fig 1).

▶ Use of the gracilis myofasciocutaneous flap for closure of ischial pressure sores is a valuable addition to the armamentarium of reconstructive surgeons. The muscle is far more expendable than is the gluteus maximus and/or hamstring, especially in those patients who retain some ability to walk with aids. The problem with its use has always been the seeming unreliability of its vascular supply. The present authors' study, basing their efforts on those described by Reddy et al,[1] has clearly shown that by widely encompassing fascia around the muscle, the vascular supply is quite predictable, and the results speak for themselves (Fig 1). I think that this study exemplifies why more attention could be paid to flaps whose blood supply seems marginal to determine if modifications in the tissues transferred might increase the reliability of said flaps.

S. H. Miller, MD, MPH

Reference

1. Reddy VR, Stevenson TR, Whetzel TP. 10-year experience with the gracilis myofasciocutaneous flap. *Plast Reconstr Surg.* 2006;117:635-639.

Trunk and Perineal Reconstruction

The Role of Intrathoracic Free Flaps for Chronic Empyema

Walsh MD, Bruno AD, Onaitis MW, et al (Emory Univ, Atlanta, GA; Duke Univ, Durham, NC; Univ of Pennsylvania Health System, Philadelphia)
Ann Thorac Surg 91:865-868, 2011

Background.—The management of chronic empyema associated with a bronchopleural fistula can be a particularly challenging problem. Successful eradication may not occur without interposition of healthy vascularized tissue. Pedicled muscle flaps for coverage on the thorax have been well described. However, secondary to trauma or previous surgical procedures, a pedicle flap may not be sufficiently sized or available. Free tissue transfer is an attractive option to provide the appropriate vascularized tissue.

Methods.—Six patients with chronic empyema-bronchopleural fistulae were reconstructed with 4 rectus abdominis myocutaneous and 2 gracilis muscle flaps. The choice of recipient vessels was dictated by existing local anatomy but included intercostal, thoracodorsal, thoracoacromial, azygous, and circumflex humeral vessels. One flap required interposition saphenous vein grafts for both artery and vein.

Results.—Patient follow-up ranged from 2 to 14 years. There were no episodes of flap loss or postoperative mortality. Empyema resolution without recurrent bronchopleural fistula was achieved in all patients.

Conclusions.—Free tissue transfer is an excellent option for vascularized tissue interposition in patients who are not candidates for pedicled muscle transfer. Multiple potential recipient vessels provide tremendous versatility, arguing for early consideration of free tissue transfer.

▶ This article reinforces the findings of earlier studies, which suggest the feasibility and the effectiveness of intrathoracic free flaps for chronic empyema. The accepted standard approach is to use pedicled muscle flaps, transferred into the thorax, to cover a surgically repaired bronchopleural fistula. When pedicled flaps are not available (eg, when previous surgery impairs the blood supply of a logical choice flap), a free flap becomes the preferred treatment. One might ask the question: Even if a pedicled flap is possible, might a free flap be better (despite the potential for significantly increased operative time)? In those circumstances in which a pedicled flap could be used but a free flap would clearly provide much more complete coverage of the fistula closure and more dead space obliteration, the free flap may indeed be the wiser choice. Monitoring of a completely intrathoracic free flap provides some challenges, but probably no more than those encountered when the business end of a pedicled flap is similarly hidden from view.

R. L. Ruberg, MD

3 Trauma

Head and Neck

Deformation of Nasal Septum During Nasal Trauma

Lee SJ, Liong K, Lee HP (Natl Univ Hosp, Singapore; Natl Univ of Singapore)

Laryngoscope 120:1931-1939, 2010

Background.—Injury to the nasal septum is commonly found in most nasal fractures. The nasal septum deforms and crumples, leading to nasal deviation and internal nasal obstruction.

Aim.—This study aims to identify the main areas of high stress concentration when a dynamic anteroposterior load is applied to the nasal tip, simulating nasal trauma. We wish to determine if the nasal septum acts as a crumpled zone, and deforms significantly during nasal trauma.

Materials and Methods.—An idealized and a patient-specified finite element model have been generated for the present study. Several models with various combinations of narrower angle at the Vomer Ethmoidal Junction (VEJ) are also constructed from this septum model. Finite element analyses are carried out to determine the deformation and stress distribution in the nasal septum when a dynamic anteroposterior load is applied to the nasal tip.

Conclusions.—The maximum stress areas in the nasal septum are in the vicinity of the bony-cartilaginous (BC) junction and the anterior nasal spine (ANS), which are consistent with clinical experience. A larger anteroposterior load, a longer loading duration, and a more acute VEJ angle would result in higher maximum stresses. The observations were identical in both idealized and patient-specific models. The findings of this analysis also suggest that the septum does function as a crumpled zone, absorbing a significant amount of stress before it is transmitted to the skull.

▶ This study uses finite element analysis to simulate the deformation of the nasal septum because of nasal trauma with an anteroposterior force to the nasal tip. Three idealized septal models, with different Vomer Ethmoidal Junction (VEJ) angles (90°, 80°, and 70°) and 1 patient-specific septal model are analyzed. One of the aims of this study is to determine if the septum acts as a crumple zone to diminish impact transmission to the underlying brain behind the VEJ.

For the 90° VEJ model, the bony-cartilaginous (BC) junction and the anterior nasal spine (ANS) were the first regions to experience higher stresses. The authors hypothesized that patients with an almost perpendicular VEJ are susceptible to nasal cavity obstruction in the lower half of the nasal septum and to dorsal septal deformities. In the 80° VEJ model, the maximum stress was higher and occurred earlier than in the 90° model, and the maximum stress region is in the lower half of the septum. In the 70° VEJ model, the maximum stress is higher than the 80° model, the maximum stress occurs earlier, the region of stress is closer to the dorsum, and there is even less stress at the VEJ. The authors report that with a more acute VEJ, there is a higher maximum stress, and the stress region becomes higher and closer to the dorsal septum. The VEJ region experiences less stress when the VEJ angle is more acute.

The patient-specific model had different stress waves because of irregular geometry, but the regions of maximum stress were similar to the idealized models.

The authors concluded that dynamic loads to the nasal tip created maximum stress areas of the septum at the BC junction and the ANS and that there is a diminished impact force at the VEJ, which supports the hypothesis that the septum acts as a crumple zone to protect the brain located behind the VEJ. This study is an interesting analysis of the mechanical behavior of the septum during nasal trauma. In addition to supporting the hypothesis that the septum is a crumble zone for protecting the underlying brain, the areas of maximum stress correlate clinical with posttraumatic septal deformities.

A. Gosman, MD

Burns

Variations in U.S. Pediatric Burn Injury Hospitalizations Using the National Burn Repository Data

Kramer CB, Rivara FP, Klein MB (Univ of Washington, Seattle)
J Burn Care Res 31:734-739, 2010

An understanding of population-specific variation in pediatric burn injuries is essential to the development of effective prevention strategies. The purpose of this study was to examine the etiology of pediatric burn injury considering age and race categories using the National Burn Repository. The authors reviewed the records of all pediatric patients (age <18 years) in the American Burn Association's National Burn Registry injured between 1995 and 2007. The authors compared patient and injury characteristics across race, age, etiology, and payor status. A total of 46,582 patients were included in this study. The etiology of burn injury varied by both age and race. Populations of color were younger, constituting 53.8% of patients younger than 5 years, whereas 53.9% of the total study population identified as Caucasian. Scald etiology was disproportionately less common in patients identifying as Caucasian (39.9 vs 61.4%, $P < .001$), and scald was a common etiology in older children identifying as African American, Asian, and Hispanic. Inhalation injuries were also higher in patients identifying as Native American (5.4%), Hispanic (4.2%), and African American (3.7%). Pediatric burn injury etiology varies with age and race. These data should encourage careful consideration of race, age, and other differences in formulating the most effective, population-specific prevention and outreach strategies.

▶ Considering their percentage of the population, the incidence of severe burn injury, inhalation injury, and mortality in minorities is disproportionately high. The lack of smoke detectors in lower income population homes explains part of the problem. The Oklahoma City project geometrically reduced burns in the minority community by installing smoke detectors. The other variables and being poor and living in substandard conditions provide less clear solutions

R. E. Salisbury, MD

Burn disasters in the middle belt of Ghana from 2007 to 2008 and their consequences
Agbenorku P, Akpaloo J, Farhat BF, et al (Kwame Nkrumah Univ of Science and Technology, Kumasi, Ghana; Komfo Anokye Teaching Hosp, Kumasi, Ghana; et al)
Burns 36:1309-1315, 2010

Aim.—To study the survival and mortality trends in four fire disasters in the middle belt of Ghana from 2007 to 2008 and to explore measures that could minimize the risk of future disasters.

Methods.—Data were collected from clinical records from the Burns Intensive Care Unit and the Casualty Unit of the Komfo Anokye Teaching Hospital, Kumasi, Ghana and from the various disaster sites and the Ghana Police Service.

Results.—A total of 212 were injured from four burn disasters; 37 (17%) died on the spot; 175 (83%) reported to the Casualty Unit out of which 46 (26%) were admitted. The victims admitted had mean age 24.6 years with male to female ratio 2.3:1; 25 (54%) of the admitted victims died. The average burned surface area of the admitted victims was 63%, with a mean survival rate of 46%. Statistical analysis for mortality when the surface area of the burn was >70% was 0.0005 (*P*-value).

Conclusion.—The four petrol-related fire disasters showed variable mortality rates. Death and severe disability of victims of future disasters can be avoided if intensive road accident preventive measures and massive public education are encouraged.

▶ The authors are to be complimented for their honesty in reporting a mortality of 46% in admitted patients. They enumerate all the challenges of caring for burns in a developing country. The reader should appreciate that we might well have similar results in a full-blown terrorist incident or natural disaster.

R. E. Salisbury, MD

A comparison of Ringer's lactate and acetate solutions and resuscitative effects on splanchnic dysoxia in patients with extensive burns

Aoki K, Yoshino A, Yoh K, et al (Hamamatsu Univ School of Medicine, Higashi-ku, Japan; Keio Univ, Tokyo, Japan)
Burns 36:1080-1085, 2010

We compared the effects of Ringer's lactate (RL) and acetate (RA) solutions on parameters of splanchnic dysoxia such as $PgCO_2$ (PCO_2 of gastric mucosa) and pH_i (pH of gastric mucosa) using a gastric tonometer, in addition to blood markers such as the serum arterial level of lactate, base excess, ketone body ratio, and antithrombin during the first 72 h of the resuscitation period in patients with burns covering 30% or more of their body surface. A prospective study was conducted in the university tertiary referral centers. There were no significant differences in the average age, TBSA (total burn surface area), and resuscitative fluid volume during the first and second 24 h between the two groups. In the RA group, PCO_2 gap values calculated employing the formula: $PgCO_2 - PaCO_2$ (arterial PCO_2), and pH gap calculated by: pH_a (arterial pH) $- pH_i$, improved to the normal ranges at 24 h postburn, which was significantly faster than in the RL group. On the other hand, there were no significant differences in blood parameters between the two groups over the course. These results suggest that fluid resuscitation with RA may more rapidly ameliorate splanchnic dysoxia, as evidenced by gastric tonometry, compared to that with RL.

▶ This article is a nicely constructed prospective study. The study is small, and more work needs to be done. Lactated Ringer solution is the gold standard for resuscitation and is less costly than acetate. Cost will always be important unless convincing evidence surfaces that mortality can be improved with a particular solution.

R. E. Salisbury, MD

Colloid Normalizes Resuscitation Ratio in Pediatric Burns

Faraklas I, Lam U, Cochran A, et al (Univ of Utah Health Sciences Ctr, Salt Lake City)
J Burn Care Res 32:91-97, 2011

Fluid resuscitation of burned children is challenging because of their small size and intolerance to over- or underresuscitation. Our American Burn Association-verified regional burn center has used colloid "rescue" as part of our pediatric resuscitation protocol. With Institutional Review Board approval, the authors reviewed children with ≥15% TBSA burns admitted from January 1, 2004, to May 1, 2009. Resuscitation was based on the Parkland formula, which was adjusted to maintain urine output. Patients requiring progressive increases in crystalloid were placed on a colloid protocol. Results were expressed as an hourly resuscitation ratio

(I/O ratio) of fluid infusion (ml/kg/%TBSA/hr) to urine output (ml/kg/hr). We reviewed 53 patients; 29 completed resuscitation using crystalloid alone (lactated Ringer's solution [LR]), and 24 received colloid supplementation albumin (ALB). Groups were comparable in age, gender, weight, and time from injury to admission. ALB patients had more inhalation injuries and larger total and full-thickness burns. LR patients maintained a median I/O of 0.17 (range, 0.08–0.31), whereas ALB patients demonstrated escalating ratios until the institution of albumin produced a precipitous return of I/O comparable with that of the LR group. Hospital stay was lower for LR patients than ALB patients (0.59 vs 1.06 days/%TBSA, $P = .033$). Twelve patients required extremity or torso escharotomy, but this did not differ between groups. There were no decompressive laparotomies. The median resuscitation volume for ALB group was greater than LR group (9.7 vs 6.2 ml/kg/%TBSA, $P = .004$). Measuring hourly I/O is a helpful means of evaluating fluid demands during burn shock resuscitation. The addition of colloid restores normal I/O in pediatric patients.

▶ This article from a leading burn center attempts to address the problem of burn resuscitation. The authors are quick to point out that it is a retrospective study and the use of colloid was subjective. Thus, one must be careful in attempting to develop conclusions. How to safely resuscitate is multifactorial. Blind use of a formula can be disastrous. For instance, 10% burn in a healthy child or adult might be resuscitated orally. Yet, the same size and depth of injury in an adult who is marginally dehydrated because of chronic diuretic usage and a failing heart is a serious resuscitation challenge. Likewise, a 10% burn in an abused child who is underweight and dehydrated is a problem that can tip into organ failure. There are multiple reasonable approaches to resuscitation practiced by burn centers getting excellent results. The key is to master one approach and all the permutations that can present clinically.

R. E. Salisbury, MD

Acticoat dressings and major burns: Systemic silver absorption
Moiemen NS, Shale F, Drysdale KJ, et al (Univ Hosps Birmingham Foundation Trust, UK; Smith & Nephew Wound Management, UK)
Burns 37:27-35, 2011

Despite widespread use of wound dressings containing silver, few studies have investigated patients' serum silver levels. An earlier study of Acticoat use in small burns showed transient elevations of serum silver. The aim of this study was to examine the serum silver profile when Acticoat is used in major burns.

A prospective study of 6 patients with burns greater than 20% total body surface area (TBSA). All burn wounds, including grafted and non-grafted areas and skin graft donor sites, were dressed with Acticoat or Acticoat Absorbent. Patients' serum silver levels, biochemistry and haematology were examined before, during and after the application of the silver dressings.

The median total wound size (including donor sites) was 46.1% TBSA. The median maximum serum silver level recorded, 200.3 µg/L, reached at a median of 9.5 days following initial silver dressing application. This decreased to a median of 164.8 µg/L at the end of the treatment period and to a median of 8.2 µg/L at the end of follow-up. One adverse event, partial skin graft loss was thought to be dressing related.

In this small study, serum silver levels were elevated but remained similar to that reported following the use of silver sulfadiazine. This study confirmed our view that Acticoat is safe to use on patients with burns, even when they are extensive.

▶ Although the numbers in this prospective study are small, the conclusions are important. Silver-based dressings have been tested clinically for many years. Deleterious effects have not been noted and these authors agree. The kernel of truth is that the burn patient is treated with a multitude of agents, often by residents with little experience. It is imperative that everyone involved in the patient's care be versed in the side effects of all the agents.

R. E. Salisbury, MD

Antibiotics and the burn patient
Ravat F, the Société Française d'Etude et de Traitement des Brûlures (SFETB) (Centre Hospitalier St Joseph et St Luc, Lyon, France; et al)
Burns 37:16-26, 2011

Infection is a major problem in burn care and especially when it is due to bacteria with hospital-acquired multi-resistance to antibiotics. Moreover, when these bacteria are Gram-negative organisms, the most effective molecules are 20 years old and there is little hope of any new product available even in the distant future. Therefore, it is obvious that currently available antibiotics should not be misused. With this aim in mind, the following review was conducted by a group of experts from the French Society for Burn Injuries (SFETB). It examined key points addressing the management of antibiotics for burn patients: when to use or not, time of onset, bactericidia, combination, adaptation, de-escalation, treatment duration and regimen based on pharmacokinetic and pharmacodynamic characteristics of these compounds. The authors also considered antibio-prophylaxis and some other key points such as: infection diagnosis criteria, bacterial inoculae and local treatment. French guidelines for the use of antibiotics in burn patients have been designed up from this work.

▶ This consensus article from the French burn centers is comprehensive and well written. While individual institutions may disagree with some indications for or against treatment, the article could serve as the basis for grand rounds. Perhaps the most important point regarding the spread of hospital-based infection not dealt with in the article is the negligence of hospital personnel in obeying infection control protocols. Simple hand washing between patient visits, gowning, and wearing gloves make a significant difference, especially in immunosuppressed patients.

R. E. Salisbury, MD

A Review of the Local Pathophysiologic Bases of Burn Wound Progression
Shupp JW, Nasabzadeh TJ, Rosenthal DS, et al (Washington Hosp Ctr, DC; Georgetown Univ School of Medicine, Washington, DC)
J Burn Care Res 31:849-873, 2010

Burn wound progression refers to the phenomenon of continued tissue necrosis in the zone of stasis after abatement of the initial thermal insult. A multitude of chemical and mechanical factors contribute to the local pathophysiologic process of burn wound progression. Prolonged inflammation results in an accumulation of cytotoxic cytokines and free radicals, along with neutrophil plugging of dermal venules. Increased vascular permeability and augmentations of interstitial hydrostatic pressure lead to edema with vascular congestion. Hypercoagulability with thrombosis further impairs blood flow, while oxidative stress damages endothelial cells and compromises vascular patency. A number of studies have investigated the utility of various agents in modulating these mechanisms of burn wound progression. However, as many of studies have used animal models of burn injury, often with administration of therapy preburn, obscuring the clinical applicability of the results to burn patients is of questionable benefit. An understanding of the complex, interrelated mediators of burn wound progression and their ultimate point of convergence in effecting tissue necrosis—cell apoptosis or oncosis—will allow for the future development of therapeutic interventions.

▶ This review article is outstanding and addresses a perplexing clinical problem. The mortality of large second-degree burns is considerably less than that of a similar-sized third-degree injury. In spite of extensive research, the progression of the zone of stasis to irreversible tissue death is poorly understood. How to prevent this phenomenon and achieve healing of the partial-thickness injury is unclear. Solving the problem would shift the mortality curve dramatically.

R. E. Salisbury, MD

A simple tool for mortality prediction in burns patients: APACHE III score and FTSA
Moore EC, Pilcher DV, Bailey MJ, et al (The Alfred Hosp, Prahran, Melbourne, Australia; Monash Univ — Clayton Campus, Melbourne, Australia; et al)
Burns 36:1086-1091, 2010

Prediction of outcome for patients with major thermal injury is important to inform clinical decision making, alleviate individual suffering and improve hospital resource allocation. Age and burn size are widely accepted as the two largest contributors of mortality amongst burns patients. The APACHE (Acute Physiology and Chronic Health Evaluation) III-j score, which incorporates patient age, is also useful for mortality prediction, of intensive care populations. Validation for the burns specific cohort is unclear.

A retrospective cohort study was performed on patients admitted to the Intensive Care Unit (ICU) via the Victorian Adult Burns Service (VABS), to compare observed mortality with burns specific markers of illness severity and APACHE III-j score. Our primary aim was to develop a mortality prediction tool for the burns population.

Between January 1, 2002 and December 31, 2008, 228 patients were admitted to the ICU at The Alfred with acute burns. The mean age was 45.6 years and 81% ($n = 184$) were male. Patients had severe injuries: the average percent TBSA (total body surface area) was 28% (IQR 10−40) and percent FTSA (full thickness surface area) was 18% (IQR 10−25). 86% ($n = 197$) had airway involvement. Overall mortality in the 7-year period was 12% ($n = 27$).

Non-survivors were older, had larger and deeper burns, a higher incidence of deliberate self-harm, higher APACHE III-j scores and spent less time in hospital (but similar time in ICU), compared with survivors.

Independent risk factors for death were percent FTSA (OR 1.03, 95% CI 1.01−1.05, $p = 0.01$) and APACHE III-j score (OR 1.04, 95% CI 1.02−1.07, $p < 0.001$). Mortality prediction based on both of these variables in combination was more specific than either individual variable alone (AUROC 0.85, 95% CI 0.79−0.92).

Likelihood of death for patients with severe thermal injury can be predicted with accuracy from APACHE III-j score and percent FTSA. Prospective validation of our model on different burn populations is necessary.

▶ Prediction of outcome with major thermal injury is important to inform clinical decision making, alleviate individual suffering, and improve hospital resource allocation. Mortality prediction tools are important to benchmark performance and identify areas for improvement but should be used cautiously for individuals. They are most valuable in comparing outcome over time and between centers.

R. E. Salisbury, MD

Adult Burn Patients With More Than 60% TBSA Involved—Meek and Other Techniques to Overcome Restricted Skin Harvest Availability—The Viennese Concept
Lumenta DB, Kamolz L-P, Frey M (Med Univ of Vienna, Austria)
J Burn Care Res 30:231-242, 2009

Despite the fact that early excision and grafting has significantly improved outcome over the last decades, the management of severely burned adult patients with ≥60% total body surface area (% TBSA) burned still represents a challenging task for burn care specialists all over the world. In this article, we present our current treatment concept for this entity of severely burned patients and analyze its effect in a comparative cohort study. Surgical strategy comprised the use of split-thickness skin grafts (Meek, mesh) for permanent coverage, fluidized microsphere bead-beds for wound conditioning, temporary coverage (polyurethane sheets, Epigard®; nanocrystalline silver dressings, Acticoat®; synthetic copolymer sheets based on lactic acid, Suprathel®; acellular bovine derived collagen matrices, Matriderm®; allogeneic cultured keratinocyte sheets; and allogeneic split-thickness skin grafts), and negative-pressure wound therapy (vacuum-assisted closure). The autologous split-thickness skin graft expansion using the Meek technique for full-thickness burns and the delayed approach for treating dorsal burn wounds is discussed in detail. To demonstrate differences before and after die introduction of the Meek technique, we have compared patients of 2007 with ≥60% TBSA (n = 10) to those in a matched observation period (n = 7). In the first part of the comparative analysis, all patients of the two samples were analyzed with regard to age, abbreviated burn severity idex, Baux, different entities of % TBSA, and survival. In the second step, only the survivors of both years were separated in two groups as follows: patients receiving skin grafts, using the Meek technique (n = 6), were compared with those without Meek grafting (n = 4). When comparing the severely burned patients of 2007 with a cohort of 2006, there were no differences for age (2007: 46.4 ± 13.4 vs. 2006: 39.1 ± 14.8 years), abbreviated burn severity index score (2007: 12.2 ± 1.0 vs. 2006: 12.1 ± 1.2) or % TBSA (2007: 72.1 ± 11.7 vs. 2006: 69.3 ± 8.7% TBSA). In these two rather small groups of severely burned patients with ≥60% TBSA, the overall survival rate of patients was 70.0% (7/10) in 2007 and 42.9% (3/7) in 2006, respectively. Almost all nonsurvivors in both years died within the first 5 days after admission. If assessing the different treatment modalities of the survivors, we found that although the Meek group patients were older (Meek 48.8 ± 13.3 vs. non-Meek 26.8 ± 11.5 years, P =.0381) and had consequentiy higher Baux scores (Meek 124.0 ± 2.9 vs. non-Meek 93.8 ± 8.5, P =.0095) than the non-Meek patients, this seemed to have no effect on length-of-stay (80.5 ± 9.7 vs. non-Meek 79.8 ± 33.0 days), hospital length-of-stay (85.7 ± 14.8 vs. non-meek 84.3 ± 26.1 days) or number of operations (6.5 ± 1.0 vs. non-Meek 7.0 ± 4.1 operations). The achieved results represent a combination of various treatment changes and, therefore, cannot be attributed to a single modality. The Meek technique is one of the technical options to choose from, to achieve permanent skin replacement; we think that it has its place if integrated in a whole treatment concept for management of severely burned patients.

▶ The incidence of total body burns greater than 60% admitted to burn centers is usually small. Thus, articles describing successful experience treating life-threatening burns are always welcome. The authors carefully describe many different techniques, including one for graft expansion (Meek technique), that warrant review. Survival is multifactorial, and the authors wisely did not attempt to draw inappropriate conclusions from the small number of patients.

R. E. Salisbury, MD

Anesthesia and Intraoperative High-Frequency Oscillatory Ventilation During Burn Surgery

Walia G, Jada G, Cartotto R (Ross Tilley Burn Centre, Toronto, Canada)

J Burn Care Res 32:118-123, 2011

High-frequency oscillatory ventilation (HFOV) is a mainstay in the ventilatory management of severe acute respiratory distress syndrome in our burn center. Many patients require burn surgery while on HFOV, potentially necessitating the use of HFOV during general anesthesia in the operating room. The purpose of this study was to describe the technique of providing and maintaining intraoperative HFOV. This is a retrospective analysis of the hospital and anesthesia records of all adult burn patients who went to the operating room on HFOV at our regional burn center between October 22, 1999, and April 30, 2009. There were 57 procedures performed on 36 patients who were receiving HFOV for severe acute respiratory distress syndrome available for analysis (age 45 ± 16 years, %TBSA burn 43 ± 14, % full-thickness burn 32 ± 19, and 69% with inhalation injury). Intraoperative HFOV settings were mean airway pressure 33 ± 4 cm H_2O, frequency 5 ± 1 Hz, and FiO_2 0.7 ± 0.2. There were no significant changes in oxygenation as measured by the PaO_2/FiO_2 ratio and the oxygenation index, but there was a transient but significant increase in $PaCO_2$ intraoperatively. Existing continuous infusions of midazolam, opioids, and neuromuscular blockers were continued during surgery and were augmented by a variety of parenteral agents, including propofol, fentanyl, and ketamine during surgery. Prone positioning was required in 16 of 57 procedures. Subanalysis of the prone cases showed no significant changes in the PaO_2/FiO_2 ratio or oxygenation index but again showed a significant but temporary increase in intraoperative $PaCO_2$. HFOV was aborted for conventional mechanical ventilation in three cases due to respiratory deterioration (2 cases) and hemodynamic instability (1 case). There were no intraoperative deaths. In-hospital mortality was 33%. Intraoperative HFOV was feasible and safe in the overwhelming majority of cases, and aside from an inconsequential period of intraoperative hypercapnia, this was not associated with any hemodynamic instability or compromise in oxygenation.

▶ The patient with acute respiratory distress syndrome still has an extremely high mortality rate, regardless of the burn center. The authors have shown 2 important points. First, high-frequency oscillatory ventilation can be administered safely. Second, skilled anesthesia support is mandatory in these patients.

Specifically, there are many options in anesthesia, but most are not applicable in these patients, requiring careful preoperative assessment.

R. E. Salisbury, MD

Use of β-Agonists in Inhalation Injury
Palmieri TL (Shriners Hosp for Children Northern California, CA)
J Burn Care Res 30:156-159, 2009

Background.—Inhalation injury causes several effects. Casts and protein-aceous materials accumulate in the airway, causing bronchoconstriction and airway hyperreactivity resembling what is seen in reactive airway diseases. If a large cutaneous burn accompanies the inhalation injury, capillary permeability in the lung and distal airway increases. The resulting pathologic condition is similar to what happens in acute lung injury (ALI), acute respiratory distress syndrome (ARDS), and reactive airway disease. Few therapies are effective in reactive airway disease and ARDS, but inhaled β_2-agonists have shown efficacy in preclinical studies of ALI/ARDS. The properties of β-agonists; the clinical effectiveness of these agents in ALI/ARDS, reactive airway disease, and inhalation injury; and the efficacy of β_2-agonists in inhalation injury were outlined.

Properties.—β_2-adrenoreceptors are found in airway smooth muscle and throughout the lung, especially in the smaller airways. Receptors occur in pulmonary epithelial and endothelial cells, type II cells, and mast cells. β_2-agonists have a preferential affinity for β_2-receptors and are designed to minimize the cardiac effects of using nonspecific β-agonists. Structural modifications decrease their metabolism by carboxymethyl transferase. Aerosolized delivery also diminishes the systemic effects of β_2-agonists on cardiac and skeletal muscle metabolism while activating β_2-receptors in the bronchi. Thus it avoids the unwanted cardiac and metabolic effects that come with systemically administered β_2-agonists. Aerosolization also produces a rapid therapeutic response. Particle size and respiratory parameters such as inspiratory flow rate, tidal volume, and airway diameter influence the effectiveness of aerosol therapy, which depends on delivering the drug to the distal airway. About 10% of the inhaled dose enters the lungs.

Some properties of β_2-agonists make them attractive for inhalation injury therapy. Their bronchodilator action improves respiratory mechanics by lowering airflow resistance and peak airway pressures, relaxes bronchial smooth muscle, and binds to and stabilizes the active form of the β-adrenergic receptor. β_2-agonists also offer anti-inflammatory properties, increase airspace fluid clearance, and can stimulate epithelial repair. All of these properties have the potential to improve the outcomes for ALI/ARDS patients and patients with inhalation injury.

Clinical Evidence.—The β_2-agonist salbutamol decreased extravascular lung water after ALI, which decreased mortality, in a randomized prospective trial. Inhaled salbutamol also decreased the duration and severity of ALI as well as the incidence of high-altitude pulmonary edema.

Use in Inhalation Injury.—Albuterol delivered via continuous nebulization has been tested in a laboratory model of inhalation injury and 40% total body surface area burn injury in sheep. Albuterol produced a 30% reduction in peak and plateau airway pressures, improved Pao_2/Fio_2 ratio and pulmonary shunt fraction, and significantly decreased lung lymph flow. Lung permeability index and lung wet-to-dry weight were also significantly diminished. Lung physiology was improved overall, with reduced pulmonary edema and lung vascular permeability to protein. Retrospective data on the use of continuous albuterol in children with inhalation injury improved oxygenation, compliance, and pH in the first 72 hours after treatment with no complications affecting cardiac, metabolic, or electrolyte status.

Conclusions.—Before β_2-agonists can be recommended for the treatment of inhalation injury they must undergo further prospective study. Albuterol, although having a proven track record in reactive airway disease, produces several side effects, such as tachycardia with high doses or hypokalemia that requires careful monitoring and quick correction. Nebulized albuterol requires consistent delivery via the ventilator circuit and monitoring by an experienced respiratory therapist. Any trial of these agents must include a standardized delivery method.

▶ Inhalation injury remains a major cause of mortality in patients with or without extensive skin injury. Clinical advances have been few, and this article, along with the one by Wolf SE,[1] nicely indicate possible local and systemic and therapeutic modalities.

R. E. Salisbury, MD

Reference

1. Wolf SE. Vitamin C and smoke inhalation injury. *J Burn Care Res.* 2009;30: 184-186.

Vitamin C and Smoke Inhalation Injury
Wolf SE (Univ of Texas Health Science Centre, San Antonio)
J Burn Care Res 30:184-186, 2009

Background.—The incomplete combustion of organic compounds can produce noxious chemicals to which the airway can be exposed, causing smoke inhalation injury. Usually the injury is confined to the upper airways, and involves an inflammatory response characterized by the recruitment of neutrophils with increased activity, degranulation, and the release of proteases and toxic oxygen free radicals. The increased neutrophil activity is related to decreased antioxidant activity. Because both inflammation and oxidative damage are involved, the administration of an antioxidant such as vitamin C may prevent further injury. Vitamin C has lessened oxidative damage in several in vitro and preclinical models outside the lungs. It decreases low-density lipoprotein oxidation, scavenges intracellular superoxide, and increases nitric acid activity. The specific effects of vitamin C in smoke inhalation injury were evaluated in a clinical trial of burned subjects; its effects on resuscitation in burned sheep and in dogs with burn injury were also studied.

Clinical Trial.—Thirty-seven subjects with burns exceeding 30% total body surface area (TBSA) were randomly assigned to receive placebo or 66 mg/kg/hr of vitamin C intravenously for 24 hours. Seventy-three percent of the subjects also had inhalation injury diagnosed by bronchoscopy at admission, with equal distribution between the two groups. Measurements included resuscitation volumes, weight, vital signs, and ventilatory parameters. The 24-hour resuscitation volume in the vitamin C group diminished by 40% compared to the placebo group. The vitamin C given in these high doses (about 4.5 gm/day over 24 hours) significantly reduced resuscitation volumes. Also, the placebo group required 21 ventilator days, but the vitamin C group only needed 12 ventilator days. Therefore both improved oxygenation and perhaps decreased lung damage were noted in the group treated with vitamin C, which may indicate its effects on lung inflammation or reflect a whole-body response.

Preclinical Trials.—Sheep received a 40% TBSA full-thickness burn and were assigned to treatment with placebo or high-dose vitamin C (10 gm in the first 500 ml of resuscitation volume followed by a 15 mg/kg infusion over 48 hours). None of the animals had smoke inhalation injury. A reduction of 49% in cumulative net fluid given to maintain equivalent urine output was seen in the vitamin C group.

Dogs with smoke inhalation injury were randomly assigned to receive an antioxidant cocktail including vitamin C or be in a control group. The treatment reduced extravascular lung water volume, pulmonary vascular resistance, carboxemia, hypoxia, and acidosis compared to the controls. Mortality for the two groups was 47.6% for the controls and 19.1% for the treated group.

Conclusions.—Giving high doses of vitamin C to patients having inhalation injury may improve outcomes. With burns and inhalation injury, vitamin C may improve oxygenation and decrease ventilator days. Preclinical studies indicate the presence of oxidant damage in the lungs after smoke inhalation injury might be diminished by the use of antioxidants such as vitamin C. Further study is needed.

▶ Inhalation injury remains a major cause of mortality in patients with or without extensive skin injury. Clinical advances have been few, and this article, along with the one by Palmiere TL,[1] nicely indicate possible local and systemic and therapeutic modalities.

R. E. Salisbury, MD

Reference

1. Palmiere TL. Inhalation therapies: use of β-agonists in inhalation injury. *J Burn Care Res.* 2009;30.

Phenylephrine Tumescence in Split-Thickness Skin Graft Donor Sites in Surgery for Burn Injury—A Concentration Finding Study

Mitchell RTM, Funk D, Spiwak R, et al (Univ of Manitoba, Winnipeg, Canada)
J Burn Care Res 32:129-134, 2011

The purpose of this study is to determine the lowest concentration of subcutaneous phenylephrine (neosynephrine) required for effective vasoconstriction in skin graft donor sites. Surgery for burn injury is associated with blood loss. Tourniquet use and tumescence with epinephrine have decreased blood loss. However, absorption of epinephrine has been reported with systemic effects. Phenylephrine, an α1-adrenergic receptor agonist, has vasoconstrictive properties similar to epinephrine's without other α-adrenergic or β-adrenergic activity. The aim of this study is to determine the lowest effective concentration of phenylephrine that will provide vasoconstriction in split-thickness graft donor sites. By using intensive care unit equivalency tables, the authors estimated a concentration of phenylephrine on the basis of current epinephrine tumescence. This concentration was titrated up or down according to an algorithm established a priori, determining the minimum concentration that achieved vasoconstriction in three consecutive patients. The primary outcome was local vasoconstriction. Secondary outcomes measured were pre-, intra-, and postoperative mean arterial pressure, systolic pressure and heart rate, graft take, and donor site healing. The subjects were six otherwise healthy adult patients (five men and one woman) with a mean age of 36 years. The average TBSA was 737.5 cm^2. Vasoconstriction was achieved at 5 μg/ml. No significant alterations in hemodynamic measures were observed. The optimal concentration of phenylephrine for prevention of bleeding in donor sites appears to be 5 μg/ml. Participants will be able to identify the effects of phenylephrine and epinephrine tumescence. They will also identify the concentration at which phenylephrine will be effective in donor sites.

▶ This is an interesting extension of some earlier work by Canepa et al.[1] That study demonstrated, as did this one, that phenylepinephrine was an effective vasoconstrictor. In the earlier study cited, performed in a rat model and testing concentrations of phenylepinephrine from 1:10 000 to 1:40 000, a concentration of 1:40 000 (much larger than the doses used in this study) significantly reduced blood loss, reduced lidocaine absorption, produced minimal reduction in tissue Po$_2$, and did not enhance bacterial invasion. In the rat study, the technique of injection of phenylepinephrine was not found to be a factor in efficacy. I encourage the authors to enlarge the scope of their studies, to include greater numbers of patients, and to consider studying local tissue effects of phenylepinephrine as well as its systemic effects.

S. H. Miller, MD, MPH

Reference

1. Canepa CS, Miller SH, Buck DC, Demuth RJ, Miller MA. Effects of phenylephrine on tissue gas tension, bleeding, infection and lidocaine absorption. *Plast Reconstr Surg.* 1988;81:554-560.

Volkmann's contracture in high-voltage electrical injury

Ahn CS, Maitz PKM (Concord Repatriation General Hosp, Rhodes, New South Wales, Australia)
Eur J Plast Surg 33:323-329, 2010

Burn injuries are a common form of trauma, it occurs in 1% of the population of Australasia each year. Of these injuries, the devastating effects of high-voltage electrical burns in deep tissue injury causing compartment syndrome and subsequent Volkmann's ischemic contracture are well documented. This report highlights the importance of early recognition of the severe electrical burn injury and its clinical consequences. Early identification through vigilant monitoring and diagnostic adjuncts, together with early intervention, whether conservative monitoring or operative management is of utmost importance in the prevention of ongoing complications and recovery from injury.

▶ High-voltage electrical injuries are not common, and thus, errors can be made easily during diagnosis and treatment. The authors are to be congratulated for their honesty in admitting their errors and discussing this case in great detail. Unfortunately, they refer to nonoperative treatment as a conservative course of care, which is incorrect. For this patient, not doing an escharotomy and a fasciotomy was radical care as the subsequent litany of problems prove. Although everyone desires firm guidelines for deciding when to do surgical decompression, there is no single infallible rule or test. It would be wise to study the reviews from major burn centers to get a background of opinions. When in doubt, it is safer to do a decompression than risking ischemia and subsequent necrosis.

R. E. Salisbury, MD

A 12-Year Comparison of Common Therapeutic Interventions in the Burn Unit

Whitehead C, Serghiou M (Shriners Hosps for Children, Galveston, TX)
J Burn Care Res 30:281-287, 2009

Although most occupational and physical therapists in an acute burn care setting use similar therapy practices, the time frames at which these therapeutic interventions are carried out vary according to the burn centers' practices. The purpose of this survey was to investigate current trends in burn rehabilitation and compare the results with a similar survey performed in 1994. The survey was designed in a similar fashion to the 1994 survey to ascertain common trends in burn rehabilitation. The survey was sent to 100 randomly selected burn care facilities throughout the United States and Canada. Content included rehabilitation interventions, including evaluation, positioning, splinting, active range of motion, passive range of motion, ambulation, as well as the cross-training of therapists. Significant increases in the percentages of burn centers initiating common therapy practices were found. Positioning (41% increase), active range of motion (48% increase), passive range of motion (52% increase), and ambulation (29% increase) were all found to have increases in the number of burn centers employing these practices in the same time frame. Overall comparison from 1994 to 2006 shows that common therapy techniques are being initiated earlier in the patient's acute burn stay. These results are consistent with recent medical trends of earlier acute discharges and more focus on outpatient rehabilitation.

▶ This article, along with the one by Finlay et al,[1] should be read together. The 12-year comparison of interventions indicates that more is being done in burn units to address rehabilitation. The study of lower limb function shows that more sophisticated work can and should be done. As standards of care improve, those units that are not in compliance might lose trauma center designation and insurance reimbursement.

R. E. Salisbury, MD

Reference

1. Finlay V, Phillips M, Wood F, Edgar D. A reliable and valid outcome battery for measuring recovery of lower limb function and balance after burn injury. *Burns.* 2010;36:780-786.

Coverage of Large Pediatric Wounds With Cultured Epithelial Autografts in Congenital Nevi and Burns: Results and Technique
Sood R, Balledux J, Koumanis DJ, et al (Indiana Univ School of Medicine, Indianapolis; Albany Med College, NY; et al)
J Burn Care Res 30:576-586, 2009

The use of cultured epithelial autografts (CEA) for the treatment of large burn wounds has gained popularity in recent years. This technique may circumvent the restrictions of limited donor site availability and hasten permanent wound coverage for large TBSA burns. The availability of a large amount of skin from a small donor site with the promise of permanent wound coverage suggests its use in other conditions such as giant congenital nevi (GCN) as well. The risk of malignant transformation of GCN to melanoma although somewhat controversial is significant enough to warrant early excision in childhood. Cultured keratinocytes may provide one-stage coverage of these large wounds, lessening the number of surgeries and the inherent staging problems of tissue expansion or auto-grafting. A retrospective single institution review was done for 29 children (20 burns and 9 patients with GCN) who underwent coverage of their large surface area wounds with CEA over an 18-year period. Excellent take rates were noted; 76.4% for burn patients and 66% for patients with GCN. Several strategies in preoperative, perioperative, and postoperative care have been standardized and have helped improve outcome. The keys to success with the CEA technique have been aggressive control of wound sepsis, surgical technique, specific use of topical antimicrobials, dressings, and the standardization of nursing and physiotherapy care. Although the cost of CEA is high, the benefits to patient care make this technique an appealing choice for large wound coverage in the pediatric population.

▶ The application of cultured epithelial autografts for treatment of large burn wounds is an accepted modality, with a track record of success. The use of this approach for giant congenital nevi is more controversial. The authors propose this approach because it allows excision of large areas of nevus-containing skin with immediate closure. They describe the advantage of this method as 1-stage coverage. However, it is important to examine the quality of this coverage. Even in cases that are shown in the article, a revision involving excision of unsightly or even unstable scar resulted in additional surgical procedures. For many patients, multiple stages of tissue expansion would clearly be more time consuming and costly, but the quality of the final result is often much more satisfactory than the coverage achieved with cultured epithelium. Therefore, the cultured keratinocyte approach could be considered more applicable to very large congenital nevi, where tissue expansion is logistically difficult or even impossible. In those cases, the protocol carefully described by the authors should yield a high rate of success.

R. L. Ruberg, MD

Acute Management of Burn Injuries to the Hand and Upper Extremity

McKee DM (Texas Tech Univ, Lubbock)
J Hand Surg Am 35:1542-1544, 2010

Background.—The management of burns depends on the depth and location of the injury as well as the patient's age. Depth, conveyed by the term *degree*, strongly influences the initial treatment of burn injuries. More critical injuries are handled first, often leaving less severe hand and upper extremity injuries until after the more serious burns have been addressed.

Classification.—The degree of damage to the epithelium, dermis, subcutaneous tissue, and deeper structures determines the classification of the burn. First-degree burns damage only the epidermis and cause no open wounds or blisters. Often these heal without scarring or surgical intervention.

Second-degree or partial-thickness burns injure the epidermis and various dermal levels. They can be superficial or deep. Superficial second-degree burns often heal through re-epithelialization with local wound care in 10 to 14 days. These burns form blisters and are painful because of damage to the nerve endings in the dermis. However, scarring is minimal because the inflammatory phase is shortened by the re-epithelialization. Minimal to no functional loss occurs if therapy and edema control measures are instituted promptly. In contrast, deep second-degree burns penetrate further into the dermal layer and destroy most epithelial cells, limiting re-epithelialization. Without functional nerve endings, these burns are insensate and nonpainful. Instead of blisters, they develop a thick eschar. Spontaneous healing produces poor re-epithelialization and extensive collagen deposits, resulting in extensive scarring and impaired function. Excision and grafting, similar to what is needed for full-thickness burns, are often required.

Third-degree or full-thickness burns damage the entire epidermis, dermis, and subcutaneous tissue. Unless they are small, they do not heal spontaneously and cause extensive scarring. Nonviable skin must be excised and skin grafts applied.

In fourth-degree burns the injury extends into structures such as muscle, tendon, and bone. These extreme injuries require staged reconstruction and possibly amputation.

Management.—Skin moisturizers and early movement are sufficient to manage first-degree burns. For superficial second-degree burns, local wound care is needed, with choices depending on surgeon preference, wound site, and patient age, among other factors. Deep second-degree burns and third-degree burns are managed with excision of nonviable tissue and early skin grafts. Tangential excision helps in controlling the debridement process. Wound coverage is usually done with split-thickness skin grafts. Surgical approaches depend on burn location, depth, and preference of the surgeon. Patients should begin occupational therapy as soon as possible, with an emphasis on active range of motion, passive range of motion, and control of edema. Presurgical, perisurgical, and postsurgical splinting is used as indicated.

▶ This article, by an orthopedic surgeon, was published in the *Journal of Hand Surgery*. Its worth lies in the tables summarizing principles of treatment. The when and how are not indicated, and the bibliography is too brief to be helpful. However, each portion of the tables deserves a full review and discussion before choices of treatment are made.

R. E. Salisbury, MD

Early excision and skin grafting versus delayed skin grafting in deep hand burns (a randomised clinical controlled trial)
Mohammadi AA, Bakhshaeekia AR, Marzban S, et al (Shiraz Univ of Med Sciences, Iran; et al)
Burns 37:36-41, 2011

Introduction.—Early excision and grafting (E&G) of burn wounds has been reported to decrease hospital stay, hospital costs and septic complications, and some purport reduced mortality while decreasing hospital costs.

In today's practice, all burn wounds unlikely to achieve spontaneous closure within 3 weeks are excised and grafted. Early studies did not demonstrate dramatic differences in cosmetic or functional results. This is particularly true with burns of the face, hands and feet. In this study, early excision and skin grafting was compared with delayed skin grafting in deep hand burns.

Materials and Methods.—From September 2006 to February 2008, 50 patients with hand burns and average burn size less than 30% total body surface area (TBSA) deep second- and third-degree were randomly divided into early E&G group (group I) and delayed grafting group (group II).

Gradual and careful limb and digit range of motion was started on about 10th–14th postoperative day. We used a questionnaire based on the Disabilities of the Arm, Shoulder and Hand (DASH) questionnaire to evaluate final functional outcome. Further, hypertrophic scar formation, contracture and deformities were followed and managed accordingly.

Results.—The most common site of involvement was the metacarpophalangeal (MCP) joint with frequency of 39% and 40% in groups I and II, respectively. There were no statistically significant differences between both groups regarding deformity severity, scar formation, sensation, major activities and overall satisfaction.

Discussion.—In treating burns of the hand, the primary goal should always be to restore the functionality of the hand. Although early surgery shortens the healing time and lessens the hospital stay, our results did not show any significant difference between these two methods regarding the function, scar formation, daily activity limitation and overall satisfaction.

▶ Perhaps the debate over proper treatment for hand burns will never be resolved. This nicely done prospective study demonstrates no superiority for early excision and grafting. The authors agree with others that a good result may be obtained either way. Poor surgery will give worse results than nonoperative management. In the delayed group, hand therapy, splinting, and control of bacterial proliferation can produce good results.

R. E. Salisbury, MD

Dermal substitution with Matriderm® in burns on the dorsum of the hand

Ryssel H, Germann G, Kloeters O, et al (Univ of Heidelberg, Germany)
Burns 36:1248-1253, 2010

Background.—Dermal substitutes are used increasingly in deep partial and full-thickness burn wounds in order to enhance elasticity and pliability. In particular, the dorsum of the hand is an area requiring extraordinary mobility for full range of motion. The aim of this comparative study was to evaluate intra-individual outcomes among patients with full-thickness burns of the dorsum of both hands. One hand was treated with split-thickness skin grafts (STSG) alone, and the other with the dermal substitute Matriderm® and split-thickness skin grafts.

Material and Methods.—In this study 36 burn wounds of the complete dorsum of both hands in 18 patients with severe burns (age 45.1 ± 17.4 years, 43.8 ± 11.8% TBSA) were treated with the simultaneous application of Matriderm®, a bovine based collagen I, III, V and elastin-hydrolysate based dermal substitute, and split-thickness skin grafting (STSG) in the form of sheets on one hand, and STSG in the form of sheets alone on the other hand. The study was designed as a prospective comparative study. Using both objective and subjective assessments, data were collected at one week and 6 months after surgery. The following parameters were included: After one week all wounds were assessed for autograft survival. Skin quality was measured 6 months postoperatively using the Vancouver Burn Skin Score (VBSS). Range of motion was measured by Finger-Tip-Palmar-Crease-Distance (FPD) and Finger-Nail-Table-Distance (FNTD).

Results.—Autograft survival was not altered by simultaneous application of the dermal matrix ($p > 0.05$). The VBSS demonstrated a significant increase in skin quality in the group with dermal substitutes ($p = 0.02$) compared to the control group with non-substituted wounds. Range of motion was significantly improved in the group treated with the dermal substitute ($p = 0.04$).

Conclusion.—From our results it can be concluded that simultaneous use of Matriderm® and STSG is safe and feasible, leading to significantly better results in respect to skin quality of the dorsum of the hand and range of motion of the fingers. Skin elasticity was significantly improved by the collagen/elastin dermal substitute in combination with sheet-autografts.

▶ A recent publication described and compared the use of the collagen-elastin matrix in over 46 patients and 69 paired wound sites over a 12-year period.[1] Most patients underwent scar and reconstructive procedures, with a smaller subset receiving the matrix for acute wound coverage. In their study, they were only able to relate an objective improvement in 2 categories: surface roughness when applied for reconstructive applications and elasticity when widely meshed autografts were used. Subjectively, patients and observers noted statistical improvement in pliability, relief, and general observer scores; however, elasticity was not statistically found to have been otherwise improved.

In this article, the authors treated 36 paired dorsal burn hand wounds (18 patients), using split-thickness skin sheet grafts on 1 hand and single-stage Matriderm (elastin-collagen matrix) and split-thickness skin sheet grafts on the contralateral hand. Patients wore pressure garments for greater than 16 hours per day, and a topical B5 vitamin moisturizer was used 3 times per day. Measured parameters were graft taken at 1 week and range of motion measurements and Vancouver Burn Skin Score (VBSS) assessment at 6 months.

The authors conclude that there was no significant difference noted in the skin graft taken and that objective skin elasticity was improved when the matrix was used. The former is a particularly gratifying result of this study, validating at least in these smaller surface area applications the potential for single stage bilaminate coverage. The latter assessment relies on VBSS assessment, a validated but subjective scale. It is here that many feel that the use of adjunctive objective assessment tools may be warranted before durable claims of intrinsic wound quality assessments might be quantified. To that end, various modalities are now generally available and consist of cutometers, colorimeters, durometers, and tonometers in addition to 3-dimensional analysis, laser Doppler, and ultrasound scanners.

Postburn scar maturation is thought to take several years. All of us in the field certainly look forward to continued objective evaluation to further appreciate the effects of time and cost on efficacy and applicability.

M. Tennenhaus, MD

Reference

1. Bloemen MC, van Leeuwen MC, van Vucht NE, van Zuijlen PP, Middelkoop E. Dermal substitution in acute burns and reconstructive surgery: a 12-year follow-up. *Plast Reconstr Surg.* 2010;125:1450-1459.

Comparison between topical honey and mafenide acetate in treatment of auricular burn

Hashemi B, Bayat A, Kazemei T, et al (Khalili Hosp, Shiraz, Iran)
Am J Otolaryngol 32:28-31, 2011

The auricle is a frequently injured part of the head and neck during thermal injury leading to ear deformity. The burned ear represents one of the most difficult problems for reconstructive surgeons. Mafenide acetate is a topical agent used routinely for these patients, but it has some disadvantages including painful application and allergic rash. Some authors have reported the healing effect and antibacterial activity of honey. The study reported here was undertaken to compare the effect of honey and mafenide acetate on auricular burn in rabbit. In our study, although the pathologic score of the honey group was better than that of the mafenide group both on 14 and 21 days after burning, it was not statistically significant. In the mafenide acetate group, deep complication of burn (chondritis) was significantly lower than that of the honey group. In conclusion, in contrast to healing and antibiotic activity reported for honey, it may have failure in preventing deep bacterial complications of wound (like chondritis). So in deep wounds, the use of honey as dressing is not recommended.

▶ This article provides an opportunity to review some basic burn principles. It is well known that mafenide impedes wound healing. The value of mafenide and Silvadene is the ability to decrease sepsis. The skin of the ear is so thin and the blood supply so fragile that uncontrolled bacterial proliferation can easily result in conversion of partial- to full-thickness wounds, ear loss, and even death.

R. E. Salisbury, MD

Burn Scar Assessment: A Systematic Review of Different Scar Scales
Brusselaers N, Pirayesh A, Hoeksema H, et al (Ghent Univ Hosp, Belgium; et al)
J Surg Res 164:e115-e123, 2010

Background.—Scars can be devastating and disfiguring, because they are clearly visible, stigmatizing, and permanent reminders of the initial accident or surgical event. Yet, there is still no consensus about the optimal *scale or tool* to assess the characteristics and evolution. Our aim was to evaluate the clinical importance of scar scales specifically developed for burn scars.

Materials and Methods.—The systematic literature search involved PubMed and the Web of Science (including Science Citation Index).

Results.—The search resulted in 29 articles (including seven reviews) dealing with a new, modified, or validated scale. Scar scales assess several characteristics, of which color, pliability, and thickness were considered the most important. Physical limitation, pain, and pruritus are often more disturbing than the appearance of the scar, and are therefore also introduced in scar evaluation, as well as the interference with daily life activities (e.g., psychologic impact).

Conclusion.—In contrast to the more objective scar assessment *tools*, scar scales usually cover more aspects of the scars and are less time-consuming in clinical practice. However, no strong conclusions can be made about their efficacy and validity. In addition to digital photography, scar scales are a valuable instrument in the clinical evaluation and follow-up of scars.

▶ As more patients survive lethal burn injuries, this subject assumes greater importance. Sadly, most professionals are speaking different languages—meaning they are using different assessment tools. The result is that people are using very different criteria for surgery and very different standards for claiming success.

R. E. Salisbury, MD

Methods and Tools Used for the Measurement of Burn Scar Contracture
Parry I, Walker K, Niszczak J, et al (Shriners Hosp for Children, Northern California, Sacramento, CA)
J Burn Care Res 31:888-903, 2010

After burn injury, scar contracture can cause significant impairment and functional deficit. Many studies have investigated the treatment and prevention of burn scar contracture, but few studies have focused on the methods for measuring contracture. The purpose of this study was to determine whether consistent and objective methods of measurement are used to quantify scar contracture in the clinical evaluation of burn patients and in burn research. A survey was administered to 407 burn therapists to determine the methods and tools used clinically to measure scar contracture, while a review of recent burn literature was conducted to determine the methods and tools used in burn research. The results of the survey indicate that there is a lack of consensus in the methods and tools used for the measurement of scar contracture, both clinically and in research. Instead, a variety of measurement methods was reported, each with varying degrees of objectivity. Clinically, the methods are rarely checked for reliability or performance competency. In burn research, the methods and tools vary, and contracture data obtained are often reported in an inconsistent manner. If the measurement of scar contracture is not done objectively and consistently, then it is difficult to determine reliability, validity, and responsiveness of the measurement methods. Development of standard protocols with reliable measures of scar contracture would improve the quality of burn care and research.

▶ An extensive survey done by the authors that merely confirms what we all know to be true therapy is valuable, but the science is thin.
 The use of compression garments has fostered a cottage industry, but the value remains questionable. Answers will only be found when major centers adopt similar measurement tools and work together.

R. E. Salisbury, MD

A new alternative for reconstruction of soft triangle defects secondary to burn injury: Superiorly based columellar flap
Ersoy B, Çelebiler Ö, Numanoğlu A (Marmara Univ School of Medicine, Uskudar, Istanbul, Turkey)
J Plast Reconstr Aesthet Surg 63:1733-1735, 2010

Nasal reconstruction following severe burn injury remains a challenge in plastic surgery. In burn patients, the external nares and the soft triangle are commonly affected subunits of the nose where local tissue deficit and scar contraction during the recovery period contribute to soft triangle deformity and alar stenosis. These patients usually have associated facial burns with varying severity, which significantly limit the availability of local flaps. Reconstruction with skin grafts often yields unsatisfactory results because of the mismatch in colour and texture in addition to the primary and secondary contraction phenomena. The use of superiorly based columellar flap, which has yielded satisfactory results on a female patient, would be a new and reliable option for reconstruction of the soft triangle deficit with alar stenosis.

▶ The results of this report are so poor in attempting to manage this problem that any case report showing some success is welcome. The case is well illustrated and warrants study.

R. E. Salisbury, MD

Post-burn philtrum restoration
Grishkevich VM (A.V.Vishnevsky Inst of Surgery of the Russian Academy of Med Sciences, Moscow, Russia)
Burns 36:698-702, 2010

One of the consequences of face burn is upper lip deformation with philtrum injury. The philtrum's absence poses severe cosmetic defects. A literature review shows no effective developed technique which allows the

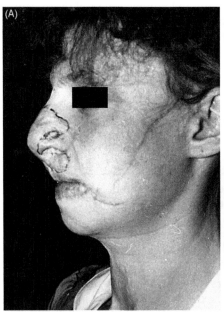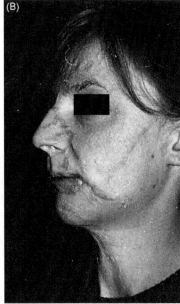

FIGURE 2.—Result of the philtrum, upper lip, and nose reconstruction. (A) Before surgery: severe deformity of the upper lip, nose, and philtrum destruction. (B) Two years after reconstruction: scars have been excised with skin grafting, the restored philtrum adorns the upper lip and the whole face. (Reprinted from Grishkevich VM. Post-burn philtrum restoration. *Burns.* 2010;36:698-702. Copyright 2010 with permission from International Society for Burn Injuries.)

surgeon to restore the upper lip and the philtrum in a single-stage procedure. The article presents a new method for burn-damaged philtrum restoration. Two scar stripes are deliberately left in place above the upper lip where the normal philtral ridges should be. The width of these two stripes (ridges) should be around 4 mm. The upper lip scars, lateral both ridges and between them, are excised forming the philtral dimple. The wound is covered with a split thickness skin graft. Two U-shaped sutures are led through the skin graft, both scar stripes and deeper through the underlying tissues between stripes. A bolster is plunged between the ridges in order to fill the dimple and is fixed by the tie-over dressing with tension. The skin transplant lying laterally to the ridges is covered with a separate tie-over dressing. The bolster is being kept in place for the duration of 7 days. As a result, the scar ridges preserve their height and the dimple keeps its depth. Good long-time follow-up results (up to 7 years) were observed in all 18 patients. In most cases the dimple can be slightly smoothed with time. The suggested method of philtrum restoration is an important component of the burned upper lip reconstruction as part of the post-burn facial resurfacing (Fig 2).

▶ Clever use of burn scars to restore a more normal central upper lip. Of course, for this technique to work, the burn scars must be mature and the color match a good one. The long-term follow-up seems to demonstrate that the scar philtral ridges retain their height.

S. H. Miller, MD, MPH

A Treatment Strategy for Postburn Neck Reconstruction: Emphasizing the Functional and Aesthetic Importance of the Cervicomental Angle
Zhang YX, Wang D, Follmar KE, et al (Shanghai Jiao Tong Univ School of Medicine, China; Duke Univ Med Ctr, Durham, NC)
Ann Plast Surg 65:528-534, 2010

The authors describe an algorithm for reconstruction of both the soft tissue and skeletal components of severe postburn neck deformities. The critical functional and aesthetic importance of the cervicomental angle is emphasized. The neck is subdivided into 3 anatomic subunits: (1) lower lip/chin subunit, (2) submental subunit, and (3) anterior neck subunit. After release of contractures, platysmaplasty is performed to prevent recurrence and to deepen the cervicomental angle. In cases where chin retrusion is present, sliding genioplasty is performed. The 3 subunits are resurfaced individually by skin grafts and free flaps. The combined scapular and parascapular bilobed free flap is an ideal flap for cases involving 2 subunits. Fifty patients with severe postburns neck contractures were treated. After excision and release of scar, 47 (94%) patients underwent platysmaplasty, and 12 (24%) patients underwent sliding genioplasty. Defects were covered with skin grafts alone in 20 (40%) patients, with free flaps only in 22 (44%) patients, and with a combination of skin grafts and free flaps in 8 (16%) patients.

▶ This article introduces a number of valuable concepts that can be combined in severe postburn contracture cases to achieve a much improved cervicomental angle and chin projection. (1) Introduction of a platysmaplasty allows deepening of the cervicofacial angle and increased bulk of tissue over the mentum. It is important to note that this is *not* the same platysmaplasty that is done for aesthetic improvement in the aging neck. In the burn cases, the entire platysma is incised transversely, and the superior portion is rotated upward to lie over the chin. (2) Addressing the skeletal structure through sliding genioplasty achieves further enhancement of chin projection. Even though the burn contracture is largely a soft tissue problem, adding a bony reconstructive component seems to be very beneficial in selected cases. (3) The authors revise the standard approach to the subunits of the neck by dividing the upper and lower neck into 2 separate units. By addressing each area individually, and not as part of a single top-to-bottom neck unit, the authors achieve further enhancement of the cervicomental angle. The postoperative results illustrated in this article effectively emphasize the value of these different components of the authors' approach.

R. L. Ruberg, MD

Combined AlloDerm® and thin skin grafting for the treatment of postburn dyspigmented scar contracture of the upper extremity

Oh SJ, Kim Y (Hallym Univ Sacred Heart Hosp, Anyang-si, Gyeonggi-do, Republic of Korea)
J Plast Reconstr Aesth Surg 64:229-233, 2011

Postburn dyspigmented scar contractures of the upper extremity often require aesthetic improvement. The ideal reconstruction of this deformity remains a challenge because the various available skin grafts and flaps result in skin colour mismatches, prominent marginal scars and donor morbidity. Postburn scar contractures and dyspigmented areas of the upper extremity can be improved by a combination of dermabrasion and Alloderm® graft over scar-releasing defect. Their raw surfaces are subsequently re-surfaced with thin split-thickness skin graft (0.005−0007 inches thick).

Twenty-seven patients with wide dyspigmented scar contractures of the upper extremity underwent the combined techniques described by us. The median patient age at burn incidents was 3 years and at operation was 24 years. Median thin skin graft area was 180 cm^2, and the median AlloDerm® graft area was 40 cm^2.

Thin skin and AlloDerm® grafts took root completely in all patients without re-grafting. Follow-up periods ranged from 30 to 67 months (average 47.6 months). Re-pigmentation was achieved in all cases and all scar contractures were adequately released and treated with an AlloDerm® graft. Paired differences between preoperative and postoperative parameters as determined by the Vancouver Scar Scale (VSS) were significant. Focal hypertrophic scar and reddish-coloured graft sites gradually improved over 3—4 years postoperatively. Graft margin and donor scars were inconspicuous. Our described combined technique was found to treat these deformities effectively.

We suggest that the use of Alloderm® and thin skin grafting be considered in patients concerned about this type of cosmetic disfigurement.

▶ This article is notable for several reasons. First, the state of the art in burn care has advanced to the point that patients desire scar improvement of extremities that could be covered by clothes. This attitude must be recognized as real and not frivolous. Second, the authors had no graft loss, demonstrating excellent technique.

R. E. Salisbury, MD

A reliable and valid outcome battery for measuring recovery of lower limb function and balance after burn injury
Finlay V, Phillips M, Wood F, et al (Royal Perth Hosp, Australia; Univ of Western Australia, Australia)
Burns 36:780-786, 2010

Introduction.—The measurement of recovery after burns to the lower limbs is hampered by an absence validated injury specific tools. This research aimed to select and validate a battery of outcome measures of recovery after lower limb burn injury (LLBI).

Method.—*Reliability study*: Reliability of the single leg stance (SLS), the Timed Up and Go (TUG) and the tandem walk (TW) tests were measured using a test—retest trial involving 28 patients with LLBI. *Validity study*: Clinical data from 172 patients with LLBI were used to compare changes in each LL outcome measure with changes in the Burn Specific Health Scale-Brief (BSHS-B).

Results.—All tests, except the SLS test with eyes closed, demonstrated excellent inter-rater reliability (ICCs = 0.81—0.93). The TUG and the TW-forwards tests were shown to be valid and to provide additional information to the BSHS-B when combined as a battery. The TW-backwards test was redundant while the SLS and ankle DF measures did not correlate highly with the BSHS-B.

Conclusion.—This study shows that the TUG test and the TWF are reliable and valid in the burns population and along with the BSHS-B form a useful test battery for measuring recovery from LLBI.

▶ This article, along with the one by Whitehead et al,[1] should be read together. The 12-year comparison of interventions indicates that more is being done in burn units to address rehabilitation. The study of lower limb function shows that more sophisticated work can and should be done. As standards of care improve, those units not in compliance might lose trauma center designation and insurance reimbursement.

R. E. Salisbury, MD

Reference

1. Whitehead C, Serghiou M. A 12-year comparison of common therapeutic interventions in the burn unit. *J Burn Care Res.* 2009;30:281-287.

Barriers Impacting Employment After Burn Injury
Schneider JC, Bassi S, Ryan CM (Massachusetts General Hosp, Boston)
J Burn Care Res 30:294-300, 2009

This study investigates the barriers to return to work after burn injury. The electronic records of burn survivors treated at a Regional Burn Center outpatient clinic from 2001 to 2007 were retrospectively reviewed. Inclusion criteria included employment at the time of burn injury and age 18 years or older. Documentation of barriers to return to work were reviewed and classified into eight categories. Logistic regression analysis was used to determine predictors of return to work at more than 1 year. Ordered logistic regression analysis was performed to determine barrier predictors of employment. The authors identified 197 patients for inclusion in the study. The age was 37 ± 0.8 (mean ± SEM) and total body surface area burned was $16 \pm 1.3\%$. Two thirds (n = 132) of subjects returned to work by 1 year. The most common barriers included pain (n = 79), neurologic problems (n = 69), impaired mobility (n = 58), and psychiatric issues (n = 51). Pain was the most frequent barrier to return to work at all time intervals. Significant predictors of return to work at more than 12 months included length of hospital stay, inpatient rehabilitation, electric etiology, and burn at work ($P < .05$). Impaired mobility was a statistically significant ($P < .05$) barrier and other medical issues showed a trend toward statistical significance ($P = .054$) in predicting return to work at more than 12 months. There are many barriers that impede return to work in the burn population, including pain, neurologic problems, impaired mobility, and psychiatric issues. Early identification of those at risk for prolonged unemployment should prompt expeditious referral to comprehensive rehabilitation services that include work hardening and vocational training programs.

▶ This article is an outstanding retrospective analysis. It emphasizes the importance of early intervention in helping survivors regain their ability to return to work. Thus, early psychiatric evaluation to identify posttraumatic stress disorder and a work hardening program are mandatory.

R. E. Salisbury, MD

4 Hand and Upper Extremity

General

What's New in Hand Surgery
Amadio PC (Mayo Clinic, Rochester, MN)
J Bone Joint Surg Am 92:783-789, 2010

Background.—The presentations at the 2009 annual meetings of the American Society for Surgery of the Hand (ASSH), the American Association for Hand Surgery (AAHS), and the American Academy of Orthopaedic Surgeons (AAOS) offered updated information in several areas. The principal findings were briefly explained.

Trauma.—War injuries involving hand amputations are receiving more attention. Innovative changes in upper limb prosthetics include targeted muscle reinnervation (TMR), in which nerves that served the amputated part are rerouted to new muscle sites. These reinnervated target muscles produce electromyographic signals that can control upper limb prostheses, producing more rapid and natural movements of the prosthetics.

Hand transplantation immunotherapy is more complex than for single-tissue organ transplantations. New immunosuppression regimens are being developed based on data from the first two hand transplantation patients, who report fair function 7 and 9 years post-transplantation. However, both have suffered episodes of rejection and other complications related to immunosuppressive medication. Skin is the primary target of rejection, and repetitive hand trauma can trigger a rejection episode. New strategies focus on reducing or intermittently eliminating immunosuppressive therapy, with the potential to greatly reduce morbidity. Post-transplant morbidity is also being more thoroughly assessed using a decision tree. A unilateral hand transplantation produces about 25 quality-adjusted life-years (QALYs) over a remaining lifespan of 40 years, and bilateral transplantation produces 22 QALYs; the transplantations would cost more than $700,000 per QALY. The QALYs for unilateral and bilateral amputations are estimated at 34 and 29 and cost per QALY is between $14,000 and $27,000. Prosthetic adaptation is therefore preferred over current hand transplantation techniques.

Radial column plating, volar plating, and external fixation were compared for the management of radial fractures. Volar plating produced better restoration of motion and function in the first 3 months, but outcomes were similar thereafter. Complications with dorsal plates included joint stiffness and extensor tendon problems, whereas with volar plates removal was needed because of screw penetration into the radiocarpal joint, which is usually only found on postoperative tomography.

Patients with distal radial fractures were more satisfied with treatment results when they recovered at least 65% of the grip strength, 87% of the pinch strength, and 95% of the wrist arc of motion of their uninjured side. Recovery of wrist function was the most important component related to satisfaction and involved a range of motion more than hand surgeons usually consider "functional." Fracture of the ulnar styloid, which may indicate distal radioulnar joint injury, apparently does not require internal fixation. However, no studies considered the Galeazzi fracture variants, where the styloid fracture is associated with instability of the distal radioulnar joint; fixation in these cases makes the reduction of the distal radioulnar joint more stable.

Carpal tunnel syndrome often accompanies distal radial fractures. Women under age 48 years with fractures where the distal fragment is translated more than 35% of the bone width have a higher risk for post-fracture carpal tunnel syndrome. Osteoporosis treatments (bisphosphonates) and delayed fracture healing may also be linked.

A treatment algorithm was developed to manage children with closed displaced phalangeal neck fractures. First, closed reduction is attempted. If that fails, percutaneous reduction using an intrafocal Kirschner wire as a "joystick" is tried, reserving open reduction for cases where percutaneous reduction is unsuccessful. In addition, malunions of phalangeal condylar fractures in children can achieve complete remodeling within 5 years without surgical intervention. Thus for pediatric phalangeal condylar and neck fractures, less treatment appears to be sufficient for good healing.

Thumb ligament injuries are generally diagnosed using a specific angular measurement or comparison with the contralateral thumb. It now appears that lack of an end point on stress testing is the best way to detect a complete ligament tear.

Activity Restrictions.—Patients often want to know when they can return to driving. A study of 30 police officers found that regardless of hand dominance, splints on the left arm caused worse driving scores. Above-the-elbow splints caused worse outcomes than below-the-elbow splints. Outcomes may be influenced by driver position.

Postoperative Pain.—Patients can suffer different amounts of perceived pain and disability postoperatively after similar operations. Function is significantly correlated with depression, pain catastrophizing, pain anxiety, and pain rating. The levels of preoperative depression and anxiety were the most predictive, supporting the practice of assessing patients' level of anxiety and depression preoperatively.

Arthritis and Degenerative Diseases.—Implant arthroplasty produced better hand function than medical treatment in rheumatoid arthritis patients. The results with joint replacement implants are not as positive for proximal interphalangeal joint arthritis. However, surgeons who perform trapezium excision arthroplasty can remove part of the flexor carpi radialis tendon for ligament reconstruction without fear of causing postoperative declines in wrist flexion motion or wrist flexion strength. Even this approach may be unnecessary, however, with no differences in pain, motion, or strength found between persons having trapeziectomy with flexor carpi radialis ligament reconstruction, Kirschner wire fixation, and 6 weeks of postoperative casting and patients having simple trapeziectomy and 3 weeks of protection in a soft bandage.

For patients who have both thumb carpometacarpal arthritis and carpal tunnel syndrome, it may be acceptable to release the carpal tunnel through the base of the trapeziectomy incision rather than make a separate incision. In addition, should resection of the distal part of the ulna fail, distal radioulnar joint arthroplasty delivers excellent results in terms of pain, stability, motion, and patient satisfaction with no stem loosening.

Nerves.—Nerve gaps may be closed by nerve mobilization or some type of bridging, usually through nerve grafts. Nerve conduits, polyglycolic acid mesh or autologous vein from the dorsal part of the hand or forearm, were compared for their effectiveness in bridging gaps measuring 4 to 25 mm. Although postoperative sensibility was comparable, the synthetic conduits suffered more postoperative complications than the vein conduits. Neurolysis and wrapping with a resorbable collagen tube may be adequate treatment for symptomatic neuromas of the radial sensory nerve, however.

Hand Tumors.—Longer term results for collagenase injections to treat Dupuytren disease are now available. The collagenase injections were especially helpful for patients with isolated metacarpophalangeal joint contractures. However, other therapies already effectively manage these cases. Short- and long-term costs, morbidity, and outcome of needle and enzyme treatments must be assessed.

▶ A very nice overview of current topics in hand surgery. This a 30 000 foot view. For those who want in-depth information, the references will be key.

D. J. Smith, Jr, MD

A Prospective Trial on the Use of Antibiotics in Hand Surgery
Aydın N, Uraloğlu M, Burhanoğlu ADY, et al (Ankara Numune Training and Res Hosp, Turkey)
Plast Reconstr Surg 126:1617-1623, 2010

Background.—Postoperative infection is a disastrous complication in the discipline of hand surgery, as it is in any field of surgery in which infection can compromise wound healing and lead to subsequent functional impairment despite the best attempts. Different results with antibiotic use by different authors have been reported. This study was planned to put forth the place of antibiotic use in hand surgery procedures.

Methods.—This prospective, randomized, double-blind study included 1340 patients who were placed in one of four groups according to the components of their hands that were injured. Half of each group received antibiotics, and the other half received placebo.

Results.—Infections among the placebo- and antibiotic-administered patients did not display significant importance ($p = 0.759$). Infections among the four groups were not statistically significant either ($p = 0.947$). Statistical significance was not found between elective and emergency procedures ($p = 0.552$). Operations longer than 2 hours had 2.5 percent infection rates in placebo patients and 3.8 percent in antibiotic patients, which was not statistically significant ($p = 0.7$). In crush/dirty wounds there was no statistical significance in development of infections between placebo and antibiotic use ($p = 1$), nor was there any statistically significant difference between crush and dirty wounds ($p = 0.929$).

Conclusions.—The authors do not support the use of antibiotic prophylaxis for surgery of the hand. Its use should be preserved for specific infections or for patients with certain types of risk factors for infection.

▶ Fact meets reality. *Fact:* This is another good study showing no benefit of preoperative antibiotics in elective and emergency procedures. It is a prospective, randomized, double blind study evaluating 1340 patients. *Conclusion:* Infections among the placebo and antibiotic-administered patients did not display significant difference. *Reality:* In our current medical environment (read that any way you want), it is highly unlikely that there will be a dramatic shift away from using preoperative antibiotics. *Frustration:* Even with strong evidence, it is difficult to change practice patterns because of outside pressures.

D. J. Smith, Jr, MD

The 'Butter Test' to guide effective tissue cleansing after high-pressure injection injury
Urso-Baiarda F, Stanley PRW (Castle Hill Hosp, Cottingham, UK)
J Plast Reconstr Aesth Surg 63:e792-e795, 2010

A case of high-pressure fingertip injury with an unknown paint primer injectate, and the use of a simple test to determine whether it is water- or solvent-based in order to guide subsequent optimal debridement, is presented. The favourable outcome achieved was felt to have resulted, in part, from the effective single debridement thus achieved.

▶ Rarely is a case report included among my commentaries, but this is a really ingenious idea. Beware, 1 case report is not an endorsement of this treatment.

On the other hand, the use of butter for emulsification and removal of the solvent is intriguing. At the very least, this should be a quick read for anyone treating injection injuries. It will make you think.

D. J. Smith, Jr, MD

Replantation of Finger Avulsion Injuries: A Systematic Review of Survival and Functional Outcomes
Sears ED, Chung KC (Univ of Michigan Health System; Ann Arbor)
J Hand Surg 36A:686-694, 2011

Purpose.—Recent studies presenting functional outcomes after replantation of finger avulsion injuries have challenged the historical practice of performing revision amputation for all complete finger avulsion injuries. The aim of this study is to conduct a systematic review of the English literature of replantation of finger avulsion injuries to provide best evidence of survival rates and functional outcomes.

Methods.—A Medline literature search yielded 1,398 studies, using key words "traumatic amputation" or "replantation", with limitation to humans and finger injuries. Inclusion criteria required that studies meet the following requirements: (1) primary data are presented; (2) the study includes at least 5 cases with either complete or incomplete finger avulsion injuries at or distal to the metacarpophalangeal joint; (3) the study presents survival rates, total active arc of motion (TAM), or static 2-point discrimination (2PD) data; (4) data for incomplete and complete avulsions are reported separately; (5) patients are treated with microvascular revascularization or replantation. Survival rates, TAM, and 2PD data were recorded and a weighted mean of each was calculated.

Results.—Thirty-two studies met the inclusion criteria. Of these 32 studies, all reported survival outcomes, 13 studies reported TAM (metacarpophalangeal, proximal interphalangeal, and distal interphalangeal), and 9 studies reported sensibility. The mean survival rate for complete finger and thumb avulsions having replantation was 66% (n = 442). The mean TAM of complete finger avulsions after successful replantation was 174° (n = 75), with a large number of patients in the included studies having arthrodesis of the distal interphalangeal joint. The mean 2PD in patients after replantation was 10 mm (n = 32).

Conclusions.—We found that functional outcomes of sensibility and range of motion after replantation of finger avulsion injuries are better than what is historically cited in the literature. The results of this systematic review challenge the practice of performing routine revision amputation of all complete finger avulsion injuries.

▶ Once again, Sears and Chung challenge traditional surgical teaching. On reviewing multiple appropriate studies, they determine that functional outcomes of sensibility and range of motion after replantation of finger avulsion injuries are better than what is historically cited in the literature. The results challenge the practice of routine revision amputation for all complete finger avulsion injuries. This article is a must read for anyone doing microsurgical replantation surgery or triaging these patients. It certainly challenges my biases.

D. J. Smith, Jr, MD

An Evidence-Based Approach to Dupuytren's Contracture
Brandt KE (Washington Univ in Saint Louis, MO)
Plast Reconstr Surg 126:2210-2215, 2010

The Maintenance of Certification module series is designed to help the clinician structure his or her study in specific areas appropriate to his or her clinical practice. This article is prepared to accompany practice-based assessment of preoperative assessment, anesthesia, surgical treatment plan, perioperative management, and outcomes. In this format, the clinician is invited to compare his or her methods of patient assessment and treatment, outcomes, and complications, with authoritative, information-based references.

This information base is then used for self-assessment and benchmarking in parts II and IV of the Maintenance of Certification process of the American Board of Plastic Surgery. This article is not intended to be an exhaustive treatise on the subject. Rather, it is designed to serve as a reference point for further in-depth study by review of the reference articles presented.

▶ As noted in the introduction to each article, "The Maintenance of Certification module series is designed to help the clinician structure his or her study in specific areas appropriate to his or her clinical practice. This article is prepared to accompany practice-based assessment of preoperative assessment, anesthesia, surgical treatment plan, perioperative management, and outcomes. In this format, the clinician is invited to compare his or her methods of patient assessment and treatment, outcomes, and complications, with authoritative, information-based references."

Anyone doing hand surgery should take advantage of this review opportunity. Furthermore, this allows each practitioner the opportunity for self-assessment and benchmarking. It is important not only for the Maintenance of Certification but also as a routine to keep one's practice current.

Also read these 2 articles: "An Evidence-Based Approach to Carpal Tunnel Syndrome" and "An Evidence-Based Approach to Metacarpal Fractures."

D. J. Smith, Jr, MD

The Treatment of Dupuytren Disease

Desai SS, Hentz VR (Newport Orthopedic Inst, Newport Beach, CA; Stanford Univ Hosp & Clinics, Palo Alto, CA)
J Hand Surg 36A:936-942, 2011

The treatment of progressive Dupuytren contractures has historically been and continues to be largely surgical. Although a number of surgical interventions do exist, limited palmar fasciectomy continues to be the most common and widely accepted treatment option. Until recently, nonsurgical options were limited and clinically ineffective. However, the commercial availability and recent approval of collagenase clostridium histolyticum now provides practitioners with a nonsurgical approach to this disease. This article presents a comprehensive review of the surgical and nonsurgical treatments of Dupuytren disease, with a focus on collagenase.

▶ This is an excellent review of both the surgical and nonsurgical treatments of Dupuytren disease. It's a thorough discussion and comparison of various surgical treatments, but with new emphasis on treatment with collagenase clostridium histolyticum. Two prospective studies show excellent initial success with relatively few major complications. I would clearly be interested in using this methodology but might be more careful and discriminating with the little finger. Long-term results are lacking, and recurrence should be anticipated.

D. J. Smith, Jr, MD

An Evidence-Based Approach to Metacarpal Fractures

Friedrich JB, Vedder NB (Univ of Washington, Seattle)
Plast Reconstr Surg 126:2205-2209, 2010

The Maintenance of Certification module series is designed to help the clinician structure his or her study in specific areas appropriate to his or her clinical practice. This article is prepared to accompany practice-based assessment of preoperative assessment, anesthesia, surgical treatment plan, perioperative management, and outcomes. In this format, the clinician is invited to compare his or her methods of patient assessment and treatment, outcomes, and complications, with authoritative, information-based references.

This information base is then used for self-assessment and benchmarking in parts II and IV of the Maintenance of Certification process of the American Board of Plastic Surgery. This article is not intended to be an exhaustive treatise on the subject. Rather, it is designed to serve as a reference point for further in-depth study by review of the reference articles presented.

▶ As noted in the introduction to each article, "The Maintenance of Certification module series is designed to help the clinician structure his or her study in specific areas appropriate to his or her clinical practice. This article is prepared to accompany practice-based assessment of preoperative assessment, anesthesia, surgical treatment plan, perioperative management, and outcomes. In this format, the clinician is invited to compare his or her methods of patient assessment and treatment, outcomes, and complications, with authoritative, information-based references."

Anyone doing hand surgery should take advantage of this review opportunity. Furthermore, this allows each practitioner the opportunity for self-assessment and benchmarking. It is important not only for the Maintenance of Certification but also as a routine to keep one's practice current.

Also read these 2 articles: "An Evidence-Based Approach to Carpal Tunnel Syndrome" and "An Evidence-Based Approach to Dupuytren's Contracture."

D. J. Smith, Jr, MD

An Evidence-Based Approach to Treating Thumb Carpometacarpal Joint Arthritis
Haase SC, Chung KC (Univ of Michigan Med School, Ann Arbor)
Plast Reconstr Surg 127:918-925, 2011

The Maintenance of Certification module series is designed to help the clinician structure his or her study in specific areas appropriate to his or her clinical practice. This article is prepared to accompany practice-based assessment of preoperative assessment, anesthesia, surgical treatment plan, perioperative management, and outcomes. In this format, the clinician is invited to compare his or her methods of patient assessment and treatment, outcomes, and complications, with authoritative, information-based references.

This information base is then used for self-assessment and benchmarking in parts II and IV of the Maintenance of Certification process of the American Board of Plastic Surgery. This article is not intended to be an exhaustive treatise on the subject. Rather, it is designed to serve as a reference point for further in-depth study by review of the reference articles presented.

▶ As noted in the introduction to this article, "The Maintenance of Certification module series is designed to help the clinician structure his or her study in specific areas appropriate to his or her clinical practice. This article is prepared to accompany practice-based assessment of preoperative assessment, anesthesia, surgical treatment plan, perioperative management, and outcomes. In this format, the clinician is invited to compare his or her methods of patient assessment and treatment, outcomes, and complications, with authoritative, information-based references."

Anyone doing hand surgery should take advantage of this review opportunity. Further, this allows each practitioner the opportunity for self-assessment and benchmarking. This is important not only for the Maintenance of Certification but also as a routine to keep one's practice current.

Also read these articles: An evidence-based approach to carpal tunnel syndrome, An evidence-based approach to metacarpal fractures, An evidence-based approach to Dupuytren's contracture, and An evidence-based approach to flexor tendon laceration repair.

D. J. Smith, Jr, MD

Management of the Septic Wrist

Birman MV, Strauch RJ (Columbia Univ Med Ctr, NY)
J Hand Surg 36A:324-326, 2011

Background.—Septic wrist joints can involve the radiocarpal, midcarpal, distal radioulnar, and carpometacarpal articulations but also extend into the carpal tunnel and subcutaneous tissues. Obtaining an appropriate diagnosis and instituting proper treatment should be done quickly. A case was described and the current evidence reviewed with respect to how to manage possible septic wrist cases.

> *Case Report.*—Woman, 62, came to the emergency department for treatment of increasing wrist pain and swelling of 2 days' duration. She reported no trauma, but her right wrist range of motion was 30°, with pain at the extreme ends of the range. The wrist was warm, swollen, and tender as well. Radiographs showed no obvious arthritic changes or fracture. Aspiration of the radiocarpal joint dorsally between extensor compartments three and four produced 2.5 ml of thick, opaque fluid that contained 65,000 white blood cells (WBCs) and 90% neutrophils. The initial Gram stain was negative and no crystals were detected. Slightly elevated erythrocyte sedimentation rate and C-reactive protein levels were seen. The patient was given broad-spectrum antibiotics intravenously and admitted to the hospital wearing a volar wrist splint for comfort. She had marked improvement in wrist pain and swelling plus increased wrist motion within 12 hours of aspiration. After 3 days, synovial cultures grew *Staphylococcus aureus* that was sensitive to oxacillin. The patient was given oral antibiotics and discharged, with follow-up in 1 week and exercises to increase wrist motion prescribed.

Evidence.—The most useful diagnostic test for septic wrist is synovial fluid analysis, including gram stain, culture, WBC count and differential, and polarizing microscopy for crystals. However, bacterial Gram stain and culture are not consistently positive in acute septic joint and may become positive only after several days. Also gonococcal septic arthritis produces a negative culture in about half of all cases. Traditionally a synovial fluid WBC count exceeding 50,000 is considered indicative of a likely septic joint, but a recent study found culture-positive septic joints with

WBC counts under 50,000 in 39% of cases, making it sensitive only 61% of the time with this threshold. A value of 17,500 is 83% sensitive and 67% specific for septic wrist. WBC counts can be inaccurate with an acute gout or pseudogout attack, which produce high WBC counts without septic joints.

Treatment options for all septic joints include needle aspiration, arthroscopic irrigation and debridement, and open irrigation and debridement. Good results were reported in 42% of patients having surgery and 67% of patients having needle aspiration even when the aspirated patients had higher rates of serious underlying illness, ongoing extra-articular infection, previous arthritis in the joint, or recent treatment with antibiotics or immunosuppressants. Aspiration produced excellent results in all septic wrists; however, it is considered definitive treatment only for idiopathic sepsis. Surgery is preferred for cases related to surgical procedures or prosthetics. Excellent results are possible with surgery, particularly when done within 10 hours of the diagnosis. Open irrigation and debridement can require repeated procedures, as can arthroscopy. The outcomes for patients with and without a second procedure were comparable.

Conclusions.—The most accurate diagnostic approach to septic wrist rests on the examiner's experience and level of clinical suspicion. Synovial fluid analysis is the preferred diagnostic test, with some guidance offered by synovial WBC counts. These are unreliable in establishing or excluding septic wrist alone. The treatment approaches are aspiration alone, arthroscopic debridement, and open debridement; none has proved itself more effective in all cases than the others. Further study is needed.

▶ Based on case evaluation, the authors outline evidence-based approach to diagnosis and treatment of the septic wrist. This is a nice review of existing literature. The bottom line is that diagnosis is empiric at best, and treatment is not standardized. Any controlled study will ultimately help clinical future treatment.

D. J. Smith, Jr, MD

Necessity of Routine Pathological Examination After Surgical Excision of Wrist Ganglions

Guitton TG, van Leerdam RH, Ring D (Massachusetts General Hosp, Boston)
J Hand Surg 35A:905-908, 2010

Purpose.—The value of routine pathological evaluation of ganglion cysts is questionable considering that the pretest odds of a wrist lesion being a ganglion cyst are usually high based on physical examination and surgical findings alone. This study evaluates the necessity of routine pathological examination of specimens derived from surgical removal of wrist ganglion cysts.

Methods.—We identified 429 consecutive adult patients who underwent surgical excision of a wrist ganglion with routine pathological examination of the specimen between 1997 and 2008. The rates of concordant, discrepant, and discordant diagnoses were reported with 95% confidence intervals. The odds of a discrepant or discordant diagnosis were calculated.

Results.—The prevalence of a concordant diagnosis was 98.6% (424 of 429; 95% confidence interval, 97.3% to 99.6%). The prevalence of a discrepant diagnosis was 1.4% (5 of 429; 95% confidence interval, 0.38% to 2.7%), and the prevalence of a discordant diagnosis was zero. The odds ratio was 0.012 for a discrepant diagnosis and zero for a discordant diagnosis.

Conclusions.—This study suggests that, in patients with the clinical diagnosis of wrist ganglion cyst, quality of care would not be compromised by abandoning the practice of routinely submitting surgical specimens for pathological examination after excision of the ganglion cyst. Discrepant diagnoses are encountered infrequently and discordant diagnoses did not occur. We recommend pathological examination only when the clear gelatinous fluid typical of a ganglion cyst is not encountered at surgery.

▶ Great study. So many times we routinely submit specimens without really thinking. The study correctly points out that the most important goal of routine pathological examination is captured in the concept of discordant diagnoses: changes in diagnoses that affect patient management. This is clearly not accomplished in the surgical excision of wrist ganglions. The recommendation for pathological examination only when the clear gelatinous fluid typical of a ganglion cyst is not encountered in surgery is rational. It would be nice to see the American College of Pathology or surgical organizations endorse this. We could stop wasting money and practicing defensive medicine.

D. J. Smith, Jr, MD

Nerve

An Evidence-Based Approach to Carpal Tunnel Syndrome

Shores JT, Andrew Lee WP (Univ of Pittsburgh School of Medicine, PA)
Plast Reconstr Surg 126:2196-2204, 2010

The Maintenance of Certification module series is designed to help the clinician structure his or her study in specific areas appropriate to his or her clinical practice. This article is prepared to accompany practice-based assessment of preoperative assessment, anesthesia, surgical treatment plan, perioperative management, and outcomes. In this format, the clinician is invited to compare his or her methods of patient assessment and treatment, outcomes, and complications, with authoritative, information-based references.

This information base is then used for self-assessment and benchmarking in parts II and IV of the Maintenance of Certification process of the American Board of Plastic Surgery. This article is not intended to be an exhaustive treatise on the subject. Rather, it is designed to serve as a reference point for further in-depth study by review of the reference articles presented.

▶ As noted in the introduction to each article, "The Maintenance of Certification module series is designed to help the clinician structure his or her study in specific areas appropriate to his or her clinical practice. This article is prepared to accompany practice-based assessment of preoperative assessment, anesthesia, surgical treatment plan, perioperative management, and outcomes. In this format, the clinician is invited to compare his or her methods of patient assessment and treatment, outcomes, and complications, with authoritative, information-based references."

Anyone doing hand surgery should take advantage of this review opportunity. Furthermore, this allows each practitioner the opportunity for self-assessment and benchmarking. It is important not only for the Maintenance of Certification but also as a routine to keep one's practice current.

Also read these 2 articles: "An Evidence-Based Approach to Metacarpal Fractures" and "An Evidence-Based Approach to Dupuytren's Contracture."

D. J. Smith, Jr, MD

American Academy of Orthopaedic Surgeons Clinical Practice Guideline on: The Treatment of Carpal Tunnel Syndrome
Keith MW, Masear V, Chung KC, et al
J Bone Joint Surg Am 92:218-219, 2010

Summary of Recommendations.—The following is a summary of the recommendations in the AAOS' clinical practice guideline, The Treatment of Carpal Tunnel Syndrome. This summary does not contain rationales that explain how and why these recommendations were developed nor does it contain the evidence supporting these recommendations. All readers of this summary are strongly urged to consult the full guideline and evidence report for this information. We are confident that those who read the full guideline and evidence report will also see that the recommendations were developed using systematic evidence-based processes designed to combat bias, enhance transparency, and promote reproducibility. This summary of recommendations is not intended to stand alone. The American Association of Neurological Surgeons and the Congress of Neurological Surgeons have endorsed this guideline.

➤ *Recommendation 1:* A course of non-operative treatment is an option in patients diagnosed with carpal tunnel syndrome. Early surgery is an option when there is clinical evidence of median nerve denervation or the patient elects to proceed directly to surgical treatment. (Grade C, Level V).

➤ *Recommendation 2:* We suggest another non-operative treatment or surgery when the current treatment fails to resolve the symptoms within 2 weeks to 7 weeks. (Grade B, Level I and II).

➤ *Recommendation 3:* We do not have sufficient evidence to provide specific treatment recommendations for carpal tunnel syndrome when found in association with the following conditions: diabetes mellitus, coexistent cervical radiculopathy, hypothyroidism, polyneuropathy, pregnancy, rheumatoid arthritis, and carpal tunnel syndrome in the workplace. (Inconclusive, No evidence found).

➤ *Recommendation 4a:* Local steroid injection or splinting is suggested when treating patients with carpal tunnel syndrome, before considering surgery. (Grade B, Level I and II).

➤ *Recommendation 4b:* Oral steroids or ultrasound are options when treating patients with carpal tunnel syndrome. (Grade C, Level II).

➤ *Recommendation 4c:* We recommend carpal tunnel release as treatment for carpal tunnel syndrome. (Grade A, Level I).

➤ *Recommendation 4d:* Heat therapy is not among the options that should be used to treat patients with carpal tunnel syndrome. (Grade C, Level II).

➤ *Recommendation 4e:* The following treatments carry no recommendation for or against their use: activity modifications, acupuncture, cognitive behavioral therapy, cold laser, diuretics, exercise, electric stimulation, fitness, graston instrument, iontophoresis, laser, stretching, massage therapy, magnet therapy, manipulation, medications (including anticonvulsants, antidepressants and NSAIDs), nutritional supplements, phonophoresis, smoking cessation, systemic steroid injection, therapeutic touch, vitamin B6 (pyridoxine), weight reduction, yoga. (Inconclusive, Level II and V).

➤ *Recommendation 5:* We recommend surgical treatment of carpal tunnel syndrome by complete division of the flexor retinaculum regardless of the specific surgical technique. (Grade A, Level I and II).

➤ *Recommendation 6:* We suggest that surgeons do not routinely use the following procedures when performing carpal tunnel release:skin nerve preservation (Grade B, Level I) epineurotomy (Grade C, Level II) The following procedures carry no recommendation for or against use: flexor retinaculum lengthening, internal neurolysis, tenosynovectomy, ulnar bursa preservation (Inconclusive, Level II and V).

➤ *Recommendation 7:* The physician has the option of prescribing preoperative antibiotics for carpal tunnel surgery. (Grade C, Level III).

➤ *Recommendation 8:* We suggest that the wrist not be immobilized postoperatively after routine carpal tunnel surgery (Grade B, Level II). We make no recommendation for or against the use of postoperative rehabilitation. (Inconclusive, Level II).

➤ *Recommendation 9:* We suggest physicians use one or more of the following instruments when assessing patients' responses to CTS treatment for research:
Boston Carpal Tunnel Questionnaire (disease-specific)
DASH — Disabilities of the arm, shoulder, and hand (region-specific; upper limb)

MHQ — Michigan Hand Outcomes Questionnaire (region-specific; hand/wrist)
PEM (region-specific; hand)
SF-12 or SF-36 Short Form Health Survey (generic; physical health component for global health impact) (Grade B, Level I, II, and III)

▶ A must read for anyone treating patients with carpal tunnel syndrome.

D. J. Smith, Jr, MD

Comparison of Longitudinal Open Incision and Two-Incision Techniques for Carpal Tunnel Release
Castillo TN, Yao J (Stanford Univ School of Medicine, Palo Alto, CA)
J Hand Surg 35A:1813-1819, 2010

Purpose.—This study analyzes the long-term postoperative symptoms and functional outcomes of patients who underwent either traditional open (single-incision) or 2-incision carpal tunnel release (CTR). Because 2-incision CTR preserves the superficial nerves and subcutaneous tissue between the thenar and hypothenar eminences, it may account for fewer postoperative symptoms and improved functional recovery.

Methods.—A retrospective chart review identified patients who underwent either open or 2-incision CTR for isolated carpal tunnel syndrome between 2005 and 2008 by a single surgeon. Patients with a history of hand trauma or confounding comorbidities were excluded. We mailed a Disabilities of the Arm, Shoulder, and Hand (DASH) Questionnaire and a Brigham and Women's Carpal Tunnel Questionnaire (BWCTQ) to all eligible participants. Data from the completed questionnaires were analyzed using independent *t*-tests and Pearson's correlation. Significance was set at p = .05.

Results.—A total of 82 patients (106 hands; 27 men and 55 women; mean age, 60.5 y) were eligible to participate. Of these, 51 patients (63 hands; 20 men and 31 women; mean age, 61.1 y) responded (62% response rate). The mean duration of follow-up was 22 months (range, 12—37 mo; SD 7.3 mo). The 2-incision group mean BWCTQ Symptom Severity Scale score (1.13, SD 0.25) was significantly lower than the open group mean Symptom Severity Scale score (1.54, SD 0.70, p = .001). The 2-incision group mean BWCTQ Functional Status Scale score (1.24, SD 0.51) was significantly lower than the open group mean Functional Status Scale score (1.71, SD 0.76, p = .008). The 2-incision group mean DASH score (5.10, SD 12.03) was significantly lower than the open group mean DASH score (16.28, SD 19.98, p = .01).

Conclusions.—Patients treated with 2-incision CTR reported statistically significantly less severe long-term postoperative symptoms and improved functional status compared with patients treated with traditional open CTR. Future prospective studies with objective measures are needed to further investigate the difference in outcomes found between these 2 CTR techniques.

Type of Study/Level of Evidence.—Therapeutic III.

▶ This is a nice study comparing the long-term postoperative symptoms and functional outcomes of patients undergoing either traditional open or 2-incision carpal tunnel release. The 2-incision group reports statistically significant less-severe long-term postoperative symptoms and improved functional status. Unfortunately, this is yet another retrospective study that concludes we need a prospective study. Time to make that leap.

D. J. Smith, Jr, MD

A Prospective Randomized Study Comparing Woven Polyglycolic Acid and Autogenous Vein Conduits for Reconstruction of Digital Nerve Gaps
Rinker B, Liau JY (Univ of Kentucky, Lexington)
J Hand Surg 36A:775-781, 2011

Purpose.—The optimal management of a nerve gap within the fingers remains an unanswered question in hand surgery. The purpose of this study was to compare the sensory recovery, cost, and complication profile of digital nerve repair using autogenous vein and polyglycolic acid conduits.

Methods.—We enrolled patients undergoing repair of digital nerve injuries with gaps precluding primary repair. The minimum gap that was found to preclude primary repair was 4 mm. Each nerve repair was randomized to the type of nerve repair with either a woven polyglycolic acid conduit or autogenous vein. Time required for repair was recorded. We performed sensory testing, consisting of static and moving 2-point discrimination, at 6 and 12 months after repair. We compared patient factors between the 2 groups using chi-square and Student's *t*-test. We compared sensory recovery between the 2 groups at each time point using Student's *t*-test and compared time and cost of repair.

Results.—We enrolled 42 patients with 76 nerve repairs. Of these, 37 patients (representing 68 repairs) underwent sensory evaluation at the 6-month time point. The median age in this group was 35 years. We repaired 36 nerves with synthetic conduit and 32 with vein. Nerve gaps ranged from 4 to 25 mm (mean, 10 mm). Study groups were not significantly different regarding age, time to repair, gap length, medical history, smoking history, or worker's compensation status. Time to harvest the vein was longer but the average cost of materials and surgery in the vein group was $1,220, compared with $1,269 for synthetic conduit repairs. These differences were not statistically significant. Mean static and moving 2-point discrimination at 6 months for the synthetic conduit group were 8.3 ± 2.0 and 6.6 ± 2.3, respectively, compared with 8.5 ± 1.8 and 7.1 ± 2.2 for the vein group. Values at 12 months for the synthetic conduit group were 7.5 ± 1.9 and 5.6 ± 2.2, compared with 7.6 ± 2.6 and 6.6 ± 2.9 for the vein group. These differences were not statistically significant. Smokers and worker's compensation patients had a worse sensory recovery at 12 months postrepair. There were 2 extrusions in the synthetic conduit group requiring reoperation; however, the difference in extrusion rate was not found to be statistically significant.

Conclusions.—Sensory recovery after digital nerve reconstruction with autogenous vein conduit was equivalent to that using polyglycolic acid conduit, with a similar cost profile and fewer postoperative complications.

▶ This is a nicely designed and executed prospective trial comparing autogenous vein graft and polyglycolic acid conduits for nerve gaps preceding primary repair. The operative time to harvest the graft seems to offset the cost of the conduit. Sensory recovery was comparable with a similar cost profile. Vein grafts had fewer postoperative complications. The numbers are relatively small but appear reliable. Obviously, use can be individualized based on case, but it appears that autogenous graft is the better choice.

D. J. Smith, Jr, MD

Tendon

An Evidence-Based Approach to Flexor Tendon Laceration Repair
Lalonde DH (Dalhousie Univ, Saint John, New Brunswick, Canada)
Plast Reconstr Surg 127:885-890, 2011

The Maintenance of Certification module series is designed to help the clinician structure his or her study in specific areas appropriate to his or her clinical practice. This article is prepared to accompany practice-based assessment of preoperative assessment, anesthesia, surgical treatment plan, perioperative management, and outcomes. In this format, the clinician is invited to compare his or her methods of patient assessment and treatment, outcomes, and complications, with authoritative, information-based references.

This information base is then used for self-assessment and benchmarking in parts II and IV of the Maintenance of Certification process of the American Board of Plastic Surgery. This article is not intended to be an exhaustive treatise on the subject. Rather, it is designed to serve as a reference point for further in-depth study by review of the reference articles presented.

▶ As noted in the introduction to this article, "The Maintenance of Certification module series is designed to help the clinician structure his or her study in specific areas appropriate to his or her clinical practice. This article is prepared to accompany practice-based assessment of preoperative assessment, anesthesia, surgical treatment plan, perioperative management, and outcomes. In this format, the clinician is invited to compare his or her methods of patient assessment and treatment, outcomes, and complications, with authoritative, information-based references."

Anyone doing hand surgery should take advantage of this review opportunity. Further, this allows each practitioner the opportunity for self-assessment and benchmarking. This is important not only for the Maintenance of Certification but also as a routine to keep one's practice current.

Also read these articles: An evidence-based approach to carpal tunnel syndrome, An evidence-based approach to metacarpal fractures, An evidence-based approach to Dupuytren's contracture, and An evidence-based approach to treating thumb carpometacarpal joint arthritis.

D. J. Smith, Jr, MD

Biomechanical Evaluation of Flexor Tendon Repair Using Barbed Suture Material: A Comparative *Ex Vivo* Study

Zeplin PH, Zahn RK, Meffert RH, et al (Wuerzburg Univ Hosp, Germany)
J Hand Surg 36A:446-449, 2011

Purpose.—Barbed suture material for tendon repair opens up the possibility of a knotless reconstruction due to an increased suture—tendon interaction. The aim of this study was to compare the tensile strength of a knotted technique with a monofilament polydioxane suture to that of a knotless technique with a barbed suture material, by using a multistrand, modified Kirchmayr-Kessler tenorrhaphy.

Methods.—Sixty human flexor digitorum tendons were randomized into 4 groups. A modified, knotted, multistrand Kirchmayr-Kessler technique with an absorbable, monofilament polydioxane suture was compared with a modified, knotless, multistrand Kirchmayr-Kessler technique with an absorbable, unidirectional barbed glycolic-carbonate suture. Tendons were distracted to failure. Mode of failure and load to failure were recorded.

Results.—The knotless 2-strand Kirchmayr-Kessler barbed suture shows a significantly lower tensile strength than the knotted 2-strand polydioxane suture (p < .001). The comparison of the maximum tensile strength of the knotless (glycolic-carbonate) technique with that of the knotted (polydioxane) 4-strand technique resulted in no significant difference in either technique utilized (p = .737). The tensile strength of the 4-strand technique was greater than that of the corresponding 2-strand technique (p < .001).

Conclusions.—The 2-strand Kirchmayr-Kessler barbed suture proved to be insufficient and significantly weaker than the 2-strand polydioxane suture, and therefore it cannot be recommended. With the knotless 4-strand Kirchmayr-Kessler technique, the barbed suture material has the potential to be used in flexor tendon surgery, but it has no advantage over the 4-strand polydioxane suture.

▶ Barbed suture material for tendon repair opens up the possibility of a knotless reconstruction because of an increased suture-tendon interaction. Unfortunately, the results are not encouraging. Initial tensile strength measurements do not support the use of barbed sutures for tendon repair. On the other hand, final analysis will depend on more physiologic evaluation. Use of the barbed suture is very enticing for knotless tendon repair. Let's hope that further studies are more encouraging.

D. J. Smith, Jr, MD

Zone-II Flexor Tendon Repair: A Randomized Prospective Trial of Active Place-and-Hold Therapy Compared with Passive Motion Therapy
Trumble TE, Vedder NB, Seiler JG III, et al (Univ of Washington Med Ctr, Seattle)
J Bone Joint Surg Am 92:1381-1389, 2010

Background.—In order to improve digit motion after zone-II flexor tendon repair, rehabilitation programs have promoted either passive motion or active motion therapy. To our knowledge, no prospective randomized trial has compared the two techniques. Our objective was to compare the results of patients treated with an active therapy program and those treated with a passive motion protocol following zone-II flexor tendon repair.

Methods.—Between January 1996 and December 2002, 103 patients (119 digits) with zone-II flexor tendon repairs were randomized to either early active motion with place and hold or a passive motion protocol. Range of motion was measured at six, twelve, twenty-six, and fifty-two weeks following repair. Dexterity tests were performed, and the Disabilities of the Arm, Shoulder, and Hand (DASH) outcome questionnaire and a satisfaction score were completed at fifty-two weeks by ninety-three patients (106 injured digits).

Results.—At all time points, patients treated with the active motion program had greater interphalangeal joint motion. At the time of the final follow-up, the interphalangeal joint motion in the active place-and-hold group was a mean (and standard deviation) of $156° \pm 25°$ compared with $128° \pm 22°$ ($p < 0.05$) in the passive motion group. The active motion group had both significantly smaller flexion contractures and greater satisfaction scores ($p < 0.05$). We could identify no difference between the groups in terms of the DASH scores or dexterity tests. When the groups were stratified, those who were smokers or had a concomitant nerve injury or multiple digit injuries had less range of motion, larger flexion contractures, and decreased satisfaction scores compared with patients without these comorbidities. Treatment by a certified hand therapist resulted in better range of motion with smaller flexion contractures. Two digits in each group had tendon ruptures following repair.

Conclusions.—Active motion therapy provides greater active finger motion than passive motion therapy after zone-II flexor tendon repair without increasing the risk of tendon rupture. Concomitant nerve injuries, multiple digit injuries, and a history of smoking negatively impact the final outcome of tendon repairs.

▶ Postsurgery rehabilitation is crucial to the successful management of zone-II flexor tendon repairs. This is a nicely conceived and carried out comparison between passive and active motion in 106 injured digits. The patients were randomized post surgery. The authors do note that there have been no prospective randomized trials comparing these 2 techniques. Hard to believe, but I didn't find any either. The results favoring active motion confirm my bias.

D. J. Smith, Jr, MD

Congenital

Index Finger Pollicization

Taghinia AH, Upton J (Harvard Med School, Boston, MA)
J Hand Surg 36A:333-339, 2011

The thumb is a specialized organ with unique functions that cannot be replicated by any other digit. The most powerful technique for construction of a missing thumb is index finger pollicization. In this article, we outline our technique for index finger pollicization. Over a 30-year period, certain technical refinements have improved the function and appearance of these transposed digits.

▶ This is an excellent review of index finger pollicization. The senior author shares his experience on technique and how his procedure has evolved. This article focuses entirely on "how to" with nothing on outcomes. For those performing this surgery, this is a straightforward complete guide to the technical refinements.

D. J. Smith, Jr, MD

5 Aesthetic

General

Nutritional Assessment of Bariatric Surgery Patients Presenting for Plastic Surgery: A Prospective Analysis

Naghshineh N, O'Brien Coon D, McTigue K, et al (Univ of Pittsburgh School of Medicine, PA)
Plast Reconstr Surg 126:602-610, 2010

Background.—Assessment of nutritional status in the growing postbariatric patient population remains controversial. Previous literature suggests that these patients have poor nutrition that may have adverse effects on surgical outcomes. The authors sought to determine the optimal method of nutritional assessment in postbariatric patients.

Methods.—One hundred patients presenting for body contouring after bariatric surgery were consecutively enrolled in an institutional review board–approved prospective study. A trained nutritionist assessed protein and calorie intake. All patients underwent baseline laboratory assessment.

Results.—Eighteen percent of subjects had less than the recommended daily protein intake. Hypoalbuminemia was observed in 13.8 percent of subjects, with hypoprealbuminemia in 6.5 percent. Nearly forty percent of all patients had evidence of iron deficiency, with vitamin B_{12} deficiency present in 14.5 percent. Ten percent of subjects (all women) were confirmed to have iron deficiency anemia. Impaired fasting glucose was seen in 6.2 percent of subjects, whereas 3.6 percent had hemoglobin A1c levels greater than 6.5. Increasing age (odds ratio, 1.07) and greater change in body mass index (odds ratio, 1.11) were predictors of low protein intake. Dumping syndrome led to 13.3 times increased odds of low albumin levels.

Conclusions.—The results suggest that inadequate nutrition is common among postbariatric patients presenting for body contouring. The lack of correlation between methods of nutritional assessment supports the combination of multiple methods in determining overall nutritional status. The presence of dumping syndrome, a large change in body mass index, and advanced age may help to identify patients with an increased risk of nutritional deficiency.

▶ Preoperative assessment of postbariatric surgery patients may be more challenging than that of other body contouring patients. While many of these patients continue to be monitored and cleared for surgery by physicians at bariatric surgery centers, some patients are only followed by their primary care physicians who may not be able to provide the same level of nutritional monitoring. Even more concerning are the patients who have no postbariatric surgery follow-up. In such cases, a preoperative referral to a bariatric physician should be strongly considered. As this study demonstrates, inadequate nutrition is common among postbariatric patients presenting for plastic surgery. A large change in body mass index, the presence of dumping syndrome, and advanced age may help identify which patients are more prone to nutritional deficiency and subsequent wound-healing complications after surgery.

K. A. Gutowski, MD

Skin, Soft Tissue, and Hair

A Randomized Controlled Trial of Skin Care Protocols for Facial Resurfacing: Lessons Learned from the Plastic Surgery Educational Foundation's Skin Products Assessment Research Study
Pannucci CJ, Reavey PL, Kaweski S, et al (Univ of Michigan, Ann Arbor; Columbia Univ Med Ctr, NY; Aesthetic Arts Inst of Plastic Surgery, NY; et al)
Plast Reconstr Surg 127:1334-1342, 2011

Background.—The Skin Products Assessment Research Committee was created by the Plastic Surgery Educational Foundation in 2006. The Skin Products Assessment Research study aims were to (1) develop an infrastructure for Plastic Surgery Educational Foundation—conducted, industry-sponsored research in facial aesthetic surgery and (2) test the research process by comparing outcomes of the Obagi Nu-Derm System versus conventional therapy as treatment adjuncts for facial resurfacing procedures.

Methods.—The Skin Products Assessment Research study was designed as a multicenter, double-blind, randomized, controlled trial. The study was conducted in women with Fitzpatrick type I to IV skin, moderate to severe facial photodamage, and periocular and/or perioral fine wrinkles. Patients underwent chemical peel or laser facial resurfacing and were randomized to the Obagi Nu-Derm System or a standard care regimen. The study endpoints were time to reepithelialization, erythema, and pigmentation changes.

Results.—Fifty-six women were enrolled and 82 percent were followed beyond reepithelialization. There were no significant differences in mean time to reepithelialization between Obagi Nu-Derm System and control groups. The Obagi Nu-Derm System group had a significantly higher median erythema score on the day of surgery (after 4 weeks of product use) that did not persist after surgery. Test-retest photographic evaluations demonstrated that both interrater and intrarater reliability were adequate for primary study outcomes.

Conclusions.—The authors demonstrated no significant difference in time to reepithelialization between patients who used the Obagi Nu-Derm

System or a standard care regimen as an adjunct to facial resurfacing procedures. The Skin Products Assessment Research team has also provided a discussion of future challenges for Plastic Surgery Educational Foundation—sponsored clinical research for readers of this article.

▶ The Obagi Nu-Derm System has been demonstrated to improve the appearance of aged facial skin. It has also been promoted as part of a skin treatment protocol for laser or chemical facial skin resurfacing despite a lack of evidence of its superiority to other treatments. This head-to-head study was unable to show that the Obagi System was superior to standard treatment using Cetaphil, sunscreen, tretinoin, and hydroquinone. The methodology used should also serve as a means for future skin treatment comparisons. Hopefully, this will allow clinicians to make more cost-effective recommendations for their skin care patients.

K. A. Gutowski, MD

Orbitofacial Rejuvenation of Temple Hollowing With Perlane Injectable Filler

Ross JJ, Malhotra R (Queen Victoria Hosp, East Grinstead, UK)
Aesth Surg J 30:428-433, 2010

Background.—Temple hollowing with soft tissue volume loss is well recognized in HIV lipoatrophy. Similar changes occur as part of aging, with skeletalization of the orbital rim and clipping of the eyebrow tail.

Objectives.—The authors report their initial experience treating temple volume loss and orbitofacial asymmetry with nonanimal stabilized hyaluronic acid (NASHA).

Methods.—This study was a retrospective, interventional case series with a patient satisfaction questionnaire and independent physician grading of results. Patients initially received approximately 1 mL of Perlane (Q-Med, Uppsala, Sweden; Medicis, Inc., Scottsdale, Arizona) injected into the superficial fascia of each temple. The filler was placed behind the frontozygomatic process to soften the bony contour of the lateral orbital rim. Outcome measures included satisfaction with injection procedure, fulfillment of expectations, satisfaction with appearance, change in self-confidence, the need for retreatment, and complications.

Results.—Twenty patients were treated, for a total of 39 temples. Mean follow-up was nine months (range, four to 14 months). Patients were primarily female (90%), all were Caucasian, and their ages ranged from 20 to 60 years. Eighteen patients had age-related temple hollowing, one had dysthyroid volume loss, and one had hollowing due to orbitotemporal neurofibromatosis. The majority had 1-mL injections to each side (range, 0.3-3 mL). One patient received 3 mL to correct asymmetry. The procedure was well tolerated with ice pack cooling and no local anesthesia. Of 16 patients who replied to the questionnaire, 13 were very or moderately satisfied and requested repeat treatment, whereas three were only mildly satisfied or ambivalent. Side effects included transient mild or moderate discomfort, superficial vein prominence, and localized bruising.

Conclusions.—This series suggests the effective and safe application of Perlane in temple hollow rejuvenation and correction of asymmetry. It offers tolerability, high patient satisfaction, few complications, and the option of reversibility.

▶ Temple hollowing because of aging is not commonly recognized by patients seeking facial rejuvenation. However, once it is pointed out to a patient and corrected, a more balanced facial appearance can be obtained. Poly-L-lactic acid (Sculptra) and polymethyl methacrylate (Artefill) have both been used for this purpose with good results. The results shown with Perlane (a high viscosity nonanimal stabilized hyaluronic acid) are also acceptable. It is important to realize that the entire hollowness does not need to be corrected, as the volume of filler material required may be very expensive. Rather, the goal is to soften the sharp demarcation along the anterior temple just behind the prominent frontozygomatic arch. A linear injection in this area of 0.5 to 1.0 cc of filler can then be molded to achieve the desired contour and provide a gradual transition from the lateral face to the temple, thereby making the hollowness less obvious. Prior to injection, the superficial temporal artery and any obvious veins should be identified to avoid needle entry and filler embolization.

K. A. Gutowski, MD

Effect of Multisyringe Hyaluronic Acid Facial Rejuvenation on Perceived Age
Taub AF, Sarnoff D, Gold M, et al (SKINQRI, Lincolnshire, IL; New York Univ; Tennessee Clinical Res Ctr, Nashville; et al)
Dermatol Surg 36:322-328, 2010

Background.—The objective of aesthetic treatments is to create a more youthful appearance. Most injectable fillers are indicated for the reduction of nasolabial folds, but the current aesthetic movement is toward volume replacement in multiple areas, known as global fillers or liquid face-lift.

Objectives.—To quantify the degree of perceived age reduction from multisyringe hyaluronic acid treatment.

Materials and Methods.—Ten women were treated with 6 to 8 mL of hyaluronic acid. Exclusion criteria were no laser for 6 months and no hyaluronic acid fillers for 6 months or semipermanent fillers for 1 year. High-resolution photographs were taken in identical lighting and position before and 2 and 4 weeks after treatment. Three blinded dermatologists rated patients' ages before and after from photographs.

Results.—The dermatologists reported an average of 6.1 to 7.3 years of reduction in apparent age at 2 and 4 weeks, respectively. The patients perceived a decrease in apparent age of 7.8 and 9 years.

Conclusion.—Multisyringe injection of hyaluronic acid filler into the aging face results in a reduction of apparent age from 6.1 to 9 years after 2 to 4 weeks. Full-face correction with hyaluronic acid is an important procedure in the armamentarium of anti-aging techniques.

▶ As clinicians gain more experience with injectable fillers, it is natural that there will be an increase in the filler volumes used in a particular patient, especially those with significant facial volume loss because of advanced aging. Unlike isolated anatomic regions like the lips (where 1 mL of filler volume can provide significant results), the cheeks, nasolabial folds, and lower third of the face will need much more than 1 or 2 mL of filler to replace the volume that has been lost. Furthermore, undercorrection by using inadequate filler volumes may lead to patient dissatisfaction because a reasonable result may not be seen despite the patient's payment for an expected improvement. To achieve better results in patients who have more significant facial volume loss, it is important to educate the patient on how much facial volume has been lost and that more than 1 or 2 syringes will be needed to reverse the loss. This, of course, will lead to high costs ($3000-$6000) to achieve an optimal result, often repeated in 9 to 12 months. There is some evidence, however, that continued hyaluronic acid filler injections may decrease the amount of filler needed over time because of stimulation of collagen synthesis.

K. A. Gutowski, MD

Subcision-suction method: a new successful combination therapy in treatment of atrophic acne scars and other depressed scars
Harandi SA, Balighi K, Lajevardi V, et al (Parsian Laser Clinic, Bandar Abbas, Iran; Tehran Univ of Med Sciences, Iran)
J Eur Acad Dermatol Venereol 25:92-99, 2011

Background.—Among therapeutic modalities of acne scars, subcision is a simple, safe procedure with a different and basic mechanism for correcting atrophic and depressed scars. Subcision releases scar surfaces from underlying attachments and induces connective tissue formation beneath the scar directly, without injury to the skin surface. Therefore, subcision is a valuable method, but due to high recurrence rate, its efficacy is mild to moderate.

Objectives.—To increase the efficacy of subcision, a new complementary treatment of repeated suction sessions was added at the recurrence period of subcised scars.

Methods.—In this before and after trail, 58 patients with mild to severe acne scars of various types (rolling, superficial and deep boxcar, pitted), chicken pox, traumatic and surgical depressed scars were treated by superficial dermal undermining, with mainly 23-guage needles. The protocol for suctioning was: start of suction on third day after subcision for flat and depressing subcised scars and its continuation at least every other day for 2 weeks.

Results.—Forty-six patients followed the protocol completely, had 60–90% improvement in depth and size of scars (significant improvement) with mean: 71.73%. 28.2% of them had '80% improvement or more' (excellent improvement). Twelve patients started suction late and/or had long interval suction-sessions, had 30–60% improvement (moderate improvement) with mean: 43.75%.

Conclusion.—Frequent suctioning at the recurrence period of subcision increases subcision efficacy remarkably and causes significant and persistent improvement in short time, without considerable complication, in depressed scars of the face. Therefore, subcision-suction method is introduced as a new effective treatment.

▶ Many of us have tried subcision as a treatment modality for depressed scars, pockmarks, and acne scars. It makes sense to release the fibrous tethers that pull down on the skin and result in a visible dimple or depression. Subcision is a minimally invasive way to do this using a 23- or 27-gauge needle and blindly cutting the fibrous attachments. However, most of us who have tried this technique have been somewhat disappointed with the long-term results. Although the release can be quite impressive initially, within 1 or 2 weeks as the internal wound starts to heal, the fibrous attachments begin to reform. Over the next few weeks, these attachments begin to contract, causing the initial depressed scar to reform. The authors of this study have come up with a clever form of physical therapy to mitigate this phenomenon by applying suction on a daily basis to pull out the skin and prevent these attachments from reforming. Their results indicate that if this is done for as little as 2 weeks, there is a substantial improvement in the results as graded by both the patient and investigators. Further study is needed in a more controlled trial, but this innovative approach holds promise for one of the unmet needs in both aesthetic and reconstructive surgery.

G. C. Gurtner, MD

A simple and effective technique for improving the appearance of pin-site scars

Thione A, Gandolfi E, Mortarino C (Plastic and Reconstructive Surgery Private Practice, Como, Italy; Aesthetic Surgery Unit, Como, Italy; Plastic and Reconstructive Surgery Private Practice, Varese, Italy)
Injury 41:e15-e16, 2010

The use of an external fixator in reconstructive surgery may leave retracted and depressed scars where pins have passed through the skin; these scars do not resolve or improve spontaneously and, at the end of the reconstructive surgery, patients complain about them.

In 1994, Saleh and Howard described a method of surgical revision combining W-plasty and a buried dermal island to improve pin scars.

In 2002, Oznur and Aycan proposed a simple elevation procedure by scissors, making a 1-cm-longitudinal incision, arguing that controlled haematoma formation helps to elevate the depressed area, having experience only with scars of the thigh.

We describe a new, simple, but really effective method based on lipofilling according to Coleman.

Our technique can be performed at an outpatient clinic under local anaesthesia.

All of the adhesions of pin-site scars are cut off with a simple needle, NoKor needle 16G 1.6 mm × 25 mm, in a blind fashion by a 2—3-mm incision made with the needle, obtaining the elevation of the dimpled area easily.

At this point, the scar area is treated with an injection of adipose tissue, usually harvested from abdominal subcutaneous fat (any fat donor site could be used), obtained by conventional superwet syringe liposuction and processed according to Coleman's technique, filling the dead space created by the needle completely with a mild overcorrection (2 4 ml of fat tissue for each scar is enough). No stitches are needed and no more scars are provoked.

Immediately at the end of the surgery, no more dimpling and retracted areas are visible, solving the major complain; moreover, the clinical appearance and subjective patient feelings after a 6-month follow-up suggest considerable improvement of skin texture and scar quality and thickness.

This technique has proven to be effective for scars on arms, thighs, leg and subcutaneous border of the tibia. No complications occurred in our six preliminary cases.

We can conclude that lipofilling is an easy and effective surgery to improve the appearance of pin-site scars.

▶ Depressed scars are a common occurrence after traumatic injury. These scars can result from external fixators, halo devices, surgical procedures performed by other services and the like. Patients who have recovered from these traumatic injuries are often quite unhappy with these constant reminders of their accident, and in many cases, these depressed scars can be quite disfiguring. When these patients come in for plastic surgery consultation, most of us feel that there is little that can be offered these patients because of the poorly vascularized scar tissue tethering the dermis to the deep tissues. This article proposes a simple approach to these minor injuries by combining needle subcision with autologous fat grafting. This procedure can be performed in the office under local anesthesia and is truly minimally invasive. Although the number of cases reported is small and the results early, this is certainly an interesting approach to these difficult problems, which may help and in any event is highly unlikely to make things worse.

G. C. Gurtner, MD

A retrospective study on liquid injectable silicone for lip augmentation: Long-term results and patient satisfaction

Moscona RA, Fodor L (Rambam Health Care Campus, Haifa, Israel)
J Plast Reconstr Aesth Surg 63:1694-1698, 2010

Various injectable fillers are used for soft-tissue augmentation, including liquid injectable silicone [LS]. This study evaluates patient satisfaction and long-term results after [LS] for lip augmentation. A total of 179 patients, who received medical grade [LS] for lip augmentation, were included in the study. The microdroplet technique was used in all cases, and not more than 1 cc per lip per session was injected. The follow-up period varied from 3 years to 7 years. The long-term results (3—7 years), satisfaction level and complications were evaluated.

As many as 171 patients had upper lip injections and most had 1 cc silicone injected. Eighty-seven had lower lip injections. Eighty-five percent of the patients considered having excellent or good results. Most (76%) patients considered their lips to be as soft as before treatment. No complications were recorded for 91.1% of the patients. Complications encountered by the rest were minor and temporary, such as ecchymoses and haematoma in 6.2% and invisible but small palpable nodules in 2.2%. In our experience, the injection of [LS] by the microdroplet technique is safe for a period of 3—7 years, gives high satisfaction to the treated persons and has minimal complications (Fig 2).

▶ The authors claim that the use of a highly purified silicone, for augmentation of the lips of patients using small doses administered by a microdroplet technique, described in their article, is effective and safe. (In Fig 2 note the redness above the vermillion in the area of cupids bow. Is that artifact or real?) The study is a retrospective one, and although the duration of the follow-up ranges from 3 to 7 years, it was performed entirely by a questionnaire without any professional evaluation. One-third of the patients treated did not respond to the questionnaire so we do not know anything about the results in 80 patients. We also do not know the numbers of patients followed in the years encompassed by the 3- to 7-year timeframe. Are small quantities of this ultrapurified silicone injected in lips in small quantities really safe in the long run or will patients develop granulomas and/or movement of the silicone as they have in other

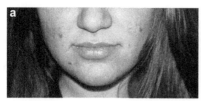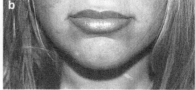

FIGURE 2.—a & b. Before and after injecting 1 cc in the upper lip and 1 cc in the lower lip. (Reprinted from Moscona RA, Fodor L. A retrospective study on liquid injectable silicone for lip augmentation: long-term results and patient satisfaction. *J Plast Reconstr Aesth Surg.* 2010;63:1694-1698, with permission from British Association of Plastic, Reconstructive and Aesthetic Surgeons.)

studies? Do we not need a major collaborative, prospective, randomized, controlled study to assess all of the fillers being used to determine which are most effective and efficacious as well as the relative costs of each? A similar, albeit larger, uncontrolled retrospective study was reported in 2011.[1]

S. H. Miller, MD, MPH

Reference

1. Hevia O. Six-year experience using 1,000-centistoke silicone oil in 916 patients for soft-tissue augmentation in a private practice setting. *Dermatol Surg.* 2009;35: 1646-1652.

Treatment of lower eyelid rhytids and laxity with ablative fractionated carbon-dioxide laser resurfacing: Case series and review of the literature
Tierney EP, Hanke CW, Watkins L (St Vincent Hosp, Indianapolis, IN; Eye Cu Group, Muncie, IN)
J Am Acad Dermatol 64:730-740, 2011

Background.—An increasing array of minimally invasive treatment modalities have evolved for periorbital rhytids. Nonablative fractional photothermolysis has been demonstrated to be effective for periorbital rhytids.

Objective.—We sought to prospectively evaluate eyelid tightening with an ablative fractional photothermolysis laser.

Methods.—We conducted a prospective, single blinded study for lower eyelid laxity in 25 subjects with a series of 2 to 3 treatment sessions.

Results.—The number of treatment sessions required for significant improvement of eyelid laxity ranged from 2 to 3, with an average of 2.44 sessions. For skin texture, the mean score decreased from 3.6 to a mean of 1.2 at 6 months posttreatment ($P < .05$) for a 62.6% mean improvement. For skin laxity, the mean score decreased from 3.3 to 1.3 at 6 months post-treatment ($P < .05$) for a 65.3% mean improvement. For rhytids, the mean score decreased from 3.5 to 1.3 at 6 months posttreatment ($P < .05$) for a 62.1% mean improvement. For overall cosmetic outcome, mean score decreased from 3.6 to 1.2 at 6 months posttreatment ($P < .05$) for a 65.7% mean improvement. Patients noted moderate postoperative erythema and edema that resolved by the 1-week posttreatment visit. Patients reported minor crusting and oozing that resolved within 48 to 72 hours.

Limitations.—This is a prospective, single blinded study in 25 patients with varying degrees of laxity and photoaging affecting eyelid skin. Additional studies assessing degree of improvement for patients with varying degrees of laxity and photoaging at variable parameters are needed.

Conclusion.—Eyelids can achieve significant improvement in skin texture and laxity with ablative fractional photothermolysis.

▶ Mild lower eyelid skin excess and rhytides without lid laxity or fat bulging can be improved nonsurgically with traditional chemical peels and laser resurfacing. Newer modalities include radiofrequency skin tightening and fractionated laser technology, which may have lower risks of complications compared with nonfractionated laser treatments. Both ablative (CO_2) and nonablative (erbium-doped:yttrium-aluminum garnet) lasers provide similar lower eyelid skin tightening, but the nonablative treatments have been shown to result in more scarring. In other studies, ablative fractional laser treatments had greater improvement in skin texture and tightening compared with treatment with nonablative fractional lasers. Because fractionated lasers do not treat the entire skin surface, the results are not as dramatic as with nonfractionated laser; however, complications seem to be less common, and downtime is significantly reduced. Multiple treatments, however, are required to yield comparable improvements. In this study, patients required 2 or 3 treatments (depending on the degree of clinical improvement with treatment) 6 to 8 weeks apart, but this seems to be a reasonable trade-off, given the fast patient recovery after each treatment. Technical considerations include only a single laser pass to the lateral canthal triangle to avoid widening the lateral opening of the eyelid and potential complications of scleral show and ectropion. However, in the crow's feet region, 3 passes on the skin may be done, as complications are unlikely in this zone. As other studies have cautioned, conservative fluences and pulse duration should be used.

K. A. Gutowski, MD

Skin Tightening with Fractional Lasers, Radiofrequency, Smartlipo
Collawn SS (Univ of Alabama at Birmingham)
Ann Plast Surg 64:526-529, 2010

Skin tightening occurs with the use of fractional lasers, radio-frequency, and Smartlipo. The fractional lasers Fraxel (1550 nm; Solta Medical, Inc., Hayward, CA) and Affirm (1440 nm, 1320 nm) (Cynosure, Westford, MA) when used in combination tighten skin and lessen solar keratoses, and improve acne scars. With radiofrequency, further tightening occurs. Smartlipo (Cynosure, Westford, MA) (1064 nm or the newer MPX with combined 1064 nm and 1320 nm) results in skin tightening and has been very helpful in improving skin tightness and smoothness on the neck either singularly or in combination with the above procedures; and with the addition of the Affirm fractional CO_2 laser (Cynosure, Westford, MA), further skin improvement and tightening occurs.

▶ For selected patients who are averse to a more invasive surgical procedure, external energy treatments (fractional lasers and radio frequency) and minimally invasive procedures (laser-assisted lipolysis) may be an option in facial rejuvenation. The combination of 3 different treatment modalities, each with a different mechanism of action, could yield a better result than any individual modality used alone. The results presented, however, are not convincing that this multimodality regimen is superior to traditional liposuction of the neck/submental area (with the addition of a chemical peel if needed). Likewise, there is no mention of the longevity of the results. The investment in these 3 modalities (both initial acquisition and maintenance costs) needs to be considered in the analysis before incorporating them into one's practice.

K. A. Gutowski, MD

Radiofrequency Ablation of Facial Nerve Branches Controlling Glabellar Frowning
Foster KW, Fincher EF, Moy RL (Central Florida Dermatology and Skin Cancer Ctr, Winter Haven; Moy-Fincher Med Group, Los Angeles, CA)
Dermatol Surg 35:1908-1917, 2009

Background.—Hyperdynamic activity of the corrugator supercilii and procerus muscles causes glabellar furrows. Recently, a novel radiofrequency device has become available that can effectively ablate the efferent nerves controlling corrugator and procerus contraction, producing clinical results that are similar to those of botulinum toxin.

Objective.—To assess the efficacy, longevity of effect, and side effects of the radiofrequency ablation device in the treatment of hyperdynamic glabellar furrows.

Materials and Methods.—Four probe entry points were used to access branches of the temporal and angular nerves. Seven and two ablations, respectively, were delivered to each temporal branch and angular nerve.

Results.—Twenty-nine patients underwent bilateral radiofrequency ablation of temporal branches of the facial nerve and the angular nerves. Abrogation of glabellar furrowing was achieved in 90% of patients. No major adverse events were observed. All patients developed mild to moderate swelling, and nine patients (31%) developed purpura in the treated areas. Sixty-nine percent of patients had effects that lasted 4 months or longer, 41% had effects that lasted 6 months or longer, and 10% had effects lasting longer than 12 months.

Conclusion.—Radiofrequency ablation of efferent branches of the temporal and angular nerves effectively eliminates corrugator and procerus contraction and concomitant glabellar furrowing.

▶ The Glabellar Frown RelaXation (GFX) nerve ablation system, renamed Relaxed Expressions (RE) consists of a radio frequency (RF) generator, a single-use ablation probe, and a footswitch. Performed in an office setting under local anesthesia, the ablation probe is placed in a nerve target area and energy is applied to cause nerve ablation. This treatment may be an alternative to botulinum toxin (BTX) neuromuscular blockade, but there are significant differences between these 2 methods. While the effects of GFX/RE treatments may last somewhat longer than BTX injections, the GFX/RE may be more expensive (because of initial device cost and use of a disposable probe), has more discomfort and swelling, and takes longer to perform the procedure. While not compared in this report, BTX may offer more versatility in selectively targeting certain portions of a muscle (ie, lateral orbicularis oculi to achieve lateral brow elevation) than GFX/RE, which targets the nerve supplying a muscle. It can be expected that RF technology will continue to evolve and may play a complementary role in reshaping the aging face and improving dynamic lines and creases.

K. A. Gutowski, MD

Eyelid

Definitive Treatment for Crow's Feet Wrinkles by Total Myectomy of the Lateral Orbicularis Oculi

de Assis Montenegro Cido Carvalho F, da Silva VV Jr, Moreira AA, et al
(Instituto Doutor José Frota de Fortaleza (IJF), Rua Barão do Rio Branco, CE, Brazil)
Aesth Plast Surg 32:779-782, 2008

Background.—A common dissatisfaction after rhytidoplasty are the remaining lateral eyelid wrinkles also known as crow's feet.

Methods.—This article presents an analysis of the enlarged myectomy of the orbicularis oculi muscle used for the definitive treatment of crow's feet in 105 patients during face lifting. Myectomy involved all the lateral portion of the orbicularis oculi muscle exposed after the undermining of the face, corresponding to about one third of the whole orbital extension of the muscle. To avoid depression in the area of the excision, a free graft from the superficial musculoaponeurotic system was performed with the blepharoplasty.

Results.—The reduction of the crow's feet was significant during the subsequent 5 years of follow-up.

Conclusion.—The enlarged myectomy allowed the treatment of a larger area in the wrinkled region without increasing the complications and with excellent results.

▶ While lateral orbicularis oculi muscle resection is not a new concept in treating lateral orbital active rhytides (crow's feet), this report shows that good results can be maintained after 5 years if the procedure is done correctly. This requires not just a limited excision or transaction of the muscle but rather a more extensive removal of the lateral muscle component from the lateral eyebrow to the malar area. Otherwise, muscle contractions may return over time and the benefits of the procedure will be lost. The recommendation of using a piece of superficial musculoaponeurotic system to fill in the depression caused by muscle excision is reasonable as the lateral orbital skin tends to be thin and less forgiving of a deeper contour deformity.

K. A. Gutowski, MD

Orbicularis Suspension Flap and Its Effect on Lower Eyelid Position: A Digital Image Analysis
Zoumalan CI, Lattman J, Zoumalan RA, et al (Manhattan Eye, Ear, and Throat Hosp, NY)
Arch Facial Plast Surg 12:24-29, 2010

Objective.—To evaluate changes in lower eyelid position using digital image analysis in patients who have undergone an orbicularis suspension flap combined with blepharoplasty.

Methods.—A total of 68 patients (136 eyes) underwent a lower eyelid orbicularis oculi suspension flap combined with blepharoplasty. Digital image analysis was used to standardize each patient's preoperative and postoperative photographs for accurate objective comparison. The photographs were analyzed for lower eyelid position.

Results.—The mean (SD) preoperative standardized distance from the center of the pupil to the lower eyelid margin (MRD2) in all procedures was 5.53 (0.74) mm. The mean (SD) postoperative standardized MRD2 was 5.22 (1.0) mm. There was a statistically significant difference in MRD2 position such that the postoperative MRD2 position decreased or the lower eyelid position was elevated by an average of 0.31 mm in comparison to the preoperative position (*P* < .001).

Conclusions.—A well-performed suspension flap can elevate the lower eyelid position to a more natural and anatomically appropriate position. By resuspending the ptotic orbicularis muscle, the suspension flap also reinforces the underlying attenuated orbital septum. Such cases may not achieve the optimum level of rejuvenation if isolated lower eyelid blepharoplasty is performed.

▶ Objective photographic documentation showed a slight increase (0.3 mm) in lower lid margin position relative to the pupil with orbicularis oculi muscle flap suspension. In a subgroup of patients followed for 1 year, the increase in elevation approached 1 mm. The effects on orbital septum tightening could not be measured, but subjective observations suggest that septal laxity may be improved also. This report adds further evidence to support the use of superotemporal orbicularis muscle suspension in lower blepharoplasty.

K. A. Gutowski, MD

Transcutaneous Lower Eyelid Blepharoplasty with Orbitomalar Suspension: Retrospective Review of 212 Consecutive Cases
Korn BS, Kikkawa DO, Cohen SR (Univ of California San Diego, La Jolla)
Plast Reconstr Surg 125:315-323, 2010

Background.—Midfacial aging is associated with increased demarcation of the nasolabial, malar, and nasojugal folds; deflation of facial soft tissues and bones; and descent of the midface. The latter is primarily attributable to attenuation of the orbitomalar ligament. Traditional surgery of the lower eyelid and midface often requires removal of excess skin, orbicularis oculi muscle, and orbital fat, which can be complicated by postoperative lower eyelid malposition. The authors describe a novel adjunct to transcutaneous lower eyelid blepharoplasty that rejuvenates the lower eyelid and midface by reconstituting the orbitomalar ligament and minimizes the development of postoperative eyelid malposition.

Methods.—This study was a retrospective, consecutive, nonrandomized, interventional case series. The authors reviewed the medical records of 212 consecutive patients who underwent transcutaneous lower eyelid blepharoplasty with orbitomalar suspension. The aesthetic outcome, patient satisfaction, and development of eyelid malposition were evaluated.

Results.—Transcutaneous lower eyelid blepharoplasty with orbitomalar suspension resulted in improved lower eyelid dermatochalasis, contour, midfacial ptosis, and appearance of the nasojugal and malar folds. All patients reported satisfaction with the aesthetic outcome. One patient (0.5 percent) developed lower eyelid retraction requiring subsequent lower eyelid tightening. Three patients (1.4 percent) developed transient lagophthalmos from lower eyelid orbicularis paresis that resolved spontaneously.

Conclusions.—Transcutaneous lower eyelid blepharoplasty combined with orbitomalar suspension is a powerful technique that can be performed concomitantly with facial rejuvenative procedures. Orbitomalar suspension addresses midfacial ptosis by restoring the natural function of the orbitomalar ligament and minimizes the development of postoperative lower eyelid malposition.

▶ Lower eyelid fat compartment preservation with fat transposition to soften the appearance of a prominent infraorbital rim and correct the tear trough deformity is useful in certain patients undergoing blepharoplasty. The addition of lateral orbicularis oculi muscle superior-lateral suspension provides additional lower eyelid support with an improvement in midface ptosis. This orbitomalar suspension variation provides superior suspension of the suborbicularis oculi fat instead of the orbicularis muscle. Based on the results shown, it is hard to judge if the effect on the lower lid and midface is better than orbicularis muscle suspension; however, the technique seems easy to perform and has minimal associated complications. Although not described, this procedure could be performed through a transconjunctival incision with a preseptal approach and a small lateral upper eyelid incision.

K. A. Gutowski, MD

Resecting orbicularis oculi muscle in upper eyelid blepharoplasty – A review of the literature

Hoorntje LE, van der Lei B, Stollenwerck GA, et al (Univ Med Centre Utrecht, The Netherlands; Dept of Plastic Surgery of the Univ Med Centre of Groningen and the Medical Centre Leeuwarden, The Netherlands)

J Plast Reconstr Aesth Surg 63:787-792, 2010

Background.—Blepharoplasty of the upper eyelids is one of the most commonly performed procedures in aesthetic plastic surgery. However, the rationale for muscle resection along with skin is uncertain.

Methods.—A PubMed search was performed using the following keywords: 'blepharoplasty' and 'muscle' as well as 'blepharoplasty' and 'orbicularis'. This yielded 419 different hits. All abstracts from English, Dutch, German or French papers were scanned for potential relevance; of which 59 papers were retrieved. The papers were considered to be relevant for our review if they described their technique for upper blepharoplasty and if they mentioned whether or not they resected orbicularis oculi muscle. Papers describing blepharoplasty combined with other surgical interventions were not included unless specific remarks about the blepharoplasty and the role of orbicularis resection were made. Studies describing a surgical technique specifically designed to create an epicanthal fold in Asians were excluded as well.

Results.—In total, 55 papers were included for review. Various reasons for muscle resection are described; most authors resect muscle without providing a reason to do so. In more recent literature, a trend towards muscle preservation is observed.

Conclusions.—A lack of consensus about what is to be done with the orbicularis oculi muscle in upper lid blepharoplasty is demonstrated. This amounts to a shortcoming, especially in training young plastic surgeons. Therefore, an algorithm is proposed.

▶ How much muscle to excise during an upper eyelid blepharoplasty? None, a thin strip, a little less than the skin excision, or the same as the skin excision? A review of the available literature does not satisfactorily answer this question. Individual surgeon's bias and opinions are not supported by comparative data, and there is no standardized method of determining which patients need or don't need muscle resection. Theoretical advantages and disadvantages are offered for each variation, but in the end, there is no consensus. Because it is unlikely that we will see the answer in a double-blind study with a single patient left-right comparison, each surgeon needs to judge his or her own results to determine if the extent of muscle excision is appropriate for an ideal aesthetic result.

K. A. Gutowski, MD

Optimizing Closure Materials for Upper Lid Blepharoplasty: A Randomized, Controlled Trial

Kouba DJ, Tierney E, Mahmoud BH, et al (Henry Ford Health System, Detroit, MI; Boston Univ School of Medicine, MA)
Dermatol Surg 37:19-30, 2011

Background.—Although upper eyelid blepharoplasty is a common procedure, subtleties in surgical technique can affect cosmetic outcomes. Suture materials commonly used include polypropylene, monofilament nylon, fast-absorbing gut, and ethylcyanoacrylate (ECA) tissue adhesive.

Objective.—To assess upper lid blepharoplasty scars in participants whose incision had been closed with 6-0 polypropylene sutures, 6-0 fast-absorbing gut sutures, or ECA.

Materials and Methods.—A randomized, split-eyelid, single-blind, prospective study of the short- (1 month) and intermediate-term (3 months) efficacy of polypropylene, fast-absorbing gut, and ECA on 36 consecutive upper lid blepharoplasties. Participants and a blinded physician evaluator evaluated cosmetic outcome 1 and 3 months after the procedure.

Results.—Three subgroups tested were ECA versus fast-absorbing gut, ECA versus polypropylene, and fast-absorbing gut versus polypropylene. At 1 month, ECA was superior to fast-absorbing gut ($p=.03$) and had a marginally better outcome than polypropylene ($p=.25$), and polypropylene had an equivalent outcome to fast-absorbing gut ($p=.46$). At 3-month follow-up, ECA remained superior to fast-absorbing gut ($p=.03$).

Conclusion.—Although sutured epidermal closure and tissue adhesive are highly efficacious for upper eyelid blepharoplasty, physicians and participants felt that cosmesis with ECA was superior to that with fast-absorbing gut.

▶ While the conclusions seem to support tissue adhesive skin closure (ethylcyanoacrylate [ECA]), the clinical differences in patient outcome are not striking. The ECA group required a deep single Vicryl suture prior to application of the ECA, and the time for skin closure was no better than the suture closure group (8 minutes vs 7 minutes, respectively). Also, the ECA group had particularly high rates of severe pruritis 1 week after skin closure. While not formally addressed, 1 vial of ECA is much more expensive than a single suture. Perhaps the only advantage of using the ECA is eliminating the need for suture removal.

K. A. Gutowski, MD

Transconjunctival Blepharoplasty for Upper and Lower Eyelids
Pacella SJ, Nahai FR, Nahai F (Scripps Clinic and Res Inst, La Jolla, CA)
Plast Reconstr Surg 125:384-392, 2010

Background.—Transconjunctival blepharoplasty remains a popular and safe technique to treat periorbital aging. In the lower lid, it can be used successfully for orbital fat excision, redistribution, or septal tightening. In the upper lid, transconjunctival blepharoplasty has a role in removal of the nasal fat pad via an isolated, direct approach.

Methods.—The authors review anatomy, indications, and surgical approaches for upper and lower lid transconjunctival blepharoplasty.

Results.—Potential complications, patient results, and the senior author's personal series are discussed.

Conclusions.—In the lower lid, this technique can be advocated in an effort to avoid lower lid complications such as sclera show or lid malposition. In the upper lid, it can be effective in treating isolated fat pads with minimal skin excess.

▶ The transconjunctival approach to the lower eyelid is applicable to most patients and can use a preseptal or postseptal dissection to access the fat pads. The preseptal variant allows for fat transposition and redraping if needed, while the postseptal and more direct route is ideal for those who just need fat removal. In either case, a direct skin excision (pinch blepharoplasty) or resurfacing (laser or chemical peel) can be added to tighten the lower lid skin. In the upper eyelid, a transconjunctival approach can be used only to remove the medial (nasal) fat pad as access to the central fat pad is blocked by the levator aponeurosis. As such, its application is much more limited and may be best for patients who only have medial upper eyelid fullness but do not need any skin excision. The anatomic descriptions and advantages of each procedure are discussed in more detail in this article. It is worth reviewing for those wishing to provide a full range of blepharoplasty options to their patients.

K. A. Gutowski, MD

Evaluation and Management of Unilateral Ptosis and Avoiding Contralateral Ptosis
Zoumalan CI, Lisman RD (New York Univ School of Medicine)
Aesth Surg J 30:320-328, 2010

Treating unilateral ptosis can be challenging and a proper preoperative evaluation may help prevent unexpected outcomes on the contralateral lid. Preoperative evaluation should include testing for Hering's law, which remains useful in understanding the phenomenon of induced contralateral eyelid retraction in the context of ptosis. Approximately 10% to 20% of patients with unilateral ptosis have some degree of induced retraction on clinical evaluation in the contralateral lid. When there is a positive

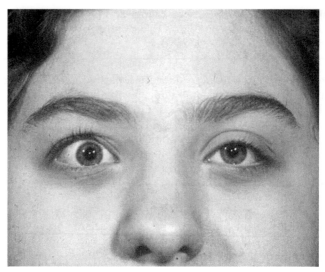

FIGURE 5.—This 17-year-old woman demonstrates pseudoretraction present in the right upper lid secondary to left upper lid ptosis. The right upper lid returned to normal position after successful ptosis repair of the left upper lid. (Reprinted from Zoumalan CI, Lisman RD. Evaluation and management of unilateral ptosis and avoiding contralateral ptosis. *Aesth Surg J*. 2010;30:320-328.)

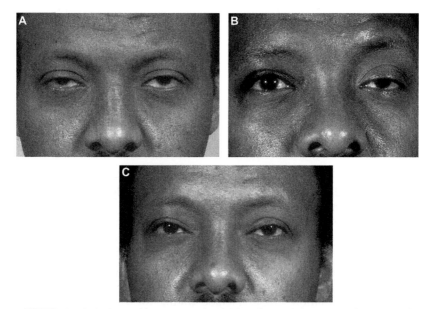

FIGURE 6.—(A) A 48-year-old man presented with bilateral congenital ptosis. (B) The patient underwent repair of the right upper lid first; note the subsequent drop in the left upper lid's position and compensatory brow elevation due to Hering's law one month postoperatively. (C) Improved lid and brow position is demonstrated five months after bilateral ptosis surgery. (Reprinted from Zoumalan CI, Lisman RD. Evaluation and management of unilateral ptosis and avoiding contralateral ptosis. *Aesth Surg J*. 2010;30:320-328.)

Hering's test on preoperative examination, the surgeon should consider a bilateral ptosis procedure. The surgical approach to unilateral ptosis depends on the severity of the ptosis and its etiology, and the surgeon should be aware of which procedure is most likely to provide the best outcome in selected instances (Figs 5 and 6).

▶ This is a nice review study outlining the authors' techniques for diagnosing the likelihood of developing contralateral ptosis after a unilateral ptosis repair and management of secondary problems, which result from the Fasanella-Servat procedure to address mild to moderate ptosis. I believe that it is imperative to evaluate not only levator function in these patients but also to test patients for hidden bilateral ptosis by manually elevating the overtly ptotic eye to overcome the effect of Hering Law and to expose the bilaterality of the ptosis. I have often used the Fasanella-Servat procedure for cases of mild ptosis and found a much lower incidence of secondary deformities requiring correction. I believe that as one stretches the indications to greater degrees of ptosis, the incidence of complications increases. Nonetheless, it is a remarkably easy procedure and for the most part, minor asymmetry and overcorrection can usually be corrected in the early postoperative period.

S. H. Miller, MD, MPH

Face, Neck, and Brow

Blinded, Randomized, Quantitative Grading Comparison of Minimally Invasive, Fractional Radiofrequency and Surgical Face-lift to Treat Skin Laxity

Alexiades-Armenakas M, Rosenberg D, Renton B, et al (Yale Univ School of Medicine, New Haven, CT; Manhattan Eye and Ear Infirmary, NY; Iridex Corp, Mountain View, CA)
Arch Dermatol 146:396-405, 2010

Objectives.—To quantify the improvements in laxity from the surgical face-lift and to perform a randomized, blinded comparison with the clinical effects of a novel, minimally invasive fractional radiofrequency (FRF) system.

Study Design.—Randomized, blinded, comparative trial.

Patients.—Fifteen sequential patients with facial skin laxity enrolled in the trial and completed FRF treatment and follow-up. Baseline and follow-up digital photographs of patients undergoing FRF were randomly mixed with 6 sets of baseline and follow-up images of patients undergoing surgical face-lift with equivalent baseline facial laxity grades.

Main Outcome Measures.—Five independent blinded evaluators graded randomized baseline and 3- to 6-month follow-up photographs using a comprehensive quantitative 4-point laxity grading scale. Quantitative changes in laxity grades were calculated and compared statistically for FRF treatment vs surgical face-lifts. Patient satisfaction and adverse events were also evaluated.

Results.—Blinded grading of unmarked, randomized baseline and follow-up photographs of patients undergoing FRF treatment randomized with baseline and follow-up photographs of patients undergoing surgical face-lift demonstrated statistically significant improvement in facial laxity, with a mean grade improvement of 1.20 for patients in the surgical face-lift group and of 0.44 for FRF-treated patients on a 4-point laxity grading scale ($P < .001$). The improvements relative to baseline were 16% for FRF treatment compared with 49% for the surgical face-lift. The mean laxity improvement from a single FRF treatment was 37% that of the surgical face-lift. Patient satisfaction was high (dissatisfied, 0%; neutral, 7%; satisfied, 60%; and very satisfied, 33%). All participants in the FRF treatment group experienced transient erythema, mild edema, and mild to moderate purpura that resolved in 5 to 10 days, and they returned to normal activities within 24 hours. There were no adverse events or complications in the FRF group. All patients in the surgical face-lift group experienced scarring at surgical margins, erythema, edema, and ecchymosis, and they returned to normal activities on suture removal at 7 to 10 days.

Conclusions.—This randomized, blinded, quantitative assessment using a validated grading scale of skin laxity improvement from the gold standard treatment, the surgical face-lift, and comparative analysis to a novel, minimally invasive FRF treatment has demonstrated 49% improvement in skin laxity relative to baseline for the surgical facelift, compared with 16% for FRF. The surgical face-lift resulted in a mean 1.20-grade improvement on the 4-point laxity grading scale. In comparison, a single, minimally invasive FRF treatment demonstrated a 0.44—laxity grade improvement, or 37% that of the surgical face-lift, without the adverse effects and complications of surgical procedures. This study provides a basis for quantifying cosmetic outcomes from novel treatments with comparative analysis to the gold standard. It also suggests that minimally invasive FRF treatment may provide an important nonsurgical option for the treatment of facial skin laxity.

▶ This well-designed study demonstrated that a standard facelift with superficial muscular aponeurotic system manipulation resulted in an almost 3-fold improvement in facial skin laxity compared with bipolar fractional radiofrequency (FRF) treatments with the Miratone system. The FRF treatments, however, had less downtime and scarring. The improvement seen with FRF is due to fractional thermal injury of deep dermal collagen, which induces dermal remodeling and generation of new collagen, elastin, and hyaluronic acid. While mild to moderate rhytides were improved with FRF, jowls had minimal improvement. Although not mentioned, it is unlikely that any significant improvement in platysmal banding would be seen. FRF may offer a nonsurgical option for mild facial rejuvenation, but longer outcomes need to be measured. As with the initial enthusiasm of laser skin tightening a decade ago, many of the dramatic results faded after 9 to 12 months.

K. A. Gutowski, MD

A Systematic Review of Comparison of Efficacy and Complication Rates among Face-Lift Techniques

Chang S, Pusic A, Rohrich RJ (Univ of Texas Southwestern Med Ctr, Dallas; Memorial Sloan-Kettering Cancer Ctr, NY)
Plast Reconstr Surg 127:423-433, 2011

Background.—The ideal face lift has the longest efficacy, the fewest complications, and ultimately, the highest patient satisfaction. With so many different techniques, there exists a need to make this comparison and to establish which approaches may work best in various groups. To date, there has been no systematic review to study the efficacy and complication rates among different face-lift techniques. This study aims to make this comparison.

Methods.—A systematic search of the English language literature listed in the MEDLINE (Ovid MEDLINE 1950 to November of 2009 with Daily Update), PubMed, and Cochrane Central Register of Controlled Trials (CENTRAL) databases yielded trials on comparison of different face-lift techniques in their efficacy and complication rates. All relevant articles' reference sections were studied for additional relevant publications.

Results.—The keyword search yielded 39 articles. Eighteen more articles were retrieved from reference sections of relevant articles. Only 10 articles made a direct comparison of efficacy between face-lift techniques, and only five articles made a direct comparison of complications between face-lift techniques.

Conclusions.—Although this systematic review revealed a lack of quality data in comparing the efficacy and safety among different face-lift techniques, it is important to review and pool the existing studies to improve patient outcomes. This analysis has also shown the need for better studies, especially randomized, prospective, controlled studies, and a need for a standardized method of efficacy analysis and patient-reported outcomes measures to allow objective comparison of face-lift techniques.

▶ With a wide array of facelift procedure options available, it is disappointing that despite a thorough systematic review of the literature, a determination of which variation is best cannot be made. More interesting is that there is scant reporting of patient satisfaction using a standardized evaluation method. Until higher quality studies are available, each surgeon should continue to objectively evaluate his/her own results and consider changing techniques without the influence of latest facelift technique fads. It may be better to focus on measuring and improving each surgeon's patient-reported outcomes (using the FACE-Q or other similar standardized validated tool) that can yield information on one of the most critical end points of any procedure—the patient's own satisfaction.

K. A. Gutowski, MD

Prevention of Acute Hematoma After Face-Lifts

Beer GM, Goldscheider E, Weber A, et al (Clinic of Aesthetic Plastic Surgery, Zürich, Switzerland; Division of Anesthesia, Lindau, Germany; Kantonspital Appenzell Innerrhoden, Switzerland)
Aesth Plast Surg 34:502-507, 2010

Acute hematoma remains one of the most frequently encountered complications after face-lift surgery. Several risk factors inherent to the patient and omission of certain intraoperative regimens are considered to cause hematoma. Significant risk factors include high blood pressure and male gender. Possible intraoperative regimens for the prevention of hematoma include tumescence infiltration without adrenaline, clotting of raw surfaces with fibrin glue, usage of drains, and application of compression bandages. However, little attention has been paid to postoperative measures. To examine whether different regimens in the postoperative phase can influence the incidence of hematoma, all face-lift patients who underwent surgery by a single surgeon in two different clinics ($n = 376$) with two different postoperative regimens were evaluated over the course of 3 years. In group 1 ($n = 308$), all postoperative medication was administered on request including medication for pain control, blood pressure stabilization, and prevention of nausea and vomiting as well as postoperative restlessness and agitation. In group 2 ($n = 68$), this medication was administered prophylactically at the end of the operation before extubation. The hematoma rate was 7% in group 1 and 0% in group 2. This study showed that the prophylactic use of medications (e.g., analgesics, antihypertonics, antiemetics, and sedatives) during the postoperative phase is superior to making drugs available to patients on request and can decrease the occurrence of acute hematoma in face-lift patients.

▶ This well-designed study strongly supports a perioperative pharmacologic protocol to minimize hypertension, pain, agitation, nausea, and vomiting. Doing so showed a significant decrease in facelift postoperative hematomas.

The prophylactic protocol included administration, before extubation, of:

1. 1 g intravenous (IV) perfalgan (an IV form of acetaminophen) for pain control.
2. 0.15 mg IV clonidine to stabilize blood pressure and prevent agitation.
3. 4 mg IV ondansetron to prevent nausea and vomiting.

Additionally, all patients were observed and monitored carefully for the first 24 hours.

Unfortunately, patients who had had open submental lipectomy or anterior platysmaplasty were excluded from this study. Because extending the facelift to include the cervical region is considered an additional risk factor for postoperative hematoma, it is difficult to know if this protocol applies to all patients with facelift. Furthermore, all patients were monitored overnight so any mild hypertension (systolic blood pressure > 130 mm Hg) was treated with additional clonidine.

Such monitoring may not be possible for patients who have outpatient surgery without home nursing care.

An important additional observation was that all patients received low-molecular-weight heparin prophylaxis starting 12 hours before the operation and continued every 24 hours until complete mobilization. In the pharmacologic protocol group, no hematomas occurred, despite the heparin use. This may alleviate concerns of pharmacologic venous thromboembolism prophylaxis in patients with facelift contributing to hematomas.

K. A. Gutowski, MD

A Comparison of Primary and Secondary Rhytidectomy Results
Funk E, Adamson PA (Univ of Toronto, Ontario, Canada)
Aesth Plast Surg 35:96-99, 2011

Background.—This study aimed to evaluate the authors' surgical experience with secondary rhytidectomy and to compare these results with those for primary rhytidectomy patients.

Methods.—A retrospective review of patients who had undergone secondary rhytidectomy was performed. In addition, an equivalent number of primary rhytidectomy patients were selected randomly. Data were collected evaluating patient age, time elapsed between rhytidectomies, type of procedure performed, superficial musculoaponeurotic system (SMAS) thickness, amount of skin resected, complications, adjunctive procedures, and patient satisfaction.

Results.—This study enrolled 21 secondary rhytidectomy patients. The average time elapsed between their previous and last rhytidectomy was 9.95 years. Using a grading scale of −4 to 4, the average SMAS thickness was 2.2 for the primary and 0.67 for the secondary rhytidectomy patients. The average skin resection was 26.6 mm for the primary and 17.6 mm for the secondary rhytidectomy patients. The complications for secondary rhytidectomy included one hematoma and one hypertrophic postauricular scar. The follow-up period ranged from 6 months to 7 years. All secondary rhytidectomy patients expressed satisfaction with their overall aesthetic result.

Conclusions.—Secondary rhytidectomy is a safe and effective procedure for the aging face. The SMAS of older patients appears to be thinner and more delicate and therefore must be handled with care. Additionally, skin resection is significantly reduced compared with that for primary rhytidectomy patients.

▶ Few articles have been written on secondary facelifts. The finding of a thinner superficial musculo-aponeurotic system (SMAS) in patients with secondary facelift supports a previous study as well as many surgeons' personal observations. The authors' approach is to do a deep plane facelift when possible for secondary cases to avoid the subcutaneous scarring that can limit the amount of tissue lift and skin redraping. This is reasonable for surgeons experienced with a deep place procedure. However, the thin SMAS may make it more diffi-cult for less-experienced surgeons. A safer and technically easier alternative is SMAS imbrication if the SMAS is found to be too thin. Other points to consider are the primary procedure incision placements and scars, tragal definition, earlobe position, and temporal tuft position, all of which may be more distorted after a secondary facelift.

K. A. Gutowski, MD

Biomechanical Analysis of Anchoring Points in Rhytidectomy
Carron MA, Zoumalan RA, Miller PJ, et al (Wayne State Univ School of Medicine, Detroit, MI; New York Univ School of Medicine; et al)
Arch Facial Plast Surg 12:37-39, 2010

Objective.—To quantify tissue tearing force at various anchoring points on the face.

Methods.—This is a prospective anatomic study using 4 fresh cadavers of persons aged 60 to 70 years at the time of death, for a total of 8 sides. Standardized 1-cm distances were measured at the various anchor points, and a single 0 Prolene suture loop was tied at each standardized anchoring point. Steady force was applied perpendicular to the plane of the face with a digital hanging scale. The scale was pulled until the suture ruptured the tissue at the anchoring point. The values at which the tissue ruptured were recorded, averaged, and compared.

Results.—The average tissue force was 7.01 kg for the root of the zygoma vs 3.44 kg for the temporalis fascia ($P < .05$). The average tissue force was 5.50 kg for infralobular tissue vs 4.09 kg for tissue of the super-ficial musculo-aponeurotic system located 1 cm anterior to the infralobu-lar tissue ($P < .05$). The force for the fascia of the sternocleidomastoid was 3.89 kg vs 5.57 kg for the mastoid fascia ($P < .05$). There was a statistically significant difference between vertical bites of the temporalis fascia at 1.90 kg vs horizontal bites of the temporalis at 5.01 kg ($P < .05$).

Conclusion.—The tissue tearing force varies by location on the face as well as suture orientation.

▶ Strength and reliability of suture fixation depend on many variables. This study provides an element of measurable differences between choices of tissue fixation points during a rhytidectomy. All else being equal, it supports the use of zygoma periosteum over temporalis fascia, immediate infralobular tissue versus 1 cm anterior to the infralobular area, and mastoid fascia versus sternocleido-mastoid muscle fascia. Sutures placed with the grain (vertical) of the temporalis fascia were more likely to pull out than sutures placed against the grain (hori-zontal) of the fascia. While suture failure is rare in rhytidectomy, it seems reasonable to use the stronger zones for tissue suspension.

K. A. Gutowski, MD

Volumetric Facelift: Evaluation of Rhytidectomy With Alloplastic Augmentation
Hopping SB, Joshi AS, Tanna N, et al (The George Washington Univ, DC; et al)
Ann Otol Rhinol Laryngol 119:174-180, 2010

Objectives.—Facial aging occurs as a result of soft tissue atrophy and resorption of the bony skeleton, which results in a loss of soft tissue volume and laxity of the overlying skin. Volumetric augmentation is a key component of facial rejuvenation surgery, and should be considered of equal importance to soft tissue lifting. Augmentation can be accomplished with synthetic fillers, autologous grafts, soft tissue repositioning techniques, and/or alloplastic implants. Only alloplastic implants, however, provide truly long-term volumetric correction. To date, there have been no large series dealing with the complications and results of implantation performed concurrently with rhytidectomy, which we have termed "volumetric rhytidectomy." We present our experience with 100 patients treated with a combination of malar and chin implants and rhytidectomy, compared to 200 patients who underwent rhytidectomy alone.

Methods.—The authors performed a retrospective review of patients treated with a combination of silicone malar and chin augmentation with rhytidectomy versus patients treated with rhytidectomy alone. Both groups of patients underwent close postoperative evaluation at 3 days, 1 week, 2 weeks, and 1 month. All patients were surveyed at 6 months to assess aesthetic satisfaction. Complication rates were noted and tabulated. Statistical analysis was performed to evaluate for any differences in the two groups.

Results.—Between 2002 and 2006, 100 patients underwent malar and chin implantation along with rhytidectomy; 200 patients underwent rhytidectomy alone. In the first group, there were a total of 6 cases in which implant removal was necessary, and 2 cases in which revision was required. There were no statistically significant differences (p < 0.05) observed between the two groups with respect to major or minor hematoma, seroma, infection, sensory nerve injury, facial nerve injury, hypertrophic scarring, dehiscence, skin sloughing, or revision.

Conclusions.—Volumetric rhytidectomy reliably augments the malar and mental areas, allows for subtle skeletal contouring, and results in successful rejuvenation. Rhytidectomy is relatively safe to perform concurrently with silicone augmentation, and does not result in an increased complication rate as compared to rhytidectomy alone.

▶ Repositioning the soft tissue during a facelift typically does not correct cheek or malar volume deficits and will not improve a chin deficiency. The addition of a chin implant may complement a facelift if it restores the harmony and proportions of the lower third of the face. In some cases, the use of extended chin implants may soften the jowls and result in a more attractive chin to neckline transition. The results of malar implants, however, are a bit more difficult to evaluate because of long-term soft tissue changes in the midface. As midface and submalar tissue is lost over time and the skin becomes thinner, some patients with malar implants will exhibit an unnatural cheek appearance highlighted by the more prominent implants. To prevent this, proper patient selection should focus on whether true malar deficiency is present and the amount of soft tissue in the submalar region. Patients with thin skin and soft tissue who are developing cheek hollowness may not be appropriate candidates for implants and may better be served with soft tissue fillers in the cheeks.

K. A. Gutowski, MD

Endoscopically assisted limited-incision rhytidectomy: A 10-year prospective study

Citarella ER, Sterodimas A, Condé-Green A (Pontifical Catholic Univ of Rio de Janeiro and the Carlos Chagas Postgraduate Med Inst, Brazil)
J Plast Reconstr Aesth Surg 63:1842-1848, 2010

The ability to bring aesthetic harmony back into the ageing face requires the blending of surgical technique, anatomic knowledge and artistic sensitivity to individualise the surgical approach for each given patient. Since the advent of endoscopic techniques for facial rejuvenation, there has been an increase in the number of patients who seek alternative facial procedures, refusing a conventional face-lift. Limited-scar rhytidectomies offer patients with mild-to-moderate facial ageing an alternative to traditional face-lift surgery. The authors present a prospective study using the endoscopically assisted limited-incision face-lifting technique.

Indications for using this technique include young patients with a relatively small amount of skin excess, older patients with thick skin and minimal skin redundancy, smokers and bald people. A set of incisions in the forehead, pre-auricular area, ear lobe and post-auricular area are done. Frontal and temporal endoscopic lifting is performed, followed by middle third and cervical undermining and transposition of a 2×5.5 cm rectangular pre-auricular superficial musculo-aponeurotic system (SMAS) flap. Overall satisfaction with the facial appearance after this procedure was rated on a scale of 1 to 5.

A total of 54 patients were operated upon during January 1997 and January 2007, which represents 13% of the total number of face-lifting procedures performed during that period. Their age ranged from 28 to 55 years old (mean 38 years), and 35% of them were men. There were two cases of haematoma formation (1%) and four patients (2%) required further liposuction of the submental region. There were no cases of nerve injury or infection. Six patients (3%) requested revision surgery after 2–4 years after the first procedure (median 3.5 years). They underwent a secondary round of face-lifting. The mean follow-up period has been 5.5 years (range 1–9 years). Sixty-nine percent reported that their appearance after limited-incision rhytidectomy was 'very good' to 'excellent' and 22% responded that their appearance was 'good'. Only 9% of patients thought their appearance was less than good.

This is not a mini-lift technique but rather a full face-lift performed through minimal incisions and assisted by the use of the endoscope. Although the endoscopically assisted limited-incision rhytidoplasty is reserved for a specific category of patients and requires a learning curve, it appears to be a procedure with a low rate of complications and a high patient satisfaction.

▶ The limited incisions used in this technique do not allow for any excision of redundant skin, hence the ideal candidates are young (mean age of 38 years) and with good skin tone. The limited access does allow for superficial musculo-aponeurotic system (SMAS) modification and tightening. While it may be a reasonable option in selected patients, the access incisions for the endoscope and instruments for SMAS dissection will still result in some of the same scars as a traditional open facelift.

K. A. Gutowski, MD

Surgical Correction of the Frowning Mouth
Parsa FD, Parsa NN, Murariu D (Univ of Hawaii, Honolulu)
Plast Reconstr Surg 125:667-676, 2010

Background.—The available perioral rejuvenation procedures only partially correct the frowning mouth deformity, which is composed of sagging of the oral commissures and frequently associated with marionette folds. The authors describe their method of surgical correction for this condition and offer a classification for frowning mouth deformity.

Methods.—Twenty-seven patients underwent correction for frowning mouth deformity from 2000 to 2009. The deformities and the corresponding methods of correction were divided into two types. In type I frowning mouth deformity, correction was performed by lentiform excisions at the vermilion border, and in type II deformity, lentiform excisions also included the marionette folds.

Results.—Correction of frowning mouth deformities, either as an isolated procedure or concurrent with face lift, was satisfactorily achieved in all 27 patients. All patients were followed for a minimum of 3 months, and 88.9 percent were followed for 1 year; 18.8 percent of the patients showed erythema and scar hypertrophy at the sites of marionette fold excision during the early postoperative period. However, all scars improved over time, with high patient satisfaction.

Conclusions.—Frowning mouth deformities are correctable by excising lentiform segments of skin through incisions placed at the vermilion border that may be extended to include the marionette folds. Proper patient selection and counseling, particularly regarding temporary or possibly permanent noticeable scar formation, is of utmost importance.

When such measures are taken, the outcome is good and patient satisfaction is high.

▶ These procedures to elevate the lateral lip and correct a frowning mouth (marionette fold excisions) are a continuation of the earlier work done individually by Austin and by Flowers to correct what typically cannot be improved with a facelift. The extended excisions described can be done in an office setting under local anesthesia and offer a natural result. The high incidence of unfavorable scarring may be because of the large Asian population in this report. Personal experience with similar techniques suggests that older patients with lighter skin may have fewer problems with scar noticeability and redness after the procedure. While a small amount of lip elevation and frown correction can be achieved with botulinum toxin and soft tissue filler injections, excisional techniques should be considered in more severe cases.

K. A. Gutowski, MD

Anterior Approach to Neck Rejuvenation
Zins JE, Menon N (Cleveland Clinic, OH)
Aesth Surg J 30:477-484, 2010

The anterior (submental) approach to neck rejuvenation has been described by multiple authors. The efficacy of the procedure depends on adequate release of cutaneous septae and cutaneous ligaments, which allows for skin contraction without skin resection as well as subplatysmal recontouring and platysma muscle tightening. With this procedure, the greatest improvement in appearance will be seen in the profile view. No improvement will occur above the mandibular border. The degree of profile improvement correlates best with skin quality. Because no skin is removed in this procedure, skin tightening is dependent upon skin elasticity. Therefore, those patients with poor skin quality will obtain lesser results. Patients are graded with regard to skin quality from grades I to IV, with grade I patients demonstrating ideal skin elasticity and grade IV patients demonstrating poor skin quality. The technique is described in detail, potential complications are noted, and technical limitations of the procedure are described.

▶ Isolated neck lifts are appropriate for patients who have such loose skin that liposuction only would not yield good results. Through the anterior approach (which may require short lateral access incisions to achieve complete skin undermining), superficial fat and intra/subplastysmal fat can be removed. If needed, digastrics muscle contouring can also be done. The plastysmal bands are easily addressed by reapproximating the medial edges in a similar fashion as the corset platysmaplasty described by Feldman. Appropriately, this article stresses that patients must be aware that no improvement can be expected above the mandible. For patients with severe skin laxity (grade IV), the addition of a facelift should be considered. For the surgeon, it is important to know that the neck skin undermining may need to be quite extensive. Otherwise, skin irregularities may result.

K. A. Gutowski, MD

Triple Suture for Neck Contouring: 14 Years of Experience

Citarella ER, Condé-Green A, Sinder R (Pontifical Catholic Univ of Rio de Janeiro and the Carlos Chagas Post-Graduate Med Inst, Brazil; Ivo Pitanguy Inst, Brazil)
Aesth Surg J 30:311-319, 2010

Background.—Preferred techniques for rejuvenation and contouring of the neck region have evolved over the past 40 years. A slender neckline is recognized as an attractive feature of youth, whereas aging of the lower face often includes ptosis of the soft tissues of the chin and banding or cording of the muscles of the anterior and lateral neck. Aesthetic rejuvenation of the face and neck involves repositioning of poorly supported soft tissues.

Objectives.—The authors review their 14-year experience with a technique incorporating standard submental liposuction with a method of triple suturing the medial platysmal bands associated with lateral plication of the superficial muscular aponeurotic system (SMAS)-platysma.

Methods.—Between 1994 and 2008, 507 patients (451 women and 56 men) were treated with this technique which consisted of placing a first line of sutures distributing tension between the medial platysmal bands and the anterior belly of the digastric muscles, a second single suture at the distal medial borders of the platysma, and a third running suture starting at the level of the thyroid cartilage up to the supramental region. In most cases, a lateral plication of the SMAS-platysma and a "stair-like" SMAS plication were performed in order to define the cervicomandibular line and treat midface flaccidity, respectively.

Results.—Mean follow-up was eight years. Complications included hematomas (4.6%) and seromas (3.6%). Four percent of patients underwent a second procedure approximately seven years after their primary procedure. Overall the majority of patients exhibited long-lasting results satisfactory to both patients and surgeons.

Conclusion.—The triple-suture technique for neck contouring creates a median vertical vector of traction, whereas lateral plication produces a lateral posterior oblique vector. The combination of these two procedures is an easily reproducible and reliable option for surgeons when patients are seeking a more youthful appearance of the neck.

▶ This variant of Feldman's corset platysmaplasty[1] includes plication of the anterior belly of the digastric muscles to correct the weakness and elongation associated with aging. The results are good, but it is hard to determine if they are superior to a standard platysmaplasty. It may be considered as an alternative to muscle belly excisional contouring for patients with prominent anterior digastric muscle bellies.

Another interesting variation described in this report is the infusion of a steroid in the subcutaneous space both at the start of the procedure and 2 weeks after surgery to decrease fibrosis sometimes seen in the cervical and submental areas. While outcomes of this were not described, the routine use of a postoperative steroid infusion may be useful to improve results.

K. A. Gutowski, MD

Reference

1. Feldman JJ. Corset platysmaplasty. *Plast Reconstr Surg.* 1990;85:333-343.

Endoscopic Brow-lift in the Male Patient

Fisher O, Zamboni WA (Univ of Nevada School of Medicine, Las Vegas)
Arch Facial Plast Surg 12:56-59, 2010

Objective.—To report our experience with the endoscopic brow-lift in male patients at a university-affiliated outpatient surgery center.

Methods.—Retrospective case series.

Results.—From 1995 to 2007, a total of 244 endoscopic brow-lift procedures were performed, 21 of which involved men. Thirteen of the male patients had receding hairlines or some degree of baldness. Two male patients had postoperative complications; 1 male patient had temporal branch neurapraxia that resolved; and 1 male patient had in-office scar revision.

Conclusions.—We have found that the endoscopic brow-lift procedure is well suited for male facial rejuvenation. Furthermore, our combined stair-step approach and suture suspension technique provides consistent results and high satisfaction regardless of the patient's hairline.

▶ Brow and forehead rejuvenation in men is different and more challenging than in women. The receding hairline, variation in hairline patterns, thin and short hair, heavier brow, and gender-specific aesthetic differences need to be taken into account when evaluating a male for a brow lift. The modifications described in this article account for some of these challenges. The stair-step technique with endoscopic-assisted visualization seems well suited for men with anterior hair loss to minimize visible scars.

K. A. Gutowski, MD

Biplanar Temple Lift for Lateral Brow Ptosis: Comparison with Uniplanar Dissection Technique

Marshak H, Morrow AA, Morrow DM (The Morrow Inst, Rancho Mirage, CA; Northwestern Univ, Chicago, IL)

Aesth Plast Surg 32:517-522, 2008

Background.—The amount of lift achievable in the temple region has been limited by traditional uniplanar dissection techniques. A biplanar temple-lifting technique (BTL), involving a biplanar dissection both deep and superficial to the superficial musculoaponeurotic system (SMAS) of the temporal region, is described. This study compares the amount of temporal lifting that can be achieved using a uniplanar dissection with that achieved using a biplanar dissection.

Methods.—Thirty-seven patients underwent bilateral temple lifting. Deep dissection was performed on the surface of the deep temporalis fascia. The skin flap was pulled in a superolateral direction and the skin overlap at the wound edge was measured. A SMAS flap was then dissected beneath the dermis from the anterior wound edge to the temporal hairline. The SMAS flap was suspended superolaterally and fixated to the deep temporalis fascia. The skin flap was again pulled in a superolateral direction and the amount of skin overlap was measured and compared.

Results.—The average potential temple skin that could be excised using the traditional dissection technique was 15.1 mm (range, 7—24 mm). The average temple skin that was excised using the biplanar dissection technique was 21.8 mm (range, 14—30 mm). The biplanar technique was shown to offer, on average, a 48% increase in lift relative to the skin-only approach. There were no cases of wound dehiscence, necrosis, or overcorrection.

Conclusion. Using the BTL technique to create a temporal SMAS flap, dissected free from overlying dermis as well as from deep temporal fascia, provides a more secure suspension of the temporal flap and significantly greater temple lift than a uniplanar dissection. The deep layering absorbs the tension of the lift, allowing for tensionless skin closure, thus decreasing the potential for scarring, hair loss, and necrosis. The increased mobility and higher suspension of the temporal flap allows for more skin excision and therefore a more pleasing lateral brow height.

▶ Most lateral brow lifts can be readily done using a subcutaneous, subgaleal, or subperiosteal dissection plane. The use of a biplanar approach allows for a greater measured intraoperative brow elevation (22 vs 15 mm). However, it is uncommon to need more than 10 to 15 mm of lateral elevation in most cases, and an overaggressive lift can cause an unnatural periorbital appearance. The biplanar technique may place less tension on the superficial scalp closure so the scarring and hair loss may be more favorable.

K. A. Gutowski, MD

Nose

Assessment of the chin in patients undergoing rhinoplasty: What proportion may benefit from chin augmentation?
Ahmed J, Patil S, Jayaraj S (Whipps Cross Univ Hosp, Leytonstone, London, UK)
Otolaryngol Head Neck Surg 142:164-168, 2010

Objective.—The chin is an important determinant of the lower third of the face, carrying much significance in an esthetically balanced facial appearance. It is, however, often neglected in patients undergoing rhinoplasty procedures in the UK National Health Service (NHS). The aim of this study was to establish the percentage of a cohort of rhinoplasty patients who may also have benefited from chin augmentation.

Study Design.—A cross-sectional study.

Subjects and Methods.—The digital preoperative pictures of the last 100 patients who underwent rhinoplasty at our institution were retrieved. Four popular methods of assessment were used to assess the chin, that is, those advocated by Silver, Legan, Merrifield, and Gonzales-Ulloa. All analyses were performed on Adobe Photoshop CS4 by two ENT registrars. Values were regarded as positive when there was interobserver agreement. Relevant angles were averaged.

Results.—A total of 94 photographs were suitable for analysis. There were 58 males. Depending on the method of assessment, the percentage of males who fulfilled criteria for augmentation ranged from 17 to 62 percent and for females the range was 42 to 81 percent. Additionally, 21 percent of males were positive on three or more of the methods utilized. The respective figure was 58 percent for females.

Conclusion.—Surgeons who practice rhinoplasty should consider making an objective assessment of the need for possible chin augmentation. Our study shows that as many as 81 percent of patients may benefit, although this figure varies with the method of assessment. In this study, the necessity for further analysis with a view to chin augmentation was more likely in women.

▶ Evaluation and chin position and potential need for chin augmentation is an essential part of any thorough rhinoplasty evaluation. Microgenia and retromicrogenia are common findings in the workup of rhinoplasty patients. These findings should be discussed with patients during the consultation process so that rhinoplasty and chin augmentation can be carried out simultaneously when desired. This article may be worthwhile to review the details of common chin assessment measurements that can determine the amount of chin correction needed.

K. A. Gutowski, MD

Asymmetric Facial Growth and Deviated Nose: A New Concept

Hafezi F, Naghibzadeh B, Nouhi A, et al (Iran Univ of Med Sciences, Tehran; Shahid Beheshty Univ of Med Sciences, Tehran, Iran; General Practitioner, Tehran, Iran)
Ann Plast Surg 64:47-51, 2010

Deviated nose correction is difficult and constitutes a very different issue from septal deviation. When correcting this deformity, traces of asymmetry can be detected. The authors demonstrate facial asymmetry accompanying deviated noses, and such asymmetry is usually ignored by surgeons who typically concentrate only on nose deformities.

A total of 5822 pre- and postrhinoplasty photographs related to 547 women and 124 men were reviewed. Out of the total population, the following 3 groups were selected: group A, gross nose and face asymmetry; group B, nose asymmetry with no facial deformity, group C, facial asymmetry with straight nose. Different measurements were applied to the selected photos, presented in Table 1. These included measurement from the lateral canthi to the lateral mouth corners (D1) and from the midface to each most lateral part of the zygomatic arch (D2). Measurements from one side were compared with those from the contralateral side to identify true anatomic differences, as presented in Figure 1.

There was a significant difference in the nose and face deformity group, as evidenced by a meaningful difference in both the D1 and D2 measurements.

We report a significant growth retardation of the midface and orbit on the concave side of the nose. This impediment may serve as the etiology for many asymmetries of the face and nose.

▶ This article brings to light a very important concept that may be frequently overlooked in practice and highlights the relationship between the asymmetric nose and the surrounding asymmetric facial structure. It is often very difficult to completely straighten a nose when it sits on an asymmetric base. Even if there is success straightening the nose on the anteroposterior view, the nose may still suffer an asymmetric cant or skew related to a foundational deficiency on 1 side. Failure to recognize this preoperatively may result in frustration for both the patient and the surgeon alike. It is an important aspect to examine preoperatively and point it out ahead of time to set the proper preoperative expectations. The authors should be commended for taking a scientific look at this common finding.

K. A. Gutowski, MD

Sonic Rhinoplasty: Sculpting the Nasal Dorsum With the Ultrasonic Bone Aspirator

Pribitkin EA, Lavasani LS, Shindle C, et al (Thomas Jefferson Univ, Philadelphia, PA)
Laryngoscope 120:1504-1507, 2010

Objectives/Hypothesis.—Rhinoplasty often requires precise, graded bone removal without damage to surrounding nasal soft tissue and mucosa. Unfortunately, current techniques are associated with decreased visualization, heat generation, mechanical chatter, and lack of surgical precision with resultant soft tissue injury. We introduce a novel technique to sculpt the nasal dorsum in a precise fashion with the ultrasonic bone aspirator and delineate its advantages over conventional techniques.

Study Design.—Retrospective chart review.

Methods.—The SONOPET ultrasonic bone aspirator (Mutoh Co., Ltd., Tokyo, Japan) utilizes ultrasonic waves to emulsify bone with concurrent irrigation and suction, enabling precise, graded bone removal under direct visualization without thermal or mechanical injury to the surrounding soft tissue or mucosa. We describe the application of this technology to dorsal hump reduction with early follow-up to 9 months. Successful reduction was determined by the senior author at postoperative follow-up appointments.

Results.—Sixty patients underwent open rhinoplasty requiring dorsal reduction with the ultrasonic bone aspirator. No individuals experienced delayed healing, infection, scarring, or major complications. Five of 60 patients had minor post surgical irregularities, which included visible nasal dorsum deformity, palpable nasal deformity, under-resection of the dorsum, and asymmetry of the nasal dorsum. No postoperative open sky deformities, inverted "V" deformities, over-resected dorsums, or skin injuries were observed.

Conclusions.—Ultrasonic bone aspiration permits safe, precise, graded bone removal without damaging surrounding nasal soft tissue and mucosa. We introduce novel applications of the ultrasonic bone aspirator in dorsal reduction that provide significant advantages over conventional techniques.

▶ This is a retrospective report of the use of an ultrasonic bone aspirator to sculpt the nasal dorsum in the course of performing open rhinoplasty. The authors claim that the results achieved including minimization of injury to the overlying skin and associated cartilage justify the increased amount of operative time (10-15 minutes per case) and the cost of the equipment (more than $100 000 for the ultrasonic aspirator and $200 for each tip). It is rather difficult to accept the conclusions in this retrospective study without at least an attempt at randomizing the authors' own patients into 2 arms, 1 group having standard rhinoplasty and the other using the ultrasonic device. Evaluating the end aesthetic result should be done by others as well as the patients. Finally, the increase in costs, associated with the purchase and the use of this equipment and whether or not the device will prove useful in other surgical specialties, needs to be clearly documented.

S. H. Miller, MD, MPH

Reconstruction of Significant Saddle Nose Deformity Using Autogenous Costal Cartilage Graft With Incorporated Mirror Image Spreader Grafts
Ahmed A, Imani P, Vuyk HD (Doncaster Royal Infirmary, UK; Tergooi Hosps, Blaricum, The Netherlands)
Laryngoscope 120:491-494, 2010

Background. Loss of septal height and tip support caused by deformities of the lower two thirds of the nose produces the classic "saddle nose" appearance. A few cases are congenital, but most result from previous septoplasty or rhinoplasty, facial trauma, or septal abscess. Cartilage filler grafts are sufficient to disguise minimal deformities and moderate ones with reasonable septal support are managed with dorsal onlay grafts plus a columellar strut and tip graft shaped from the patient's remaining septal or conchal cartilage. For major deformities, significant structural restoration, often with homologous or autologous rib costal cartilage, is needed. Warping of the costal cartilage is a major complication of the process and can produce postoperative deformities. A technique to overcome the potential for warping was proposed.

Technique.—A standardized rhinoplasty approach that preserves the remaining septal mucosa is used to skeletonize the nasal cartilages and bones. If the remaining septal cartilage is insufficient, a 4-cm long sixth rib graft is obtained through a 4- to 5-cm incision. The entire circumference of the cartilaginous rib can be dissected from its perichondrial covering, or a strip of cartilage can be left interiorly to maintain the rib's continuity. The mid-cartilage area is carved equally on each side to obtain proper neoseptal shape. Released interlocked stressed will warp away these outer slices. The shaved longitudinal strips from the costal cartilage's outer aspects are sculpted symmetrically to produce spreader grafts.

Two small bur holes are drilled tangentially through the anterior nasal spine (ANS) along with one through the caudal protruding edge. The caudal end of the septal part of the reconstruction is secured to the ANS. The neoseptum is sutured to the ANS using 3/0 Vicryl passed through the bur holes, achieving stable fixation. The inferior neoseptal area rests on the ANS. The maxillary crest is beveled to allow the free caudal border to lie between the medial crura at a 120-degree angle. Medial crural support comes from the ventral graft area. The caudal extension of the septal graft allows tip repositioning through tongue-in-groove fixation of the medial crura to the septal graft.

Next the longitudinal costal cartilage spreader grafts are placed between the septum and the separated upper lateral cartilages. Mattress sutures are used to secure them to the costal cartilage neoseptum in parallel positions. This neutralizes their tendency to warp. The grafts' superior ends are attached to both sides of a dorsal septal strut near the keystone area, then fixed to project above the free edges of the collapsed alar cartilages. This heightens the nose's mid third. A slight overlap of the reconstructed neoseptum is achieved caudally. The resulting laminated longitudinal midline structure strongly supports the entire lower two thirds of the nose.

The dorsal aspect of the composite neoseptum and spreader grafts are sutured securely to the upper lateral cartilages. Mattress sutures fix the septal mucosa to the neoseptum. Shaped and bruised cartilage grafts or soft tissue grafts will hide minor dorsal deformities, and the nose tip can be further refined. Incisions are closed and the neoseptum supported by light nasal packs and an external nasal splint.

Results.—Of 14 patients undergoing this procedure, none developed deformity related to graft warping, resorption, visibility, or displacement. The warping forces inherent to shaped rib grafts were sufficiently harnessed to avoid these problems and create a strong L-shaped midline support for these saddle nose deformity cases.

Conclusions.—The complete pathogenesis of the warping phenomenon in saddle nose repairs is not understood, but the technique described has achieved good results without postoperative deformity.

▶ This article highlights the fact that saddle nose deformities can come in complex forms and may involve the caudal septum. If such a deformity is diagnosed, reconstruction of the caudal septum to restore tip support and position is essential. As the authors point out, this can be done in conjunction with bilateral rib cartilage spreader grafts or may also be done in conjunction with a dorsal cartilage camouflage graft. Spreader grafts alone may be useful in mild deformities, however, a dorsal cartilage graft may provide more significant results in cases of major deformity. While spreader grafts will certainly optimize internal nasal valve function, the internal nasal valve may also be opened when using a dorsal cartilage graft by suturing the upper lateral cartilages to the undersurface of the dorsal graft. It is also important when correcting any saddle nose deformity to ensure to the extent possible that the etiology of the deformity has been treated and stabilized.

K. A. Gutowski, MD

Cartilage Grafts in Dorsal Nasal Augmentation of Traumatic Saddle Nose Deformity: A Long-Term Follow-Up
Mao J, Carron M, Tomovic S, et al (Wayne State Univ School of Medicine, Detroit, MI)
Laryngoscope 119:2111-2117, 2009

Objectives/Hypothesis.—To document the long-term advantages and disadvantages of cartilage grafts used to correct traumatic saddle nose deformity. Additionally, to demonstrate functional improvement and cosmetic satisfaction with the use of this graft.

Study Design.—Retrospective chart review and prospective follow-up telephone survey of 20 patients after dorsal augmentation of saddle nose deformity secondary to trauma.

Methods.—This is a single-surgeon, single-institution investigation within an academic tertiary care medical center. All patients presented for correction of saddle nose deformity after trauma, and cartilage grafts were used for augmentation of the dorsum. Minimum postoperative follow-up period of 1 year was required. A modified and expanded Nasal Obstructive Symptoms Evaluation survey, which included questions pertaining to the appearance of their nose, was used to assess both functional and cosmetic changes after surgery.

Results.—Only 1 of the 20 patients was dissatisfied with the overall outcome. Three (15%) were extremely satisfied, 12 (60%) were very satisfied, three (15%) were somewhat satisfied, and one (5%) was indifferent. In terms of function, four (20%) experienced excellent relief in nasal obstruction, five (25%) moderate relief, four (20%) mild relief, and seven (35%) noted no difference. Regarding cosmesis, two (10%) noted excellent improvement, three (15%) moderate improvement, nine (45%) mild improvement, and five (25%) noted no significant change. One (5%) patient reported worsening due to tip edema. Mean follow-up time was 6.8 years.

Conclusions.—Autogenous cartilage grafts are useful in the correction of mild to moderate traumatic saddle nose deformity. The graft is readily available, preserves long-term structural stability, and achieves functional and cosmetic satisfaction in most patients.

▶ This retrospective report of using septal and conchal cartilage grafts for correction of saddle nose deformity, through an intercartilaginous or marginal incision, is somewhat limited because of the small sample size and recall bias. However, the author's technique of using conchal and septal cartilage for dorsal nasal augmentation is a useful tool. It is interesting that the authors did not use costal rib cartilage in any of their reconstructions. In general, septal cartilage grafts can be usefully implemented for dorsal depressions less than 5 mm. These cartilages can be stacked, if necessary, as the authors point out. The curved, irregular, soft nature of conchal cartilage tend to make this cartilage source less desirable, but it can be used to fill small defects. Costal cartilage grafts tend to be more useful in depressions greater than 5 mm, and when carved properly, can result in a smooth and consistent result. Functional results can also be improved in the saddle nose deformity when the upper lateral cartilages are sutured up to a strong costal cartilage graft, which may increase subjective functional breathing scores.

K. A. Gutowski, MD

Applications of GORE-TEX Implants in Rhinoplasty Reexamined After 17 Years

Conrad K, Torgerson CS, Gillman GS (Univ of Toronto, Ontario, Canada)
Arch Facial Plast Surg 10:224-231, 2008

Objective.—To determine the efficacy of GORE-TEX (W. L. Gore & Associates Inc, Flagstaff, Arizona) alloplast in rhinoplasty.

Design.—A 17-year retrospective medical chart review at a teaching hospital, community hospital, and private facial cosmetic surgery center. A total of 521 patients (122 male and 399 female; age range, 13-70 years) were followed for 12 months to 17 years. All patients had undergone GORE-TEX implantation rhinoplasty (685 implants in 158 primary procedures and 508 secondary procedures) performed by 1 surgeon. Patient satisfaction, expressed with respect to desired cosmetic benefit and functional outcome, and physician assessment, based on aesthetic improvement, technical considerations, and complications, were evaluated. Results were assessed according to the follow-up notes in the medical chart reflecting patients' and surgeon's comments and full preoperative and postoperative photographic documentation.

Results.—GORE-TEX alloplasts, 1 to 10 mm thick, implanted in the nasal dorsum (n = 264), lateral nasal wall (n = 252), supratip dorsum (n = 85), and premaxilla (n = 84) showed excellent stability and tissue tolerance. Biological complications that required implant removal occurred in 1.9% of patients and included infection, soft tissue swelling, migration, and extrusion.

Conclusions.—With the exception of the nasal tip, columella, or problems in which corrections would require rigidity of the grafted or implanted material, the GORE-TEX alloplast is a safe, inexpensive, and predictable alternative to autografts. In the present series, more than 95% of implants used were 1 to 4 mm thick. In the remaining 5%, 6 implants ranged from 8 to 10 mm thick, and we found them acceptable. It is our opinion that for both primary and secondary rhinoplasty with adequate endonasal and external soft tissue coverage, GORE-TEX should be strongly considered for major and minor corrections of the nasal wall and bridge in properly selected patients.

▶ Surgeons who follow their rhinoplasty results long-term know that there are changes that can take place well after the 1-year mark. The article appropriately discusses the pros and cons of cartilage grafting versus alloplastic grafting, citing that cartilage grafts can indeed warp and may not provide enough strength or proper shape. The results from this study indicate that alloplastic material can be a useful alternative to cartilage grafting in properly selected patients and properly selected anatomic sites using careful sterile technique. The surgical complication rates were acceptably low and would be similar to complications seen with cartilage grafting, such as malposition and overcorrection. The infection rate is also low in this study; however, it is interesting that the majority of biologic-related complications were salvaged with cartilage grafts, underscoring the fact that infection rates are higher with alloplasts than with autogenous grafts. Rhinoplasty surgeons should still use caution when using alloplasts for this reason, as the incidence of warping, asymmetry, and suboptimal cartilage size and shape can be minimized with proper surgical technique and proper selection of cartilage source.

K. A. Gutowski, MD

Nose Elongation: A Review and Description of the Septal Extension Tongue-and-Groove Technique
Ponsky DC, Harvey DJ, Khan SW, et al (Case Western Univ, Cleveland, OH)
Aesth Surg J 30:335-346, 2010

Several articles have been published about the short nose, many of which begin with a statement about the difficulty and complexity that this deformity poses for the rhinoplasty surgeon. Regardless of the challenges, many surgeons have undertaken the task of elongating the short nose and have subsequently shared with the rhinoplasty community the subtle techniques they have developed through their experience. The authors present a review of the literature that has contributed to the understanding of the etiology, evaluation, assessment, and operative procedures in the reconstruction of the short nose, specifically with regard to septal extension grafts. Additionally, the senior author's (BG) technique and experience of nearly 30 years of practice is described.

▶ This is an excellent review article worthy of careful study. The authors take the reader through the necessary diagnostic and planning steps for correction of these difficult deformities. Variations of the septal extension tongue-and-groove technique as proposed by the senior author have been successfully used by others and us. While use of rib cartilage and bone is occasionally warranted when correcting the short and depressed nose, donor site morbidity may be unacceptable and alternative techniques such as the use of Gore-tex or cadaver bone graft should be considered.

S. H. Miller, MD, MPH

Nasal Base Modification in Asian Patients
Oh S-H, Kim D-A, Jeong JY (Chungnam Natl Univ, Daejeon, South Korea; PLUS Aesthetic Surgery Clinic, Daejeon, South Korea)
J Oral Maxillofac Surg 68:686-690, 2010

The nasal characteristics of white persons and Asian persons represent the extremes of a spectrum. Typically, the common complaints of Asian patients include a dorsum that is wide and lacks anterior height and a tip that projects poorly and is not well defined. Large amounts of subcutaneous fat, thick skin, and a wide, flattened crura contribute to poor tip projection. Asians also have more excessive alar flaring and a wider nasal base.

As a consequence of these characteristics of the nasal base, more aggressive and wider surgical approaches must be used. If the conventional method of alar rim resection alone is used to correct an Asian nasal base, it can cause many problems, such as a conspicuous external scar, an unattractive change in nostril shape, tip projection disturbance, and a blunt alar-facial angle.

We were able to preserve the advantages of this method and overcome its disadvantages by combining a modification of alar rim resection and an alar cinching suture in nasal base correction. We describe our experience with narrowing the alar base in cases with a wide nasal base and alar flaring using a procedure that combines alar rim resection and an alar cinching suture.

▶ Assessment of the alar base and potential need for alar base reduction is an integral part of every rhinoplasty evaluation. Options for correction include both excisional techniques and cinching suture techniques. Each of these techniques has considerable potential and each also has potential limitations. The authors describe their techniques for capitalizing on the benefits of both techniques. As the authors point out, very wide alar bases may require both excisional and suturing techniques. Excisional techniques can be used to change both nostril shape and size as well as a reduction in the columellar-to-alar base distance. When using excisional techniques to reduce alar base distance, care must be taken to preserve the alar-facial groove and also the natural curve of the alar base. This can be done by making the incision just above the alar groove and within the crease of the alar base-upper lip junction and performing the excision within the nasal vestibule rather than the lateral curve of the ala.

K. A. Gutowski, MD

Trunk, Genitalia, and Extremities

Abdominoplasty and Its Effect on Body Image, Self-Esteem, and Mental Health

de Brito MJA, Nahas FX, Barbosa MVJ, et al (Federal Univ of São Paulo School of Medicine (UNIFESP-EPM), Brazil; Federal Univ of São Paulo (UNIFESP), Brazil)
Ann Plast Surg 65:5-10, 2010

The impact of abdominoplasty on the quality of life of abdominoplasty patients was assessed 1- and 6-months postoperatively. Forty women aged 25 to 60 years were divided into study group (25 patients who underwent abdominoplasty) and waiting-list control group (15 patients). Three questionnaires (Body Shape Questionnaire [BSQ], Rosenberg Self-Esteem Scale [RSE/UNIFESP], and Short Form 36 Health Survey Questionnaire [SF-36]) were administered to the study group (preoperatively, 1- and 6-months postoperatively) and control group (on 2 occasions 6 months apart).

A significant positive impact on body image, self-esteem, and mental health was found 1- and 6-months postoperatively. Significant differences were observed in role physical, role emotional, and vitality 1-month postoperatively. In the control group, significant differences were found for vitality. There was a significant improvement in Comparative perception of body image (6-month assessment) in the study group compared with controls. Abdominoplasty improved body image, self-esteem, and mental health.

▶ Many plastic surgeons have witnessed the apparent improvement in self-esteem in breast augmentation patients. It is reasonable to believe that the same is true for body contouring patients, particularly those undergoing an abdominoplasty. The decrease in negative thoughts, feelings, and behaviors related to a patient's appearance after abdominoplasty may challenge the notion that "beauty is only skin deep." We should keep in mind that an improvement in self-esteem is an important factor in motivating patients to see a plastic surgeon and that a therapeutic benefit can be achieved.

K. A. Gutowski, MD

Abdominoplasty: Same Classification and a New Treatment Concept 20 Years Later
Bozola AR (FAMERP - Medicine School of São José do Rio Preto, São Paulo, Brazil)
Aesth Plast Surg 34:181-192, 2010

Twenty years after my first paper on abdominoplasty, I find that the classification of abdominoplasty remains the same, but new operative techniques allow for accentuated improvement of the results through more liposuction, less undermining in tunnels, and reduction of skin traction. I use the same classification of diagnoses proposed in 1988, dividing the aesthetic alterations into five groups, and describe my experience during a 6-year period with 502 patients. I used vibroliposuction and performed plicature of the muscular aponeurosis through tunnels (where there are no important muscular perforator vessels), without damaging the vascularization. I propose an appropriate ratio of 1/1.5 between infra- and supraumbilical segments for uses in diagnosis and treatment, and the same ratio between the perimeter of the waist and the hips up to 1/1.618, known as the golden or divine proportion. According to this new treatment concept, vibroliposuction is used in GI. Vibroliposuction and suprapubic fusiform skin resection with an indigenous canoe shape are used in GII. Vibroliposuction, fusiform skin resection, and plicature of the external oblique muscle aponeurosis through two lateral tunnels are used in GIII. Vibroliposuction, fusiform skin resection, plicature of the rectus muscles aponeurosis through a medial tunnel, and detachment of the umbilicus aponeurotic implantation and reattachment in a maximum proportion of 1/1.6 between the infra- and supraumbilical skin segment with a bolster stitch are used in GIV. In GV, all the infraumbilical skin and a subcutaneous segment are removed after vibroliposuction, then a median tunnel from the umbilicus to the xiphoid process and a plicature of the rectus muscle aponeurosis from the pubis to the xiphoid process are made, and then the umbilicus is transposed. When necessary, a plicature of the oblique external muscle aponeurosis through two lateral tunnels is made resulting in three tunnels.

▶ The continued evolution of trunk contouring includes more aggressive lipo-suction and tissue excision but with less tissue undermining. The concepts and graduated approach to the different classifications discussed in this single author's experience are worthwhile to review.

- Use of narrow tunnels (instead of wide undermining) for muscle aponeurosis plication to preserve vascularity
- Addition of narrow lateral tunnels to correct external oblique laxity
- Treatment of the circumferential trunk (instead of only the anterior abdomen)
- Incorporation of incisions in the inframammary crease when appropriate
- Detachment and reimplantation of the umbilicus in selected cases

K. A. Gutowski, MD

Fleur-de-Lis Abdominoplasty: A Safe Alternative to Traditional Abdominoplasty for the Massive Weight Loss Patient
Friedman T, O'Brien Coon D, Michaels JV, et al (Univ of Pittsburgh Med Ctr, PA)
Plast Reconstr Surg 125:1525-1535, 2010

Background.—Traditional abdominoplasty techniques often fail to adequately correct the complex contour deformities in the massive weight loss patient. To address these deformities, addition of a vertical skin resection to the traditional horizontal excision has become a popular procedure. The authors analyzed the impact of vertical (fleur-de-lis) excision on complications when compared with traditional transverse excision.

Methods.—A review of massive weight loss patients enrolled in an institutional review board—approved prospective registry was performed on consecutive patients undergoing abdominoplasty by a single surgeon. Patients were included if they underwent at least 50 pounds of weight loss. Demographic information, procedural data, and outcome measures were studied. Logistic regression and *t* tests were performed to analyze differences in complication rates for both procedures and identify risk factors for complications.

Results.—Four hundred ninety-nine patients met inclusion criteria, of whom 154 (31 percent) had a fleur-de-lis vertical component. The overall abdominal complication rate for all patients was 26.3 percent, with a 5.0 percent rate of major complications. Transverse-only and fleur-de-lis abdominoplasty had similar rates of complications with the exception of a higher rate of wound infection in the fleur-de-lis group on multivariate analysis. Risk factors for abdominal wound complications with either procedure included male sex, high body mass index, concurrent component separation, and previous subcostal scars.

Conclusions.—Fleur-de-lis abdominoplasty can be safely performed with complication rates comparable to those of traditional abdominoplasty techniques. Ideal candidates are patients with upper abdominal skin laxity who may not achieve an adequate aesthetic result with transverse-only excision.

▶ The addition of a vertical skin excision to a horizontal abdominoplasty incision (inverted T) is not a new concept but has become more used because of the extensive abdominal wall deformities seen in massive weight loss patients. It is particularly useful in patients with additional skin excess/rolls at the level of the mid and upper abdomen, where a horizontal excision alone may not offer optimal results. It can be offered to patients with upper abdominal scars as the scar may be incorporated into the vertical incision. An added benefit is the improvement in the waistline. Patients need to understand that the trade-off is an additional scar with the potential for more wound-healing problems at the junction of the 2 incisions. Wound-healing complications may be minimized by avoiding lateral undermining, tension at the incision junction, and careful tissue handling. Attention needs to be paid to the amount of upper abdominal tissue excised to minimize dog-ear formation in the epigastric area. However, incisions extending to the inframammary crease can be used to work out skin excess if needed (and discussed with the patient preoperatively).

In this study, subcostal scars were not correlated with wound-healing problems other than skin infection (because of conservative undermining and intentional perforator sparing). However, concomitant component separation for hernia repair was correlated with an increased risk of minor wound necrosis (most likely because of the undermining required to perform fascial release). The authors suggest performing component separation with a traditional transverse abdominoplasty procedure and deferring the vertical skin component to a later time if both are required. Because the authors attempted to exclude these procedures on smokers, the low complication rate should not be extrapolated to tobacco users

K. A. Gutowski, MD

A Case for the Safety and Efficacy of Lipoabdominoplasty: A Single Surgeon Retrospective Review of 173 Consecutive Cases
Weiler J, Taggart P, Khoobehi K (Louisiana State Univ Division of Plastic Surgery, New Orleans)
Aesth Surg J 30:702-713, 2010

Background.—The combination of liposuction and abdominoplasty has been slow to be accepted, primarily due to a perceived higher incidence of complications associated with the procedure. There has also been extensive debate about the combined procedure's effects on flap vascularity and viability and the extent to which liposuction may be performed in conjunction with surgical abdominoplasty.

Objective.—The authors present data from their four-year experience supporting lipoabdominoplasty as a safe and effective procedure for body contouring.

Methods.—The authors retrospectively reviewed a case series of lipoabdominoplasties performed between 2004 and 2008 by the senior author (KK). A total of 173 consecutive patients who presented for abdominal contouring were included in the study. Each patient underwent a combined procedure beginning with liposuction utilizing the superwet technique, followed by an inverted V-pattern abdominoplasty.

Results.—Of the patients included in this study, 171 (98.8%) were women and two (1.2%) were men. The average age of the patients was 41.53 years, and the average body mass index was 26. The average amount of total lipoaspirate from the flanks was 2166.09 mL, and the average specimen weight resected was 972.80 g. Complications included partial dehiscence/skin necrosis (12 patients; 6.9%), infection requiring antibiotic therapy and/ or intervention (13 patients; 7.5%), suture spitting (one patient; 0.5%), seroma (six patients; 3.4%), major fat necrosis requiring local debridement (one patient; 0.5%), and skin flap necrosis requiring readvancement of the abdominal flap (two patients; 1.1%). There was a revision rate of 8.0%: two patients required additional liposuction to smooth out unevenness, five patients required scar revision, and seven patients had dog-ears requiring intervention. All revisions were performed under local anesthesia. There were also five instances of confirmed deep vein thrombosis (2.8%) and two cases of pulmonary embolism requiring hospitalization (1.1%).

Conclusions.—The senior author's (KK) lipoabdominoplasty technique, combined with his current preoperative and postoperative protocols, is believed to be a safe procedure that results in excellent cosmetic results. In contrast to some of the current literature, the data show a reduction of overall complications as compared to historical norms.

▶ Additional evidence is provided to support anterior abdominal flap liposuction during abdominoplasty. The key technical point is to perform minimal dissection superior to the level of the umbilicus, not to exceed the medial edges of the rectus fascia (maximum 8-10 cm in width). This should be just enough to allow for correction of any rectus diastasis. Although the study was not focused on venous thromboembolism (VTE), the 2.8% deep venous thrombosis and 1.1% pulmonary embolism incidence are concerning and suggest that lower extremity sequential compression devices may not be enough for VTE prophylaxis in this patient population. Surgeons should strongly consider adding pharmacologic VTE prophylaxis and refer to the recent Caprini guidelines.[1]

K. A. Gutowski, MD

Reference

1. Pannucci CJ, Bailey SH, Dreszer G, et al. Validation of the Caprini risk assessment model in plastic and reconstructive surgery patients. *J Am Coll Surg.* 2011;212: 105-112.

Prevention of Seroma After Abdominoplasty

Beer GM, Wallner H (Univ Zürich-Irchel, Winterthurerstrasse, Switzerland; Division of Plastic, Aesthetic, and Reconstructive Surgery at Landesklinikum Feldkirch, Austria)
Aesth Surg J 30:414-417, 2010

Background.—Seroma is one of the most troubling complications after abdominoplasty; incidence rates of up to 25% have been reported. If it is correct that shearing forces between the two separated abdominal layers play a key role in the development of seroma, postoperative immobilization of the patient until the layers are sufficiently adhered may be a solution to the problem.

Objective.—The authors examine the association between length of immobilization and the development of seroma.

Methods.—This retrospective study included 60 patients; half were immobilized for 24 hours (group 1) and the other half were immobilized for at least 48 hours (group 2). For thromboembolism prophylaxis, all patients received low molecular weight heparin and compression stockings. Postoperative follow-up for detection of seroma continued for at least three months.

Results.—Mobilization after 24 hours led to a seroma rate of 13%, whereas immobilization of at least 48 hours decreased the seroma rate to 0%.

Conclusions.—For abdominoplasty patients with a low or moderate thromboembolic risk, the data suggest that immobilization for at least 48 hours with chemical and mechanical thromboembolism prophylaxis significantly reduces the risk of seroma.

▶ Although 2 days of bed rest after an abdominoplasty may decrease seroma rates, it is not a practical solution, given the cost of inpatient surgery and hospitalization and the risk of venous thromboembolism. A better approach may be the use of progressive tension sutures, which are now supported by multiple independent studies.

K. A. Gutowski, MD

Reducing Seroma in Outpatient Abdominoplasty: Analysis of 516 Consecutive Cases

Antonetti JW, Antonetti AR (Private practice in Dallas, TX)
Aesth Surg J 30:418-425, 2010

Background.—Over the past 30 years, the preferred techniques and settings for abdominoplasty have evolved considerably, but controversy remains regarding the surgical and postoperative approaches that best limit serious complications such as seroma.

Objective.—The authors evaluate their 28-year experience with abdominoplasty and suggest a technique (progressive tension sutures without placement of drains) for reducing the overall complication rate, most significantly with regard to seroma.

Methods.—A retrospective review was conducted of 517 consecutive abdominoplasty cases in the senior author's clinic. The cases were divided into five groups based on operative setting, postoperative care, and surgical technique. Concurrent procedures and complications were also reviewed.

Results.—The authors found that the last group of patients, in whom abdominoplasty with progressive tension sutures (but without drains) was performed as an outpatient procedure, had the lowest incidence of seroma. Specifically, the incidence of clinically significant seroma formation requiring aspiration was 9.6% in early groups, when abdominoplasty was performed as an inpatient procedure; the rate was 24% when it was performed as an outpatient procedure without the placement of progressive tension sutures, but was then reduced to 1.7% with the placement of progressive tension sutures and no drains.

Conclusions.—Abdominoplasty can be safely performed with other concomitant procedures (such as liposuction) in a strictly outpatient setting when surgical time is limited. Despite controversy in the previous literature, the authors' data support the conclusion that the placement of progressive tension sutures without drains dramatically decreases overall complication and seroma rate during abdominoplasty.

▶ This large series further supports the use of progressive tension sutures, as described by Pollock and Pollock,[1] to minimize seromas after abdominoplasty.

K. A. Gutowski, MD

Reference

1. Pollock H, Pollock T. Progressive tension sutures: a technique to reduce local complications in abdominoplasty. *Plast Reconstr Surg.* 2000;105:2583-2586.

Scarpa Fascia Preservation during Abdominoplasty: A Prospective Study

Costa-Ferreira A, Rebelo M, Vásconez LO, et al (São João Hosp, Porto, Portugal; Univ of Alabama at Birmingham)

Plast Reconstr Surg 125:1232-1239, 2010

Background.—Preservation of the Scarpa fascia has been suggested as a way of lowering complications associated with conventional abdominoplasty. Objective evidence regarding this strategy is lacking. The purpose of this investigation was to evaluate the effect of preserving the Scarpa fascia in the infraumbilical area during a full abdominoplasty.

Methods.—A prospective study was performed at a single center from November of 2005 to November of 2007 of the patients submitted to abdominoplasty with umbilical transposition. Two groups were identified: group A, classic full abdominoplasty; and group B, full abdominoplasty with preservation of infraumbilical Scarpa fascia. Several variables were determined: age, body mass index, previous surgical procedures, comorbid conditions, specimen weight, time to suction drain removal, total volume of drain output, and length of hospital stay.

Results.—A total of 208 full abdominoplasties were performed (group A, 143 patients; group B, 65 patients). There was no statistically significant difference between groups with respect to body mass index, previous abdominal operations, comorbid medical conditions, or weight of the surgical specimen ($p > 0.05$). The group with preservation of the Scarpa fascia had an average reduction of the total amount of drain output of more than 50 percent ($p < 0001$). This group also had an average reduction of 2.0 days until the time to drain removal ($p < 0.001$) and 1.9 days of the hospital stay ($p < 0.001$).

Conclusion.—Preservation of the Scarpa fascia during abdominoplasty has a beneficial effect on patient recovery, as it reduces the total drain output, time to drain removal, and length of hospital stay.

▶ Many strategies are offered to decrease drain output after abdominoplasty. Perhaps the most effective is the use of progressive tension sutures (PTS), which eliminates the use of drains altogether. In this series, Scarpa fascia preservation did decrease the length of drain use (but did not eliminate it as do PTS). The 2-day decrease in length of hospitalization is artificial because the author's institutional policy is to discharge patients only after all drains are removed. In the United States, however, it is very common to perform abdominoplasties as an outpatient procedure regardless of drain use.

If Scarpa fascia preservation is done, it is possible that lymphatic drainage is less disturbed. (Anatomical studies show that abdominal wall lymphatic structures seem to be preferentially located in the area deep to the Scarpa fascia.) If so, it would be interesting to measure if there is an improvement in postoperative edema when these structures are preserved.

K. A. Gutowski, MD

Rectus Diastasis Corrected with Absorbable Suture: A Long-Term Evaluation

Nahas FX, Ferreira LM, Ely PB, et al (Federal Univ of São Paulo/EPM, Brazil; et al)

Aesth Plast Surg 35:43-48, 2011

Background.—Correction of rectus diastasis (RD) is performed during most abdominoplasties. This study aimed to evaluate the long-term result of RD correction when the plication of the anterior rectus sheath is performed with an absorbable suture.

Methods.—Abdominoplasty was performed for 12 women who presented with Nahas' type A musculoaponeurotic deformity. The RD was measured preoperatively with two computed tomography (CT) scan slices at two levels: 3 cm above and 2 cm below the umbilicus. The bony levels at which the slices were taken served as a reference for the postoperative CT scans. During the operation, the RD was measured with a ruler at the same levels as the preoperative CT scan slices. The force necessary to bring the medial edge of the rectus muscle to the midline was measured on both levels with a dynamometer. Plication of the anterior rectus sheath was performed using a double-layer 0-PDS (polydioxanone) suture. Postoperative CT scans were performed 3 weeks after the operation. A long-term follow-up CT scan was performed 32–48 months postoperatively for every patient.

Results.—The 3-week postoperative CT scan proved that the correction of RD was achieved by the procedure. Despite the fact that there were different abdominal wall resistances and that the average weight gain during this period was 4.5 kg, the long-term CT-scans showed no recurrence of RD for any patient of this series in either the superior or inferior abdomen.

Conclusion.—Plication of the anterior rectus sheath with PDS suture to correct RD seems to be a long-lasting procedure.

▶ This prospective study supports the use of long-lasting absorbable sutures in place of permanent sutures for correction of abdominal rectus diastasis. Although permanent sutures are usually not a source of problems, in thin patients the knots may be palpable. In some cases, granulomas and suture abscesses have been seen years after an abdominoplasty procedure. Long-acting absorbable (polydioxanona suture) sutures appear to allow for permanent correction of rectus diastasis with perhaps fewer problems than when using permanent sutures.

K. A. Gutowski, MD

Wide Abdominal Rectus Plication Abdominoplasty for the Treatment of Chronic Intractable Low Back Pain

Oneal RM, Mulka JP, Shapiro P, et al (Univ of Michigan Med Ctr, Ann Arbor; St Joseph Mercy Hosp, Ann Arbor, MI; Mayo Clinic, Rochester, MN)

Plast Reconstr Surg 127:225-231, 2011

Background.—A previous report demonstrated that the wide abdominal rectus plication abdominoplasty is an effective treatment modality in select patients with low back pain who failed to achieve relief with conservative therapy.

Methods.—The authors studied eight female patients who presented with chronic low back pain and marked lower abdominal wall muscular laxity. All had failed to respond to conservative management for their chronic back pain. They all underwent wide abdominal rectus plication abdominoplasty. Patient selection and details of the procedure are discussed.

Results.—There were no significant complications in this series, and all the patients had prompt and prolonged alleviation of their back pain. Length of follow-up ranged from 2 to 11 years.

Conclusions.—Changes in the biomechanics of the lower abdominal musculature as a result of the wide abdominal rectus plication abdominoplasty are discussed in the context of increasing spinal stability, leading to an alleviation of chronic low back pain. An argument is made that this abdominoplasty procedure produces a spine-stabilizing effect by (1) tightening the muscles of the lateral abdominal complex and thus increasing intraabdominal pressure and (2) increasing the efficiency of these muscles so that their effectiveness as spine stabilizers is increased. Even though this is a small series, the fact that all the patients sustained long-term alleviation of their preoperative chronic back pain suggests that the wide abdominal rectus plication abdominoplasty should be considered as an option for patients with weak lower abdominal muscles and intractable low back pain who have failed conservative management.

▶ This study supports another small report and the unpublished observations of some plastic surgeons whose patients noticed improvement in low back pain after correction of a wide abdominal diastasis. Interestingly, patients showed almost immediate relief that was sustained on long-term follow-up and were able to resume their same level of normal physical activity experienced before the onset of their preoperative low back pain. The wide abdominal plication involves more than a typical abdominoplasty, as in most cases, the lateral borders of the rectus muscle were drawn together to the midline. The patient's intra-abdominal pressure (using a bladder catheter) and lower extremity venous pressure (using a venous catheter) were monitored during the plication. While it may be too early to offer wide abdominal plication as a treatment for chronic lower back pain, in patients who have been appropriately evaluated and selected, this may be an option if all other treatments have failed. The authors' selection criteria include the following: (1) The patient has intractable back pain that is unresponsive to all conservative measures, (2) the patient exhibits marked lower abdominal wall laxity and weakness, and (3) there is no acute radiographic or clinical evidence of progressive neurologic damage being caused by an identifiable structural lesion in the spine.

K. A. Gutowski, MD

Low Scar Abdominoplasty with Inferior Positioning of the Umbilicus
Colwell AS, Kpodzo D, Gallico GG III (Massachusetts General Hosp, Boston)
Ann Plast Surg 64:639-644, 2010

Miniabdominoplasty with umbilical free float has received little attention in the literature in 15 years and has been criticized for an abnormally low umbilicus. We hypothesized the umbilicus in women presenting for abdominal contouring is positioned higher than ideal and thus may benefit from lowering. In addition, we felt modifications of the original umbilical float technique would improve aesthetic results. A retrospective review identified 60 patients aged 34 to 56 who had abdominoplasty with umbilical fascial transection and inferior positioning. Technical modifications included low placement of a full transverse abdominal scar, abdominal flap undermining to the rib cage, more inferior umbilical repositioning, flank liposuction, and plication of diastasis recti from xiphoid to pubis. Patients did not have enough excess skin to allow traditional abdominoplasty without a high-transverse or vertical midline scar. No umbilical or incisional skin necrosis occurred. To assess optimal umbilical position, plastic surgeons were asked to draw the ideal position on pre- and postoperative photographs from 5 patients. The mean ideal umbilical position was 2.2 cm lower than the actual position ($P < 0.01$) in preoperative photographs and was close to the true position in postoperative photographs. In conclusion, lower abdominoplasty with inferior umbilical positioning is an excellent choice for the middle age, postpartum woman with excess abdominal skin and full length diastasis recti but a normal body mass index.

▶ This procedure may be applicable to massive weight loss patients who have significant upper abdominal skin laxity and are undergoing a mastopexy or breast reduction with an inframammary fold (IMF) incision. Attention must be paid to proper IMF reconstruction to avoid lower pole breast distortion. If combined with a lower incision abdominoplasty or circumferential abdominoplasty, limited abdominal undermining should be performed to maintain vascularity to the abdominal skin.

K. A. Gutowski, MD

Neoumbilicus in abdominoplasty: points of finesse
Sinha M, Vijh V (Selly Oak Hosp, Birmingham, UK)
Eur J Plast Surg 33:189-191, 2010

Most of the scar and resulting 'dog ears', as a result of abdominoplasty, are inconspicuous and can be well hidden in the clothing. Neoumbilicus is often at display and an aesthetically pleasing umbilicus heightens the patient satisfaction from such a procedure. This paper discusses our technique of restoration of the umbilicus. The neoumbilical site is marked 1 cm inferior to the projected stalk. A small ellipse is excised and a core of adipose tissue is excised in a conical fashion underneath it. The umbilicus is anchored to the rectus sheath at 3, 9 and 6 o'clock points in the described manner. We then discuss the importance of the vector of pull on the umbilical stalk and relate this to production of an aesthetically pleasing superior hood. The technique creates an aesthetically pleasing umbilicus that is sited in a gentle depression, with a superior hood. The technique has been used on 40 patients in the last 4 years who have been followed up for at least 6 month. The various points of finesse and the details of the senior author's technique are presented by means of illustrations and photographs.

▶ Of the many techniques available to inset the umbilicus during abdominoplasty, maneuvers that create a superior hood and a slightly vertical umbilical orientation seem to provide the best aesthetic results. The key points of the described technique are the following:

1. The site for the neoumbilicus is marked on the abdominal wall 1 cm below the umbilical stalk (be sure to leave a slightly longer umbilical stalk when performing the initial umbilical stalk incision and dissection)
2. Thinning the fat of the abdominal flap in the area around the neoumbilicus.
3. Three-point sutures in the 3-o'clock, 6-o'clock, and 9-o'clock positions.
4. Fast-absorbing skin sutures to minimize suture marks.

K. A. Gutowski, MD

Transversus Abdominis Plane Block Reduces the Analgesic Requirements After Abdominoplasty With Flank Liposuction
Araco A, Pooney J, Araco F, et al (Dolan Park Hosp, Bromsgrove, Birmingham, UK; Univ of Rome Tor Vergata, Italy; et al)
Ann Plast Surg 65:385-388, 2010

Introduction.—The transversus abdominis plane (TAP) block is a technique of locoregional anesthesia that blocks the sensorial afferent nerves localized between the transversus abdominis muscle and the internal oblique muscle. We describe results obtained with a case control study between patients undergoing abdominoplasty with the TAP block compared with a similar group of patients not receiving the block.

Materials and Methods.—Medical notes were reviewed, and patients were classified according to the presence of TAP. Outcomes evaluated were the requirements of morphine in the first postoperative hour and the number of co-codamol tablets administered afterward.

Results.—Seventy-five patients were screened. No intra- or postoperative complications were recorded. TAP+ patients required significantly less analgesia during the first 12 postoperative hours ($P < 0.001$). The patients with increased body mass index and large flap resected were more likely to fail the anesthetic block and required postoperative analgesia.

Conclusions.—In aesthetic abdominal surgery, the TAP block is safe, is performed without ultrasound guidance, and markedly reduces the requirement of postoperative opioid analgesia. Future studies will now confirm these results and evaluate the consequences in terms of postoperative nausea, vomiting, and overall satisfaction of patients.

▶ The rationale for this block is that most of the sensory fibers that innervate the anterior abdominal wall are located in the plane between the internal oblique and transversus abdominis muscles. Studies of pain control after other operations show that the block provides significant pain relief and reduces the postoperative consumption of opioid analgesics. Therefore, it may be useful in providing immediate comfort in abdominoplasty patients and decreasing narcotic use postoperatively. The transversus abdominis plane block is simple to perform by the plastic surgeon during an abdominoplasty. After the abdominal flap is elevated but before muscle fascia plication, a 2-cm oblique incision is made on both sides of the fascia, 3 cm medial and 4 to 5 cm superior to the anterior superior iliac spines. The external oblique muscles are identified, and the fibers of the external and internal oblique muscles are separated by blunt dissection until the transversus abdominis muscle is visualized. Bupivacaine hydrochloride (total dose 2 mg/kg) is injected bilaterally with a blunt needle in the plane between the internal oblique and the transversus abdominis muscles. The oblique external muscle fascia is then repaired, and the abdominoplasty procedure is continued.

K. A. Gutowski, MD

Painless Abdominoplasty: The Efficacy of Combined Intercostal and Pararectus Blocks in Reducing Postoperative Pain and Recovery Time
Feng L-J (Case Western Reserve Univ School of Medicine, Pepper Pike, OH)
Plast Reconstr Surg 126:1723-1732, 2010

Background.—Reducing postoperative pain following abdominoplasty is essential for shortening the length of recovery time, reducing the use of narcotics, promoting quicker return to normal activities, and maximizing overall patient satisfaction. The extended use of narcotics and pain pumps is often unacceptable because of nausea, restriction of normal activities, and inconvenience. When the recovery process is not too lengthy and debilitating for the patients, they are more likely to refer the procedure to others and to return for additional elective procedures.

Methods.—The charts of 209 patients undergoing abdominoplasty over a 10-year period were reviewed. The control group ($n = 20$) received no blocks, whereas the treatment group ($n = 77$) received a combination of nerve blocks, using bupivacaine, tetracaine, and Depo-Medrol. Recovery room data and patient questionnaires were used to evaluate clinical efficacy. Patient procedures were classified into four severity classes for analysis.

Results.—The treatment group had significantly less pain across all severity classes and required significantly less narcotics and less time in the recovery room. Pain scores continued to be significantly lower at home. Patients had significantly less nausea, took less pain medication, and resumed normal activities significantly sooner than the control group.

Conclusions.—This is the first study showing successful long-term relief of pain associated with abdominoplasty using a combination of intercostal, ilioinguinal, iliohypogastric, and pararectus blocks. This pain-block procedure significantly reduces the recovery time and allows the patient to return to normal activities and work much sooner.

▶ The addition of anesthetic blocks to abdominoplasty procedures seems reasonable given the significant reduction in postoperative pain they provide. The dramatic improvement in pain following nerve blocks persisted for a week after surgery. Other pain reduction techniques are also useful but limited by duration of effect (tumescent fluid) and the need to use additional devices (pain pumps). The blocks used in this series should add minimal time to the procedure (less than 10 minutes) and cost less than a pain pump. These techniques can be incorporated into clinical practice by working with the same anesthesia provider on a regular basis, one who is willing to assist with the intercostal nerve blocks if needed. Everyone involved will see the benefit of reduced recovery room time, faster discharge to home, and better patient comfort.

K. A. Gutowski, MD

Abdominoplasty Combined with Cesarean Delivery: Evaluation of the Practice

Ali A, Essam A (Ain Shams Univ, Cairo, Egypt)
Aesth Plast Surg 35:80-86, 2011

Abdominoplasty is an aesthetic surgical procedure that restores abdominal contouring. Repeated pregnancy usually leads to lower abdominal skin redundancy and excess fat accumulation. Delivery via Cesarean section adds weakness to the lower abdominal wall muscles and yields a lower transverse Cesarean scar. Recently and in some cultures, abdominoplasty is requested at the same time of Cesarean delivery. Those women usually want to get the benefit of undergoing the abdominoplasty combined with Cesarean delivery in the same setting, thus avoiding a future surgery. This study was designed to evaluate the aesthetic outcome of combined abdominoplasty with Cesarean delivery. The study included 50 pregnant women from February 2008 to December 2009 with an average follow up period of 6 months. Nine patients (18%) developed wound infection; three of them (9%) developed wound dehiscence. Six patients (12%) developed lower abdominal skin necrosis; three of them (6%) were treated conservatively and healed by secondary intention, while surgical debridement and secondary sutures were needed in the other three patients (6%). Residual abdominal skin redundancy in 9 patients (18%), outward bulging of the abdomen and lack of waist definition in 16 patients (32%), and outward bulging of the umbilicus in 12 patients (24%) were the reported unaesthetic results. The results were compared with results of 80 abdominoplasties in nonpregnant women. The study concluded that abdominoplasty combined with Cesarean delivery carries a higher incidence of complications and does not give the desired aesthetic outcome. The authors do not recommend this practice.

▶ The authors confirm what many plastic surgeons have already observed when combining abdominoplasty with a cesarean delivery—complications are more frequent and the results are less dramatic. It is not surprising that it is harder to tighten the abdominal wall muscles in the presence of an enlarged uterus. While patients may desire a combined procedure for their convenience and cost savings, they should be advised that the outcomes may be less than those achieved by postponing the abdominoplasty for 6 to 12 months.

K. A. Gutowski, MD

Management of Upper Abdominal Laxity After Massive Weight Loss: Reverse Abdominoplasty and Inframammary Fold Reconstruction

Agha-Mohammadi S, Hurwitz DJ (Hurwitz Ctr for Plastic Surgery, Pittsburgh, PA)
Aesth Plast Surg 34:226-231, 2010

Background.—Central to body contouring after weight loss surgery is treatment of the abdominal region, often through a circumferential abdominoplasty. This procedure, however, neglects the laxity of the lower thoracic/upper abdominal region. A reverse abdominoplasty with reconstruction of a new inframammary fold (IMF) corrects this deformity through removal of excess skin along the IMF. Since 2002, we have performed 88 reverse abdominoplasty procedures within the context of a single or staged total-body lift (TBL).

Methods.—A retrospective chart review of 129 TBL cases indicated that 88 patients had a combined or staged reverse abdominoplasty and circumferential abdominoplasty. Complication rates were noted as localized or generalized.

Results.—Fifty-three of our patients had combined reverse abdominoplasty and circumferential abdominoplasty and 35 had the reverse abdominoplasty during a second stage. The complication rates for both groups were about 5% per patient per procedure with differences that were not statistically significant. Also, the revision rates for reverse abdominoplasty and circumferential abdominoplasty were similar for both groups, indicating patient satisfaction with the procedures.

Conclusion.—In selected patients, effective treatment of the abdominal region demands correction of both the upper and lower abdominal laxity and contour. This can be performed safely, effectively, and reliably by a reverse abdominoplasty with IMF reconstruction independently or simultaneously with circumferential abdominoplasty.

▶ This procedure may be applicable to massive weight loss patients who have significant upper abdominal skin laxity and are undergoing a mastopexy or breast reduction with an inframammary fold (IMF) incision. Attention must be paid to proper IMF reconstruction to avoid lower pole breast distortion. If combined with a lower incision abdominoplasty or circumferential abdominoplasty, limited abdominal undermining should be performed to maintain vascularity to the abdominal skin.

K. A. Gutowski, MD

Aesthetic and functional reduction of the labia minora using the Maas and Hage technique
Solanki NS, Tejero-Trujeque R, Stevens-King A, et al (Cambridge Univ, UK; Addenbrooke's Univ Hosp, Cambridge, UK)
J Plast Reconstr Aesth Surg 63:1181-1185, 2010

Introduction.—Enlarged labia minora can cause functional, aesthetic and psychosocial problems. There are many reported techniques for their surgical correction in both the gynaecological and surgical literature suggesting that no one method is superior to the others. The problem is compounded because an individual surgeon's experience is likely to be small given the infrequent request for surgery. For these reasons it is important that existing techniques are validated by independent surgeons rather than describing yet another variation.

Methods.—Patients who underwent surgical reduction of their labia minora from 2001—2008 were retrospectively reviewed. All cases were performed by the same surgeon using the Maas and Hage technique of a running interdigitating W-shaped excision.

Results.—12 patients aged from 15 to 52 years underwent reduction labioplasty for idiopathic hypertrophy. Postoperatively there were no wound dehiscences or infections. One patient developed a painful haematoma 2 h after surgery necessitating surgical evacuation while another went into postoperative urinary retention relieved by overnight catheter-isation. Both made uneventful recoveries. All patients were satisfied with their 'natural looking' cosmetic results and have returned to their normal activities without recurrence of their presenting symptoms. The mean follow up was 14 weeks but none have subsequently required or requested revisional surgery.

Conclusions.—The running W-shaped resection was found to be an easy and effective method of reducing the labia minora by a single operator in a small series of cases. This independent review demonstrates the repro-ducibility of this technique and the favourable aesthetic and functional outcomes for the patient.

▶ Labial reduction procedures appear to be growing in popularity. These authors show the results of the running W-plasty technique to be quite accept-able, and their patient satisfaction rate is very high. This is a small series compared with other reports in the past, but it has one interesting feature: Many of the patients do not have labia minora enlargement, which meets the accepted definition of labial hypertrophy; nevertheless, they requested the surgery and were pleased with their results. This finding probably reflects the growing trend among women for enhanced labial aesthetics. The patient doesn't need to meet an arbitrary standard of hypertrophy to qualify for, and to be satisfied with, labial reduction surgery.

R. L. Ruberg, MD

Mons Pubis Ptosis: Classification and Strategy for Treatment
El-Khatib HA (Weill Cornell School of Medicine, Doha, State of Qatar)
Aesth Plast Surg 35:24-30, 2011

Background.—Obesity and massive weight loss cause bulging and ptosis of the mons pubis. The pubic area can cause an embarrassment to patients. In some cases, the deformity can be seen even under clothing. Ptosis of the mons usually is addressed during abdominoplasty. The author presents a new clinical classification of mons deformity based on the amount of adipose tissue deposit and the degree of ptosis. A strategy of treatment to achieve a proper rejuvenation of mons deformities is provided.

Methods.—Between 2004 and 2009, a total of 132 patients with pendu-lous bellies and mons pubis deformities underwent abdominoplasty and lifting of the mons. A technique using a dermal-fascial suspension with permanent sutures to hang the weight of the mons skin and subcutaneous tissues on the musculoaponeuretic system of the lower abdomen is described. The age of patients undergoing the operation ranged from 20 to 53 years. During the follow-up period (12—38 months), all the patients by the author, who reviewed their medical charts. A Likert scale and an evaluation ques-tionnaire were used to assess the aesthetic outcome of mons lifting.

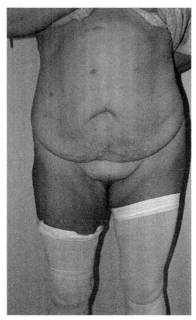

FIGURE 12.—Preoperative view (after massive weight loss) of grade 4 mons deformities with partial covering of the genitalia. Note the abdominal scars of laparoscopic gastric banding. (Reprinted from El-Khatib HA. Mons pubis ptosis: classification and strategy for treatment. *Aesth Plast Surg.* 2011;35:24-30, with kind permission from Springer Science+Business Media.)

Results.—All the patients who underwent lifting of the mons pubis were free of postoperative contour deformities and had a long-lasting outcome. At this writing, patient satisfaction has remained high.

Conclusion.—The clinical classification and treatment guidelines reported are designed to provide simple procedures with minimal complications that have tremendously rejuvenated the mons (Figs 12 and 13).

▶ This is a report of a large number of patients who have undergone reduction and repositioning of the mons pubis. The clinical classification provided by the author and his recommendations for dealing with the deformities should prove useful to other surgeons dealing with this issue. The major contribution of this author to previous work is tacking the fascial-dermal tissues of the mons to the rectus sheath.[1] Obviously, care has to be exercised to avoid displacing the urethral meatus, labia majora, and the hairline of the mons pubis.

S. H. Miller, MD, MPH

Reference

1. Alter GJ. Management of the mons pubis and labia majora in the massive weight loss patient. *Aesth Surg J.* 2009;29:432-442.

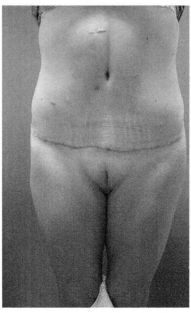

FIGURE 13.—Postoperative view of grade 4 mons deformities with partial covering of the genitalia. Note the abdominal scars of laparoscopic gastric banding. (Reprinted from El-Khatib HA. Mons pubis ptosis: classification and strategy for treatment. *Aesth Plast Surg.* 2011;35:24-30, with kind permission from Springer Science+Business Media.)

L-Brachioplasty: An Adaptable Technique for Moderate to Severe Excess Skin and Fat of the Arms

Hurwitz DJ, Jerrod K (Univ of Pittsburgh Med Ctr, PA)
Aesth Surg J 30:620-629, 2010

The L-brachioplasty is an L-shaped pattern of excision with the long limb from the elbow to the axilla and the short limb extending at right angles through the axilla and along the lateral chest. The width of the excisions through the arm, axilla and chest is based on preoperative assessment through anatomical point locations followed by pinch and gathering maneuvers. The following modifications have improved aesthetics and reduced complications: 1) improved geometric design, 2) anchor fixation of the posterior V-shaped advancement flap to the deltopectoral fascia, 3) excision site liposuction (ESL), and 4) and barbed suture closure.

The free hand markings are followed by measuring equal anterior and posterior incision distances. The subcutaneous fat within the excision site is completely suctioned. After the perimeter is incised, the skin resection begins full thickness from the chest and through the axilla and then the skin only through proximal to distal arm skin. An anchor suture advances the posterior triangular flap to the deltopectoral fascia. A long-lasting absorbable barbed suture is passed through as a running horizontal mattress, starting from the center of the wound. A second continuous rapidly absorbing barbed intradermal suture completes the closure.

Over the past 30 arms, only one seroma was aspirated on one occasion. There have been no lymphoceles. Appreciable swelling is over within a month. Incision dehiscence was limited to less than one centimeter in five patients. Tip necrosis of the V advancement flap occurred in three arms, leaving small wounds in the axilla to heal secondarily. Minor secondary skin reduction is rare. There were no contractures across the axilla. The women appreciated the reduced hair and axillary hollow. In most cases the skin laxity was corrected and the contour from the arm across the axilla to the lateral chest was excellent. No patient expressed regret over their scar.

▶ Similar to the posterior brachioplasty, the L-brachioplasty uses liposuction. In this case, however, in an effort to preserve lymphatic and neurovascular structures, liposuction is used to debulk the area of tissue excision. The L-brachioplasty excision allows for extension onto the lateral chest wall, as does the posterior approach. The L-brachioplasty may allow for better axillary contouring and excision of axillary hair—bearing skin, which may have migrated inferiorly in massive weight loss patients. The scars, however, may be more prone to hypertrophy.

K. A. Gutowski, MD

Liposuction-Assisted Posterior Brachioplasty: Technical Refinements in Upper Arm Contouring

Nguyen AT, Rohrich RJ (Univ of Texas Southwestern Med Ctr, Dallas)
Plast Reconstr Surg 126:1365-1369, 2010

Background.—Brachioplasty has increased 4059 percent from 2000 to 2008 in the United States, with 14,059 upper arm lift procedures performed in 2008. Numerous variations in the evolution of brachioplasty have been described to improve on complications and outcomes. Liposuction-assisted posterior brachioplasty is the next step in the series of refinements in upper arm contouring.

Methods.—The authors present a series of 21 patients who underwent upper arm contouring with liposuction-assisted posterior brachioplasty, and include an operative video detailing the enhancements. After anatomical analysis of the posterior arm, noting skin and fat redundancy, appropriate patients were selected for this procedure. Operative markings, liposuction technique, and the unique excisional technique are presented with intraoperative video footage.

Results.—Patients tolerate liposuction-assisted posterior brachioplasty very well, with minimal complications and good results. One post—bariatric surgery patient experienced a small wound dehiscence, and one non—bariatric surgery patient developed a slight hypertrophic scar in one arm. No other complications were noted. No revisions were performed.

Conclusions.—Liposuction-assisted posterior brachioplasty is an efficient and reproducible procedure in selected patients with generalized inferior arm skin and fat redundancy. It simplifies the markings and resection. It provides a safe procedure by preserving lymphatics, blood loss, and nerves. It produces reliable and predictable results with optimal outcomes. This technique offers another refinement in the evolution of upper arm contouring.

▶ Liposuction can frequently be combined with brachioplasty, particularly in the zone over the biceps muscle, to achieve an improved contour. Ideal patients are those with moderate arm fat excess and moderate skin excess along the entire arm and/or upper arm. The described technique uses a posterior tissue excision approach, which has several advantages:

1. Less risk of cutaneous nerve injury
2. No skin flap undermining
3. Less scar hypertrophy (but the scar is not hidden in the medial arm)
4. Better preservation of the lymphatics

The positioning is somewhat different than for a medial incision brachioplasty, but this can be easily accomplished with the aid of a self-retaining retractor frame or an assistant. While this series used ultrasound-assisted liposuction, the same results can be achieved with traditional or power-assisted liposuction.

K. A. Gutowski, MD

Gluteoplasty: Anatomic Basis and Technique
Serra F, Aboudib JH, Cedrola JPV, et al (Univ of the State of Rio de Janeiro, Brazil)
Aesth Surg J 30:579-592, 2010

Background.—Although the placement of implants for gluteal augmentation is becoming more common, the procedure still faces strong resistance from patients and some surgeons as a result of unsatisfactory outcomes in the past.

Objective.—The authors describe easily-identifiable anatomic reference points that can assist the surgeon in the performance of gluteoplasty, making the procedure simpler and safer.

Methods.—Based on a literature review, an anatomic study was performed of dissections of the gluteal region in seven formalinized and fresh cadavers. This study allowed the authors to observe anatomic details and propose bony reference points to guide gluteoplastic surgery. Between July 2006 and February 2009, 105 patients underwent gluteoplasty according to the guidelines resulting from the cadaveric study.

Results.—All patients were female, ages 22 to 50 years. The surgical procedure, once refined, resulted in a low complication rate. In the final

50 patients in the series, there was only one seroma, one wound infection, and no cases of dehiscence. Bruising on the side of the thigh was encountered in four of the total 105 cases (3.8%). The clinical photos demonstrate the positive aesthetic results of this technique.

Conclusions.—When gluteoplasty is performed utilizing a systematic strategy based on bone anatomy references, it can be a predictable procedure with reproducible results and minimal complications.

▶ Gluteal augmentation with implants is an uncommon procedure in the United States but is getting more attention, particularly in certain ethnic groups and in some patients with massive weight loss. Key technique points include proper pocket selection, safe pocket dissection, and avoidance of postoperative complications. The subcutaneous pocket may be more prone to long-term implant descent, as skin becomes lax over time. The submuscular pocket places the sciatic nerve at risk both during pocket creation and after implant placement. Both the subfascial and intramuscular pockets are then reasonable alternatives for implant placement. The intramuscular technique described minimizes risk to the sciatic nerve, even in cases of nerve anatomic variations. The proper pocket size and depth are important to prevent implant herniation through the gluteus muscle. This article should be reviewed by surgeons who are planning to add this procedure to their practice. Of course, the alternatives of fat grafting in place of implants should also be considered in appropriate patients (ie, those who could benefit from liposuction).

K. A. Gutowski, MD

A New Technique for Gluteal Lifting Using Deepithelialized Dermal Flaps
Handschin AE, Mackowski M, Vogt PM, et al (Med School Hannover, Germany; Mang Med One Clinics, Hamburg, Germany)
Aesth Plast Surg 34:96-99, 2010

Background.—Gluteal ptosis may result from sagging of redundant skin and fat below the infragluteal fold. The correction of gluteal ptosis and the definition of gluteal prominence can be obtained by several gluteal lifting techniques. We present a new technique to correct gluteal ptosis using deepithelialized dermal flaps.

Methods.—Eight female patients (39 ± 4 years old) with gluteal ptosis were included in the study. Six patients had been previously operated on elsewhere (liposuction, body lift). Gluteal lifting is performed using a crescent-shaped deepithelialized flap. The cranial two-thirds of the flap is sutured to the gluteal fascia, thus creating the new gluteal curvature and the position of the new infragluteal fold. The lower third of the flap is then sutured back toward the two-thirds flap within the first suture line, resulting in a doubling of the deepithelialized area.

Results.—The mean operating time was 100 ± 20 min (range = 75–110 min). There were no complications in the study group. An analysis of postoperative results revealed a very good aesthetic aspect in all patients. All patients showed an improved definition of the infragluteal fold, with a symmetric shape of the gluteal region. All patients judged the outcome as very good.

Conclusion.—The use of a deepithelialized double dermal flap is a safe and new way to obtain excellent results in rejuvenation of the gluteal region. Our technique allows for the creation of a stable and long-lasting infragluteal fold with an aesthetic buttock curvature and a defined border to the thigh region.

▶ Based on the postoperative results, this procedure offers less of a gluteal lift and more of an inferior gluteal fold reshaping with an improvement in the infragluteal (banana roll) area. It may be considered for patients who wish more definition to their gluteal fold but are not candidates for liposuction.

K. A. Gutowski, MD

Internal Suture Technique for Improving Projection and Stability in Secondary Gluteoplasty

Jaimovich CA, Almeida MWR, de Souza Aguiar LF, et al (Pontifical Catholic Univ of Rio de Janeiro Med School, Brazil; Ivo Pitanguy Inst, Rio de Janeiro, Brazil)

Aesth Surg J 30:411-413, 2010

The most common indication for primary gluteoplasty is the aesthetic correction of gluteal hypoplasia; secondary gluteoplasty is directed toward asymmetry from misplaced implants, trauma or infection of the implant, and treatment of congenital and acquired deformities. In this study, the authors describe a new suture maneuver designed to improve the result in secondary gluteoplasties. To reduce the empty pocket spaces and guarantee the stability of the new (smaller) implants, anchoring circular interlocking sutures are placed into the two sheets of the fibrotic capsule, which makes it possible to place the implant in a more favorable position.

▶ As in breast implant surgery, occasionally gluteal implants need to be exchanged for a smaller size. If the implant pocket is too large for the new smaller implant, poor results will follow. Similar to reducing the breast implant pocket by capsule suture manipulation, the described technique uses sutures to reduce the size of the gluteal implant pocket. In this case, the gluteal capsule was not cut, nor were raw capsule edges created for suturing the capsule. The results were satisfactory in this example, but based on experience with breast implant capsule manipulation, it may be better to actually cut the capsule and suture the raw edges to achieve better and longer lasting correction of the gluteal implant pocket.

K. A. Gutowski, MD

Liposuction, Fat Transfer, and Tissue Fillers

The American Society for Aesthetic Plastic Surgery (ASAPS) Survey: Current Trends in Liposuction
Ahmad J, Eaves FF III, Rohrich RJ, et al (Plastic Surgeon in Private Practice in Ontario, Canada; Plastic Surgeon in Private Practice in Charlotte, NC; Univ of Texas Southwestern Med Ctr, Dallas)
Aesth Surg J 31:214-224, 2011

Background.—The emergence of new technologies necessitates a study of current trends in liposuction and other methods for fat removal.

Objective. The American Society for Aesthetic Plastic Surgery (ASAPS) conducted a survey of its members to gain valuable information from Board-certified plastic surgeons about their experience with new technologies for fat removal and managing complications after liposuction.

Methods.—The ASAPS Current Trends in Liposuction Survey was emailed to 1713 ASAPS members. Data were tabulated and examined to determine current trends in liposuction and other fat removal techniques performed by ASAPS members.

Results.—The response rate for the survey was 28.7% (n = 492). Most ASAPS respondents reported performing between 50 and 100 liposuction procedures annually. Most plastic surgeons currently employ or have previous experience with suction-assisted lipectomy/liposuction (SAL), ultrasound-assisted liposuction (UAL), and power-assisted liposuction, but fewer reported experience with laser-assisted liposuction (LAL), mesotherapy, or external, noninvasive devices. SAL was the preferred method of fat removal for 51.4%. UAL, LAL, and SAL were most commonly associated with complications. Only 10.5% of ASAPS members employ LAL; 38% have treated a patient with complications secondary to LAL.

Conclusions.—Valuable information about current trends in liposuction and other fat removal techniques has been gained from this survey. Although many studies have been published that review issues related to safety, morbidity, aesthetics, and recovery after different methods of fat removal, more prospective studies with standardized objective outcome measures comparing these techniques, particularly newer modalities, are needed to continue improving safety-related standards of care.

▶ With current marketing efforts that bypass well-designed comparative clinical trials, it would seem that traditional liposuction (suction-assisted liposuction [SAL]) has been replaced by more high tech (and more expensive) modalities. However, at least for now, more than half of those plastic surgeons who perform liposuction seem to prefer SAL, and most of the remaining surgeons use ultrasound-assisted liposuction (UAL) or power-assisted liposuction (PAL). Not surprisingly, those who no longer used PAL or UAL cited cost and time as the most common reasons for abandoning these devices. Of those who use the new laser-assisted liposuction (LAL), only half perform more than 25 LAL procedures per year, which questions the return on investment for those who invested in LAL machines but use them only for a few cases per year. For those who use LAL infrequently, per-use rental agreements may be a better option. When asked why they preferred LAL over other modalities, 65% reported a marketing advantage (perhaps reflecting the competitive nature for aesthetic procedures in their markets), whereas 49% reported an easier recovery for the patient, and 45% felt that it produced a better aesthetic result (although these 2 claims have yet to be demonstrated objectively). Based on self-reported preferences, it seems that for most patients, plastic surgeons don't seem to feel that newer liposuction devices offer a significant advantage over SAL. Although UAL and PAL seem to work better under certain circumstances (firm tissue such as the back, chest, and for revisions), SAL has not been abandoned as the primary liposuction technique.

K. A. Gutowski, MD

Treatment of Iatrogenic Abdominal Contour Irregularities
Pereira LH, Sterodimas A (Luiz Haroldo Clinic, Rio de Janeiro, Brazil; Pontifical Catholic Univ of Rio de Janeiro and the Carlos Chagas Post-Graduate Med Inst, Brazil)
Aesth Plast Surg 34:129-135, 2010

In many countries, liposuction is the most frequently performed aesthetic procedure. The procedure is promoted as a safe, easy-to-learn, outpatient procedure. The increasing number of liposuction procedures, often performed by inadequately trained physicians, has led to a growing number of iatrogenic postliposuction contour deformities and skin irregularities. This report describes a treatment protocol for iatrogenic abdominal contouring deformities. For patients who present with contour deformities but no skin flaccidity, the type 1 treatment plan (syringe-assisted lipectomy and lipografting) is the suggested approach. In cases of contour deformities and infraumbilical skin flaccidity, the type 2 treatment plan (minilipoabdominoplasty and lipografting procedures) is used. Finally, in the case of contour deformities as well as supra- and infraumbilical flaccidity, the type 3 treatment plan (lipoabdominoplasty and lipografting procedures) is indicated.

▶ Contour deformities after liposuction are not uncommon and can frequently be improved in an office setting with fat grafts and minor liposuction. The progressive algorithm described is reasonable and offers significant improvement by combining fat grafting, recontouring with liposuction, and if needed, tissue excision. Whenever possible, revisions should wait until at least 6 months after the primary procedure to allow for edema resolution, proper tissue deformity assessment, and internal scar softening. When performing fat graft injections, it is worthwhile to release any fibrotic areas around the tissue depressions. This can be done with a narrow cannula or sharp large bore needle. In moderate to severe deformities, the patient should be instructed that complete improvement may not be possible and that repeat treatments may be needed. In a patient who is already distressed because of a poor liposuction outcome, setting realistic expectations is critical before offering a corrective procedure.

K. A. Gutowski, MD

Surgical complications of lipoplasty — management and preventive strategies
Thomas M, Menon H, D'Silva J (The Cosmetic Surgery Inst, Mumbai, India)
J Plast Reconstr Aesth Surg 63:1338-1343, 2010

Background.—Lipoplasty and its associated complications are well researched and documented. In most articles, the focus has been on the major life threatening complications of liposuction. Most of these major complications are related to conditions other than surgical trauma *per se*, namely anaesthesia, hypothermia, long duration of surgery and fluid overload. With the exception of pneumothorax and abdominal perforation, surgical trauma does not cause major complications.

Although most surgical complications are classified as minor, they present as major events for patients and the treating physician. All efforts to prevent even minor complications to enhance patient satisfaction are needed.

This article presents a review of only the surgical-trauma-related complications of lipoplasty and discusses their management and preventive strategy.

Methods.—A review of 200 consecutive cases of lipoplasty, performed between July 2006 and December 2007, including large-volume liposuctions (LVLs) and combined liposuction abdominoplasties, was undertaken. Complications relating only to the surgical trauma of liposuction were analysed.

Results.—Complications such as hyperpigmentation of access points, postoperative fluid collection, asymmetry, irregularity, external genital swelling and haematoma were noted.

Postoperative fluid collection and haematoma required active intervention. Drainage of fluid collection using a liposuction cannula was effective and prevented recurrence and the need for repeated aspirations. Major surgical complications such as pneumothorax and abdominal wall perforations could be avoided by following simple rules.

Conclusions.—Major complications related to surgery can be avoided by following well-known safety guidelines.

To enhance patient satisfaction, minor complications related to surgical trauma need to be addressed aggressively. This article discusses methods to lower the incidence of most surgical complications.

▶ Most complications after liposuction are considered minor and can be resolved with only a brief office procedure. As such, treatment and prevention of these problems are not frequently discussed. In 200 consecutive liposuction patients, the complications and their respective percentages were seroma

(3.5%), irregularity (2.5%), hematoma (0.5%), asymmetry (2.0%), hyperpigmentation (> 1 year) (15.0%), and external genital swelling (4.0%).

Because these events may detract from patient satisfaction, the prevention and avoidance techniques described are worth considering, especially for those with limited experience with liposuction. Based on personal experience, seromas/fluid collections, hematomas, and some irregularities are frequently due to overaggressive liposuction technique. In addition to placing incisions in skin creases and hidden areas, the access site hyperpigmentation may be avoided by making sure the incision is large enough to prevent repetitive trauma from the liposuction cannula.

K. A. Gutowski, MD

Analysis of Postoperative Complications for Superficial Liposuction: A Review of 2398 Cases
Kim YH, Cha SM, Naidu S, et al (Hanyang Univ, Seoul, Korea; the Sein Aesthetic Clinic, Seoul, Korea; Natl Univ Hosp, Singapore; et al)
Plast Reconstr Surg 127:863-871, 2011

Background.—Superficial liposuction has found its application in maximizing and creating a lifting effect to achieve a better aesthetic result. Due to initial high complication rates, these procedures were generally accepted as risky. In a response to the increasing concerns over the safety and efficacy of superficial liposuction, the authors describe their 14-year experience of performing superficial liposuction and analysis of postoperative complications associated with these procedures.

Methods.—From March of 1995 to December of 2008, the authors performed superficial liposuction on 2398 patients. Three subgroups were incorporated according to liposuction methods as follows: power-assisted liposuction alone (subgroup 1), power-assisted liposuction combined with ultrasound energy (subgroup 2), and power-assisted liposuction combined with external ultrasound and postoperative Endermologie (subgroup 3). Statistical analyses for complications were performed among subgroups.

Results.—The mean age was 42.8 years, mean body mass index was 27.9 kg/m^2, and mean volume of total aspiration was 5045 cc. Overall complication rate was 8.6 percent (206 patients). Four cases of skin necroses and two cases of infections were included. The most common complication was postoperative contour irregularity. Power-assisted liposuction combined with external ultrasound with or without postoperative Endermologie was seen to decrease the overall complication rate, contour irregularity, and skin necrosis. There were no statistical differences regarding other complications.

Conclusion.—Superficial liposuction has potential risks for higher complications compared with conventional suction techniques, especially postoperative contour irregularity, which can be minimized with proper selection of candidates for the procedure, avoiding overzealous suctioning of superficial layer, and using a combination of ultrasound energy techniques.

▶ When performing trunk and extremity liposuction, passing of cannulas in the superficial plane may cause grooves and contour irregularities that are difficult to correct, even when using the smaller 2- or 3-mm cannulas. Although this series shows reasonable results with low complication rates for superficial liposuction, the patients also had ultrasound and Endermologie applied as part of the protocol. This adds another variable and additional cost to the treatment. The few before and after pictures provided seem to show results that would be possible with only traditional deep and intermediate plane liposuction and without the need for additional ultrasound treatment. Based on the results provided, the use of superficial liposuction does not seem warranted and may result in skin necrosis (which is very rare with traditional nonsuperficial liposuction).

K. A. Gutowski, MD

Safety and Efficacy of UltraShape Contour I Treatments to Improve the Appearance of Body Contours: Multiple Treatments in Shorter Intervals
Ascher B (Paris Academy, France)
Aesth Surg J 30:217-224, 2010

Background.—The UltraShape Contour I System (CE 0344; UltraShape Ltd., Yoqneam, Israel) is a noninvasive fat reduction and body contouring system currently approved for use outside the United States that utilizes focused ultrasound to selectively disrupt adipocytes.

Objective.—To evaluate the clinical safety and efficacy of the Contour I system when the intervals between treatments are shortened.

Methods.—Twenty-five healthy Caucasian women were selected from the patient population at two clinics in Paris, France, and received three 30- to 90-minute Contour I treatments in the abdominal region at two-week intervals. Safety parameters evaluated included adverse events, local skin reaction, and pain. Efficacy parameters evaluated included treatment area circumference, body weight, and comparison of before and after photos. Untreated thigh areas served as an internal control. Subjects were followed for 84 days after the last treatment (day 112).

Results.—No adverse events occurred. The majority of subjects (n = 23; ~90%) reported no pain. Mean midline circumference (2 cm below midline) was reduced by 2.47 cm ($P < .001$) on day 14 after the first Contour I treatment, 3.51 cm ($P < .001$) on day 56, and 3.58 cm ($P < .001$) on day 112. Peak midline circumference reduction was 3.12 cm on day 112. Most patients (n = 14; 63%) reported a positive change in body contour. Mean thigh circumference (the control area) was unchanged; the relative change between treated and untreated areas of the abdomen was significantly different at all time points. Circumference and weight reduction were significantly correlated ($r = 0.42$-0.71) at all time points; mean weight decrease was not statistically significant. Circumference reduction on day 112 positively correlated with patients' subjective satisfaction scores.

Conclusions.—Our data showed that successive Contour I treatments at two-week intervals were safe and tolerable and also significantly reduced treatment area circumference.

▶ Noninvasive body contouring options continue to be offered with variable results. The UltraShape Contour I System applies focused ultrasound energy through the skin and claims to selectively destroy subcutaneous fat cells without damaging other structures.

The procedure can be performed in an office setting without anesthesia or sedation. A prior controlled study showed an average circumference reduction of about 2 to 4 cm without any severe side effects. While these results may not match those of liposuction, this technology may fill the void for patients who are unwilling to consider more invasive body contouring treatments, want minimal downtime, and are willing to accept somewhat more limited results.

K. A. Gutowski, MD

Determinants of Patient Satisfaction With Ultrasound-Assisted Liposuction

Lari SJM, Roustaei N, Roshan SK, et al (Iran Univ of Med Sciences, Tehran)
Aesth Surg J 30:714-719, 2010

Background.—Liposuction is one of the most common aesthetic procedures and a number of options are available to practitioners in terms of surgical technique. One of those options is ultrasound-assisted liposuction (UAL), which has garnered considerable attention in the literature and from patients themselves. Because the role of ultrasound in body sculpting is continuing to increase over time, the authors believe that a comprehensive assessment of patient satisfaction after the procedure is essential. Currently, there are very few reports in the literature examining patient satisfaction with UAL, and to the authors' knowledge, no reports in the literature have successfully outlined the determinants and predictors of long-term satisfaction with the procedure.

Objective.—The authors examine the correlates and predictors of patient satisfaction after UAL.

Methods.—The authors conducted a prospective cross-sectional study on 609 consecutive patients who underwent UAL from 2002 to 2008. One hundred and sixty (54%) out of 300 patients with whom the authors could make contact agreed to answer a standardized questionnaire regarding their overall satisfaction.

Results.—Nearly 80% of the patients were completely or mostly satisfied with UAL. Seventy-five percent reported that they had or would recommend UAL to others. Women ($P = .009$), patients who did not gain weight after their UAL procedure (*P* <.001), patients who were content with their body appearance (*P* <.001), patients whose dress sizes decreased after UAL (*P* =.001), and patients with confidence in their body (*P* <.001) showed statistically significant higher rates of satisfaction with UAL. Among these correlates, confidence in body (odds ratio [OR] = 24.4; 95% confidence interval [CI]: 6.8-83.3) and contentment with body appearance (OR = 5.5; 95% CI: 1.5-19.4) were found to be reliable independent predictors of patient satisfaction.

Conclusion.—Most patients were satisfied with UAL, but certain patient responses were more highly correlated with overall satisfaction than others and therefore can be considered predictors of long-term patient satisfaction with this procedure. The results of this study may provide plastic surgeons with valuable clues that can enhance preoperative planning and therefore enable further improvement of patients' satisfaction with UAL.

▶ Not surprisingly, most forms of liposuction have high patient satisfaction rates. Patients who do not alter their lifestyle (diet and exercise) are at higher risk for negating the improvements after liposuction and are more likely to report less satisfaction after the procedure. Patient education and continued postliposuction discussions should encourage positive lifestyle modifications to increase the rate of long-term patient satisfaction.

K. A. Gutowski, MD

A Safety and Feasibility Study of a Novel Radiofrequency-Assisted Liposuction Technique

Blugerman G, Schavelzon D, Paul MD (Ciudad Autónoma de Buenos Aires, Argentina; Univ of California, Irvine)
Plast Reconstr Surg 125:998-1006, 2010

Background.—The feasibility, safety, and efficacy of a novel radiofrequency device for radiofrequency-assisted liposuction were evaluated in various body areas.

Methods.—From July to December of 2008, 23 subjects underwent radiofrequency-assisted liposuction using the BodyTite system. Information regarding aesthetic results and local and systemic complications was collected immediately after the procedure and at 6- and 12-week follow-up.

Results.—The mean age of the patients was 38.8 ± 12.4 years, and 87 percent were women. Radiofrequency-assisted liposuction was performed successfully in all cases; volume aspirated per patient was 2404 ± 1290 ml, whereas operative time was 158 ± 44 minutes. All patients underwent liposuction at the hip and low abdominal areas, bilaterally. Body contour improvement was observed postoperatively in all patients and there were no severe systemic or local complications, although postoperative pain was minimal in all patients. Weight and circumference reductions were significant at both 6-week and 3-month follow-up. Skin tightening was judged optimal by the surgeon in all patients.

Conclusions.—The authors' study suggests that the removal of moderate volumes of fat with concurrent subdermal tissue contraction can be performed safely and effectively with radiofrequency-assisted liposuction. Additional benefits of this technique are excellent patient tolerance and fast recovery time. Nonetheless, a larger sample is required to confirm the authors' results and guarantee the efficacy and safety of the procedure. Direct comparison with traditional liposuction or energy-assisted liposuction techniques may provide some insights to tailor future indications of this novel technique.

▶ Radiofrequency (RF) technology is being applied to skin tightening and nerve ablation to achieve improved cosmetic outcomes; however, results have shown only modest improvements. The application of RF to body contouring may offer an advantage if true tissue contraction is achieved. RF-assisted liposuction dissolves fat cells and is believed to cause immediate contraction of the collagen fibers and subdermal remodeling. Unlike traditional liposuction, the BodyTite system uses a computer and a bipolar RF handpiece with an internal and external electrode that has an imbedded thermal sensor to measure skin temperature. The surgeon determines the amount of energy applied to the tissue, and the skin temperature needs to be monitored during the procedure. The actual extraction of the liquefied fat is done by traditional aspiration with a cannula.

In this small series, tissue contraction was determined by measuring the difference in distance between 2 fixed points before and after the procedure. Unfortunately, this does not differentiate between contraction and tissue deflation. The short follow-up period does not allow for long-term assessment of the improved skin contraction. Furthermore, the pre- and postoperative images show results that could be achieved with traditional liposuction alone. In addition to the additional cost of adding RF technology to liposuction, it seems that it also increases the length of the procedure as the average procedure time was more than 2.5 hours to remove an average of less than 2.5 L of aspirate. While RF technology may have promise in achieving better body contouring outcomes, more data are needed before recommending it over traditional liposuction.

K. A. Gutowski, MD

Three-Dimensional Radiofrequency Tissue Tightening: A Proposed Mechanism and Applications for Body Contouring
Paul M, Blugerman G, Kreindel M, et al (Univ of California, Irvine; Buenos Aires, Argentina; Invasix Corp, Toronto, Ontario, Canada; et al)
Aesth Plast Surg 35:87-95, 2011

The use of radiofrequency energy to produce collagen matrix contraction is presented. Controlling the depth of energy delivery, the power applied, the target skin temperature, and the duration of application of energy at various soft tissue levels produces soft tissue contraction, which is measurable. This technology allows precise soft tissue modeling at multiple levels to enhance the result achieved over traditional suction-assisted lipectomy as well as other forms of energy such as ultrasonic and laser-generated lipolysis.

▶ Noninvasive radio frequency (RF) has been proposed for skin tightening by means of tissue heating resulting in collagen contraction. However, results may take months to see, and there are concerns of tissue damage and burns because of the high temperatures produced during treatment. This study demonstrated separate ex vivo contraction of dermal, fascial, and septa/adipose tissue from human abdominoplasty samples treated with an internal RF source (BodyTite). In the in vivo part of the study, 24 patients were treated with RF-assisted liposuction (using the BodyTite device), and immediate 8% to 15% tissue contraction was seen and maintained for up to 24 weeks. At 6 months, linear tissue contraction was between 12% and 47% depending on patient and treatment variables. If consistent and lasting results can be demonstrated, RF-assisted liposuction may be useful for patients who would otherwise be suboptimal candidates for liposuction because of skin laxity.

K. A. Gutowski, MD

Randomized, Blinded Split Abdomen Study Evaluating Skin Shrinkage and Skin Tightening in Laser-Assisted Liposuction Versus Liposuction Control
DiBernardo BE (Surgeon in Private Practice in Montclair, NJ)
Aesth Surg J 30:593-602, 2010

Background.—Laser-assisted liposuction has shown great potential in facilitating fat removal, improving patient recovery time, and decreasing postoperative side effects. Clinical experience has indicated superior skin tightening after laser-assisted liposuction than with liposuction alone.

Objectives.—The aim of the present study was to obtain quantitative, objective data for comparing tissue shrinkage and skin tightening achieved by laser-assisted liposuction versus liposuction alone.

Methods.—Ten female subjects from the author's private practice with unwanted abdominal adiposity and mild to moderate skin laxity were enrolled. On the abdominal skin of each patient, the corners of four rectangular regions (approximately 5 × 5 cm each) were tattooed with India ink and randomly assigned to treatment with laser-assisted liposuction (Smartly MPX laser, Cynosure, Inc., Westford, Massachusetts) or with liposuction alone. The laser system permits individual as well as sequential emission of 1064-nm and 1320-nm wavelengths. Skin shrinkage was quantified by calculating the changes in surface area of the regions. Skin tightening was quantified by changes in the skin stiffness index measured in the treated regions.

Results.—One month and three months after treatment, the mean skin shrinkage ratios were significantly higher on the laser-treated side than on the suction side. One month after treatment with or without laser, the mean skin stiffness and skin tightening showed no statistically significant difference from baseline. Three months after treatment, the mean skin stiffness and skin tightening were significantly higher on the laser-treated side.

Conclusions.—Laser-assisted liposuction has a statistically significant effect on skin shrinkage and tightening of the skin in the abdominal area when compared to liposuction alone.

▶ This well-designed study is the first to show quantitative skin improvement after laser-assisted liposuction (LAL). Care should be taken before applying the conclusions to all patients because the enrolled patients had mild to moderate skin laxity without structural ptosis. The treatment end point was when epidermal temperature (observed with a thermal camera) reached a uniform 40°C to 42°C. If these temperature levels are not reached, there may not be enough collagen stimulation to achieve dermal improvement. Because there is risk of skin damage from the laser, extra care and monitoring must be used compared with traditional liposuction. Although these results look promising, the LAL devices require additional procedure time, monitoring, and cost. The practical applications and patient satisfaction with cost versus outcome are not known.

K. A. Gutowski, MD

Contouring the Gluteal Region With Tumescent Liposculpture
Avendaño-Valenzuela G, Guerrerosantos J (Plastic Surgeon in Private Practice in Naucalpan, Mexico; Univ of Guadalajara, Mexico)
Aesth Surg J 31:200-213, 2011

Background.—For quite some time, plastic surgeons have experimented with novel techniques for enhancing the gluteal region. However, all of the previously-described techniques have the disadvantage of postoperative scarring, most of which is visible. As an alternative, fat injection in the gluteal region has been shown to have permanent and satisfactory results.

Objectives.—The authors discuss the results of liposuction and lipoinjection in the gluteal region.

Methods.—Between March 2000 and March 2007, 300 female patients who presented with lipodystrophy of the gluteal and paragluteal regions underwent liposuction with a modified tumescent technique. The treated sites were classified into six anatomical zones, and the patients were retrospectively grouped into types based on the frequency of treatment in each zone.

Results.—The patients ranged in age from 16 to 54 years. The follow-up period ranged from six to 36 months. Fifty percent of patients underwent liposuction in Zone I, 90% in Zone II, 0% in Zone III, 40% in Zone IV, 30% in Zone V, and 75% in Zone VI. The largest percentage of patients underwent treatment in Zones I, II, and V, with subsequent lipoinjection. Comparison of pre- and postoperative photographs and measurements revealed gluteal lifting in all patients at the point of greatest projection. Improved contour was shown in Zones I, II, and IV when all zones were treated in a combined form.

Conclusions.—The concept of refining techniques for liposuction and lipoinjection according to individual anatomical zones is essential to the evolution of the procedure. In this series, the results indicated that improving the intraoperative treatment of the hip region resulted in improved aesthetic contouring. Therefore, the authors believe that this technique can reduce the need for more aggressive surgical procedures, which thereby decreases the risk of complications, recovery time, and sequelae.

▶ The buttock has been considered a challenging area for contouring with liposuction because of unpredictable tissue contraction and subsequent buttock ptosis. The classification and treatment plans described in this large patient series show nice improvements in gluteal aesthetics. Most improvement is because of treatment of the flanks (zone II) and lateral trochanteric area (zone IV). Zone III, the region between zone I and II, was not treated in any of the patients, as it is considered a zone of adherence where contour irregularities are likely to result after liposuction. Improved buttock projection resulted from intramuscular injection of 180 to 380 mL of gravity-separated lipoaspirate. This fat redistribution technique offers an alternative to implant buttock augmentation in selected patients and may allow for better control of buttock projection. While it may not be a substitute for an excisional buttock lift in patients with massive weight loss, the result appears to be predictable in patients with good to fair skin tone. This patient series also included considerable buttock improvement in cases of congenital gluteal deformities.

K. A. Gutowski, MD

Tumescent Liposuction: Efficacy of a Lower Lidocaine Dose (400 mg/l)
Böni R (White House Ctr for Liposuction, Zürich, Switzerland)
Dermatology 220:223-225, 2010

Background.—Local anesthesia has been widely accepted as the standard of care in liposuction. Anesthesia is achieved with a standard tumescent solution, and lidocaine is most often used at a concentration of 500 mg/l.

Objective.—To evaluate the efficacy of a 400 mg/l lidocaine concentration in tumescent liposuction.

Methods.—We performed a randomized clinical trial on 200 consecutive patients undergoing lipoaspiration. Patients were divided into two groups: group A (n = 100) received tumescent solution with a lidocaine concentration of 500 mg/l, in group B (n = 100) lidocaine levels were reduced to 400 mg/l. Pain was assessed twice during the procedure, at infiltration and while liposuction was performed. Patients rated their pain level on a numeric rating scale from 0 to 10, with 10 being the worst possible pain.

Results.—Tumescent solution containing a lidocaine concentration of 400 mg/l provided effective local anesthesia during lipoaspiration. There was no statistically significant difference in the pain level between the two groups.

Conclusion.—We propose the use of a lower lidocaine concentration of 400 mg/l in the tumescent solution compared to the originally described solution containing 500 mg/l. This is of particular interest when multiple body parts or larger areas are to be treated to avoid lidocaine toxicity.

▶ Any effort to improve patient safety should be encouraged. In this case, lowering the lidocaine concentration in liposuction tumescent fluid resulted in the same amount of fluid being used and no change in patient-scored pain levels. The median total dosage of lidocaine, however, decreased from 41 mg/kg to 33 mg/kg. It seems that using a lower concentration of lidocaine (400 mg/L vs 500 mg/L) can be recommended.

K. A. Gutowski, MD

Efficacy of tumescent local anesthesia with variable lidocaine concentration in 3430 consecutive cases of liposuction
Habbema L (Medisch Centrum 't Gooi, Bussum, The Netherlands)
J Am Acad Dermatol 62:988-994, 2010

Background.—Lidocaine toxicity is a potential complication related to using tumescent local anesthesia (TLA) as the exclusive form of pain management in surgical procedures.

Objective.—We sought to determine the minimum concentration of lidocaine in the tumescent solution required to provide adequate anesthesia in patients undergoing liposuction using TLA exclusively.

Methods.—Liposuction using TLA exclusively was performed in 3430 procedures by the same surgeon. The initial concentration of 1000 mg/L lidocaine in the tumescent solution was gradually reduced to find the minimum required for adequate anesthesia.

Results.—Adequate anesthesia was achieved using a lidocaine concentration of 500 mg/L saline in all areas treated and 400 mg/L saline for most of the areas treated.

Limitations.—Data are based on the specific TLA technique used by the same surgeon. Lidocaine serum levels were not analyzed.

Conclusion.—For patients undergoing liposuction using TLA exclusively, the concentration of lidocaine in the normal saline solution required for adequate anesthesia is 400 mg/L for most body areas and 500 mg/L for some sensitive areas.

▶ This study confirms the findings of Boni that adding 40 cc of 1% lidocaine to 1000 cc of tumescent fluid can be just as effective as adding 50 cc of lidocaine. However, the technique included true tumescent infiltration (with probably higher volumes of fluid used per region than that used by most plastic surgeons who use the superwet technique) and a 30- to 60-minute waiting period to allow for fluid diffusion and prior to staring liposuction. It is possible that the total dose of lidocaine delivered may not be lower if higher amounts of fluid are infiltrated.

K. A. Gutowski, MD

Viability of Fat Cells Over Time After Syringe Suction Lipectomy: The Effects of Cryopreservation

Son D, Oh J, Choi T, et al (Keimyung Univ Dongsan Med Ctr, Daegu, South Korea; GaGa Aesthetic Plastic Surgical Clinic, Daegu, South Korea; Seoul Natl Univ College of Medicine, Korea; et al)
Ann Plast Surg 65:354-360, 2010

The purpose of this study was to determine the late decline in viability of fat cells over time for fat tissue stored at $-15°C$ and $-70°C$ after harvest from abdominal liposuction. A total of 16 females were recruited for this study. The viability of fat cell specimens was measured after freezing for 1, 3, 7, 14, 28, and 56 days. A number of viable mature adipocytes were evaluated by fluorescence microscopy after staining with fluorescein diacetate and propidium iodide. The glycerol 3 phosphate dehydrogenase activity was measured in lipoaspirates before digestion and the XTT reduction assay was performed. In addition, the XTT reduction assay was also performed on isolated lipocytes and preadipocytes.

The viability of mature adipocytes was very low for both the $-15°C$ and $-70°C$ samples after 1 day of freezing (13.3% ± 7.4% and 12.6% ± 6.3%, respectively). There was no statistically significant difference between the samples stored at the 2 temperatures. The GPDH activity of the lipoaspirates frozen, for 1 day, at $-15°C$ and $-70°C$ was 25.1% ± 10% and 28.7% ± 11%, respectively. For the XTT test, the fractional enzyme activity of the lipoaspirates frozen, for 1 day, at $-15°C$ and $-70°C$ was 30.0% ± 10.9% and 36.1% ± 12.3%, respectively. In addition, the adipocytes had low activity from day one: 15.4% ± 7.2% at $-15°C$ and 11.5% ± 5.6% at $-70°C$. Furthermore, the preadipocytes had a low activity of 8.0% ± 6.0% at $-15°C$ and 8.6% ± 3.8% at $-70°C$. At 8 weeks, there were few viable mature adipocytes and the activity of the cells was very low by XTT and GPDH testing.

The results of this study showed that the viability of adipocytes declined rapidly after frozen storage for 1 day at both $-15°C$ and $-70°C$, and decreased gradually in storage after 8 weeks; at which time only approximately 5% of the fat cells were alive. These findings suggest that the present fat preservation storage techniques using a $-15°C$ freezer or a $-70°C$ deep freezer are both inadequate to maintain the viability of fat cells.

▶ Although some technical aspects of fat grafting are still being debated, there is enough evidence that cryopreservation of fat cells (without the use of a cryoprotectant such as dimethyl sulfoxide) leads to significant loss of fat cell viability. For clinical practices that don't have proper cell cryopreservation capability, storage of fat grafts is not recommended.

K. A. Gutowski, MD

6 Breast

Mastopexy and Reduction

The Role of Antibiotics in Reduction Mammaplasty

Veiga-Filho J, Veiga DF, Sabino-Neto M, et al (Universidade Federal de São Paulo, Brazil, Universidade do Vale do Sapucaí Pouso Alegre, Brazil)
Ann Plast Surg 65:144-146, 2010

This prospective study was conducted to assess the influence of antibiotics use on surgical site infections (SSI) rates after reduction mammaplasty. Patients undergoing reduction mammaplasty were assigned to group 1 (n = 50), which received intravenous cephalotin pre- and postoperatively, besides oral cephalexin for 6 days after discharge, or to group 2 (n = 50), which received no antibiotics. Patients were followed up weekly for 30 days, regarding to SSI, by a blinded surgeon. The Centers for Disease Control and Prevention definitions and classification of SSI were adopted. There was no statistical difference between the groups in regard to age, body mass index, duration of operation, and total resection weight. SSI rates were 2% and 14% in groups 1 and 2, respectively ($P = 0.03$). In group 2, older patients and those with higher resection weight had significant higher SSI rates ($P = 0.02$ and $P = 0.04$, respectively). We observed that antibiotics use decreased SSI rates after reduction mammaplasty.

▶ This study demonstrated that perioperative antibiotics followed by 6 days of postoperative antibiotics decreased infection rates in breast reduction compared with no antibiotics. However, this study did not include a patient group that received only appropriate perioperative antibiotics (which is the minimum standard of care) without postoperative doses. Hence, it did not answer this question: Are postoperative antibiotics needed if a single dose is given within 1 hour before the start of the procedure? Until more information is available, routine postoperative antibiotics after breast reduction may not be useful.

K. A. Gutowski, MD

Occult Carcinoma in 866 Reduction Mammaplasties: Preserving the Choice of Lumpectomy

Slezak S, Bluebond-Langner R (Univ of Maryland School of Medicine, Baltimore)
Plast Reconstr Surg 127:525-530, 2011

Background.—Occult breast carcinoma is occasionally found in reduction mammaplasty specimens. Historically, these patients were treated with mastectomy because the exact location of the tumor was unknown. Currently, breast conservation is the treatment of choice in 50 to 85 percent of breast cancers. The authors present a technique of routine specimen marking that allows localization of the tumor and preservation of the choice of lumpectomy.

Methods.—This is a retrospective review of 866 patients who underwent reduction mammaplasty performed by a single surgeon between 1990 and 2009. Data were collected for patients who had occult cancer found in their specimens, including age, cancer risk factors, abnormality, nodal status, selected treatment, and survival status. Specimens were marked and oriented and then sent in separate bags to the pathologist.

Results.—There were 10 cases of occult carcinoma among the 866 women (1.15 percent) who underwent reduction mammaplasty. Six cancers were found in patients undergoing reduction for symptomatic macromastia [$n = 629$ (0.95 percent)]. Four new cancers were found in the group of patients with a personal history of cancer [$n = 237$ (1.69 percent)]. All 10 patients had normal preoperative mammograms. Location, size, and margin status were easily identified and patients were offered the choice of lumpectomy or mastectomy.

Conclusions.—This article demonstrates that careful marking of reduction specimens in high-risk patients or in women older than 40 years allows the pathologist to orient, localize, and further section tissue for margin status. Communication among plastic surgeon, pathologist, oncologist, and radiation therapist preserves the choice of breast conserving therapy for early cancers.

▶ The authors of this article present a worthwhile addition to the technique of reduction mammaplasty. The addition does not represent a change in surgical technique but instead represents a more careful way of handling and marking the tissue that is removed. As a result of this approach, the patient who is found to have an occult carcinoma of the breast becomes eligible for breast conservation treatment, lumpectomy plus radiation, instead of a more disfiguring mastectomy, if desired. The validity of lumpectomy plus radiation for breast cancer has been confirmed in many recent studies. In addition, lumpectomy through a reduction mammaplasty approach, followed by radiation, has been advocated in selected cases in which the patient is already seeking breast reduction surgery. However, this approach requires prior identification of the tumor and a careful design of the reduction incisions to permit an adequate lumpectomy. The authors' approach extends this therapeutic option to women who are found incidentally to have carcinoma of the breast in their reduction specimens. Clearly, this approach requires a bit more effort on the part of the operating surgeon, and perhaps a lot more effort on the part of the pathologist. However, the incidence of occult carcinoma of about 1% of all reductions in the experience of a single surgeon (10 cases) would seem to justify the extra effort on the part of the physicians involved in cases that meet the selection criteria described in the article.

R. L. Ruberg, MD

Augmentation and Silicone

Autologous Augmentation-Mastopexy After Bariatric Surgery: Waste Not Want Not!

Thornton DJA, Fourie LR (Pinderfields General Hosp, Wakefield, UK)
Aesth Plast Surg 34:519-524, 2010

Background.—The escalating trend in obesity is having major impact on health and the economy. As a result of NHS policies to reduce obesity, the number of patients losing weight following bariatric surgery is increasing rapidly. In addition to the systemic benefits to their general health, dramatic weight loss leads to marked changes in body habitus, with many patients seeking further "aesthetic" surgery to improve their appearance. We present our technique of autologous augmentation-mastopexy to address the problems of both skin excess and insufficient breast volume.

Methods.—Our chosen method for mastopexy uses the Wise-pattern skin excision. Augmentation of the breast deficient in volume is provided by a pedicled subcutaneous lateral thoracic perforator-based flap raised via a vertical continuation of the lateral mastopexy incision superiorly, often in continuity with a simultaneous brachioplasty incision.

Results.—Thus far, six patients have undergone autologous augmentation mastopexy following massive weight loss (range = 36–79 kg, mean = 61 kg). Follow-up of these patients ranged from 1 to 18 months (mean = 12.5 months). Postoperative complications included a donor site seroma, haematoma, and scar contracture. All patients tolerated the procedure well and they felt that the improvement in breast and chest wall contour more than compensated for the donor site scar on the lateral chest wall.

Conclusion.—Autologous augmentation-mastopexy provides a robust augmentation, giving more natural ptotic breasts while avoiding the cost and potential complications of implant augmentation. The increased lateral flank scarring is well tolerated by these patients, with the additional benefit of reducing flank fullness.

▶ Autoaugmentation is now a useful adjunct to body contouring after bariatric surgery. This article adds another technique for transposing excess tissue, which might ordinarily be discarded, to achieve breast enlargement. The technique has some of the same features as the spiral flap described by Hurwitz but probably has a more reliable blood supply than the spiral flap. The flap described in this article relies on a lateral thoracic artery perforator, as opposed to the Hurwitz approach, which uses de-epithelialized skin plus underlying fat for augmentation. The actual rotation of both of these flaps, once created, is very similar. Adding this flap to the usually performed mastopexy creates additional scar, but the overall aesthetic result (as shown in several examples in the article) is actually quite good. And in fact, a more thorough body contouring procedure would likely involve excising this tissue through a comparable incision anyway.

R. L. Ruberg, MD

Breast augmentation: Part I — a review of the silicone prosthesis
Berry MG, Davies DM (Inst of Cosmetic and Reconstructive Surgery, London, UK)
J Plast Reconstr Aesthet Surg 63:1761-1768, 2010

The present importance of breast augmentation (BA) is shown by year-on-year increases: with 8439 augmentations performed by BAAPS members in 2007 the UK still lags America where 307,000 were performed. Having survived an almost hysterical media reaction to perceived silicone health risks in the 1990s, a growing body of evidence attests to the demonstrable benefits of BA. Improved implant design coupled with surgical advances mean that high quality results with few complications can now be expected in the majority and a précis of progress is perhaps timely. This article forms part of a series that has been written to provide a 'state-of-the-art' review of contemporaneous BA practice.

▶ This is an excellent and current review of the history of breast augmentation primarily as performed using silicone implants. It encompasses a fairly comprehensive bibliography and should be one of those articles that remains in the library of all surgeons performing breast augmentation. About the only quibble I would have is that although the authors decry the knee-jerk nonscientific responses to the antisilicone paranoia that resulted in the development of ill-advised nonsilicone fillers, they fail to adequately address the failure of the plastic surgical community to scientifically study and address the concerns which were raised about silicone implants. Hopefully, we have learned that it is incumbent upon all plastic surgeons who use new devices, novel techniques, and/or medications to document the outcomes achieved and carefully record and study any adverse events and to do so with the manufacturing community that has produced them.

S. H. Miller, MD, MPH

Breast Prostheses and Connective Tissue Disease (CTD): Myth or Reality?
Bassetto F, Vindigni V, Scarpa C, et al (Univ of Padova, Italy)
Aesth Plast Surg 34:257-263, 2010

Since their first appearance, breast prostheses have been criticized as being both responsible for and giving rise to systemic disease. The literature contains many reports on the subject, and theories were controversial from the 1980s to the 2000s. The aim of this review was to gather together the most important studies on breast prostheses and systemic disease, with particular attention to connective tissue disease (CTD), in order to verify any relationship between silicone breast implants and the occurrence of pathologies.

► An historical review with a fairly complete bibliography makes this article worthwhile for those who remain interested in the controversy of whether or not silicone breast implants can cause systemic disease. It has been interesting to see the progression from an era where the causal nature of silicone-related connective tissue disease seemed highly likely to a more recent era when it was not. The author brings up 2 very recent studies, which demonstrate findings that once again suggest a relationship between silicone and systemic disease. In one study, several proinflammatory proteins have been found on silicone implants and in another study other proteins, including antipolymer antibodies and procollagen II, have been associated with fibrosis and length of time implants have been in place. Neither specifies that patients in fact had developed systemic disease but that their findings required clinical correlation. One can't fault that advice, providing we do not regress into pseudoscientific chaos again. It is obviously critical to actually identify that the proteins involved actually do cause human disease and are not just a laboratory finding. Is it possible that in some few genetically or otherwise predisposed patients, silicone can result in an inflammatory systemic disease state?

S. H. Miller, MD, MPH

Contemporary Decision Making and Perception in Patients Undergoing Cosmetic Breast Augmentation
Walden JL, Panagopoulous G, Shrader SW (Lenox Hill Hosp/Manhattan Eye, Ear, and Throat Inst, NY)
Aesth Surg J 30:395-403, 2010

Background.—Today's breast augmentation (BA) patient obtains information from a variety of sources that may positively or negatively influence her decision.

Objectives.—The authors evaluate the decision-making process of patients undergoing BA, including how they seek information regarding the procedure, potential complications, the medical device itself, referral sources, and surgeon(s).

Methods.—A written 36-item, blinded survey developed for this study was administered to all patients who underwent aesthetic primary BA by the senior author (JW) over a 12-month period in her metropolitan private practice. Patients were included only if they had undergone surgery after Food and Drug Administration approval of silicone implants and had at least four months of follow-up. Patients were excluded if they underwent reconstruction, revision, augmentation/mastopexy, or implant exchange. Data were analyzed utilizing descriptive statistics; frequencies of responses were calculated with SPSS (version 16).

Results.—Of 153 mailed surveys, 100 respondents returned completed questionnaires (65%). Mean age was 30 years (range, 20-50 years). Eighty-eight patients were in the workforce, eight were students, and three were homemakers. Thirty-three percent had completed some graduate work or had a graduate degree, and 41% had a college degree. In terms of how patients began their informational searches, 41% began with Google, 18% began with a BA portal Web site, and 1% went through referral from a primary care provider (PCP)/OB-GYN. The primary influence in a patient's decision to have BA was her own desire to change her appearance (36%), and second was her plastic surgeon's Web site (16%). On a graded scale of 10 factors ranking importance (1 = *not at all* and 5 = *extremely*), 52% said that their plastic surgeon's Web site very much or extremely influenced their decision. Of respondents, 82% had silicone implants (18% saline). The most influential factor in choosing implant filler was the feel of the silicone versus saline implants (for 41%), followed by the plastic surgeon's explanation of the difference (29%) and recent FDA approval (13%). Primary sources of information for possible complications were the plastic surgeon and BA portal sites. When asked what the worst complication could be, patients reported capsular contracture (37%), implant rupture or leak (22%), and infection (20%). The most powerful influence on choice of surgeon for BA was the plastic surgeon's Web site (49%); meeting the doctor in consultation was next (14%), followed by BA portal sites (9%). Thirty-six percent of respondents consulted with a psychiatrist or psychologist at some point in their lives, with depression, anxiety, and stress management as top-ranked reasons (in that order).

Conclusions.—The Internet (specifically Google, the plastic surgeon's Web site, and portal Web sites) is very important to patients ages 20 to 50 in their search for information on BA. Educational and reality TV may have less influence on this particular group than was previously thought. Patients are well educated, are part of the workforce, and seem to be independent and private thinkers when it comes to their decision making. Referral sources such as the PCP assume a much smaller role in the search for information than in days past.

▶ This article provides valuable data about patients' current attitudes toward various aspects of breast augmentation and about the sources that patients use to obtain information regarding this procedure. What may be most interesting is not the findings themselves but the observation that the principal information source for these patients is constantly changing. Although relatively recent studies showed that patients learned most about breast augmentation from various advertisements and reality-type television programs, the most up-to-date finding is that internet sites and the surgeon's own web site have now become the primary information sources. As might be expected, referral from the patient's primary care physician has become almost irrelevant. Therefore, a major message of this study is that surgeons seeking to inform patients about a contemporary elective procedure should use an approach that is most consistent with the latest information-gathering strategies of their target audience. Of course, these results can only be considered specific for the patients included in this study (most of whom reside in a major metropolitan area). But extrapolation to the entire population of women seeking breast augmentation is probably appropriate.

R. L. Ruberg, MD

Preoperative Sizing in Breast Augmentation
Hidalgo DA, Spector JA (Weill Cornell Med College, NY)
Plast Reconstr Surg 125:1781-1787, 2010

Background.—Implant size selection in breast augmentation patients is one of many variables to be determined before surgery. Few methods exist today that allow the patient to participate in this process and accurately determine optimal size. The authors describe a simple method of preoperative sizing using silicone implant samples.

Methods.—A total of 567 patients underwent breast augmentation: 297 had surgery before implementation of preoperative sizing and 270 patients were sized preoperatively. Sizing consisted of fitting the patients with various size silicone implants in a larger bra at least twice before surgery to determine desired size. Surveys were sent to both groups to inquire about overall satisfaction, how many preferred a different size postoperatively, and how many ultimately underwent size change surgery.

Results.—One hundred two responses (34.3 percent) were obtained from the control group and 142 (52.6 percent) were obtained from the sized group. Sized patients received smaller implants (average, 276.6 cc nonsized versus 246.4 cc sized; $p < 0.001$). Four patients (1.4 percent) in the control group underwent a size change procedure compared with none in the sized group. In the sized cohort, 69 percent believe they are the size that the process predicted, 21 percent are smaller, 9 percent are larger, and 1 percent did not answer the question.

Conclusions.—Sized patients were more satisfied than controls and fewer were interested in having a different size implant postoperatively. Sized patients indicated that preoperative sizing was both helpful and reasonably accurate in predicting final breast size.

▶ This study gives support to the notion that patients are more likely to be satisfied with the size of their breasts after augmentation mammaplasty if they have an opportunity to participate personally in the implant size selection through direct preoperative visual assessment of the potential final effect of the surgery. I think a very important part of the authors' method, and a key reason for their success, is the requirement that this visual assessment is done at least twice before a final size determination is made. Other authors suggest using various anatomic measurements to determine the optimal implant size. But in truth, the optimal size is not necessarily the one that gives the most natural-looking breast but is in fact the size that the patient herself regards as optimal, even if the surgeon may not agree. Many studies have shown that one of the most common reasons for revision surgery after augmentation mammaplasty is dissatisfaction with size. It is therefore impressive that in this series, none of the patients in the group undergoing preoperative sizing chose to undergo subsequent surgery for implant size change, even though some were not completely happy with their final size. The technique for preoperative sizing is not nearly as important as the simple act of allowing some type of direct visual assessment by the patient.

R. L. Ruberg, MD

A meta-analysis of optimum plane placement and related morbidity in primary breast augmentation

Hand F, Barry M, Kell MR (Mater Univ Hosp, Dublin, Ireland)
Eur J Plast Surg 33:241-244, 2010

Despite extensive clinical experience of breast implants, there is continued controversy regarding the optimum placement of the prosthesis. More importantly, there is insufficient data to accurately determine whether subglandular (SG) or submuscular (SM) placement of the prosthesis diminishes postoperative complications. A search of published trials ($n=34$) examined complication rates following SG and SM implant placement was conducted. Pubmed (MEDLINE) database was used and the available data was then cross-referenced. Eligible trials ($n=6$) were then reviewed and selected data extracted. Primary outcomes measured were postoperative haematoma, infection, capsular contracture and implant migration. 3603 patients were identified from relevant trials examining postoperative complication rates for both subglandular and submuscular implant planes. The submuscular implant plane was associated with a higher incidence of postoperative haematoma (OR 2.87, 95% CI, 1.44-6.11). The incidence of capsular contracture (OR 4.77) is more common when a subglandular plane is used. No significant difference was noted in the rate of postoperative infection (OR 1.20, 95% CI 0.57-2.58) or implant migration (OR 1.56, 95% CI 0.12-87.4) between the two groups. This meta analysis confirms that subglandular augmentation results in lower short-term morbidity; however, submuscular placement appears to provide the best long-term outcome in terms of morbidity. In the absence of randomized controlled trials comparing these two techniques, this meta analysis provides evidence to guide surgeons to achieve the best outcomes for their patients.

▶ The choice regarding the optimal location for breast implants (subglandular vs submuscular) is one that is highly dependent on surgeon bias. There is no prospective randomized trial upon which to base a rational conclusion that one position is better than another. This study at least provides the surgeon with reasonably reliable data about the relative incidence of 2 important complications (hematoma and capsular contracture) with different implant positions. The surgeon can then decide which of the 2 complications is more important to avoid and then select the more appropriate implant position based on the data in this study. However, there are several aspects of this study that make the data less than totally convincing. First of all, the study considered both subglandular and subfascial placement as subglandular and both total submuscular and dual-plane position as submuscular. There certainly could be significant differences between all 4 of these various approaches, but the study doesn't permit extraction of that information. Secondly, there is no attempt to sort out differences encountered with different types of implants (smooth vs textured surface, gel density, etc.). But at least the surgeon could use this information both in determining a personal bias for implant position and in counseling the patient about consequences of different approaches.

R. L. Ruberg, MD

Form Stability of the Style 410 Anatomically Shaped Cohesive Silicone Gel–Filled Breast Implant in Subglandular Breast Augmentation Evaluated with Magnetic Resonance Imaging

Weum S, de Weerd L, Kristiansen B (Univ Hosp North Norway, Tromsø, Norway)
Plast Reconstr Surg 127:409-413, 2011

Background.—In this study, the authors evaluated the form stability of the Style 410 anatomically shaped cohesive silicone gel-filled breast implant after subglandular implantation.

Methods.—Nine women who had undergone bilateral subglandular breast augmentation using Style 410 implants were examined in the prone and supine positions with magnetic resonance imaging.

Results.—In the supine position, the dimensions of the implants were similar to those specified by the manufacturer. In the prone position, there was a mean increase of 29.5 percent (range, 9.7 to 53.3 percent) in implant projection. All implants had their point of maximal projection positioned in the lower pole in both positions.

Conclusions.—The Style 410 implant is described as a form-stable, anatomically shaped, cohesive, silicone gel–filled implant. However, its shell and the degree of silicone gel cohesivity allow for a change in form depending on body posture. Compared with the supine position, there was a marked increase in implant projection in the prone position. The Style 410 implant keeps its lower pole fullness after subglandular implantation in both the supine and prone positions.

▶ This study provides us with some information about anatomically shaped cohesive gel—filled breast implants that we expected, and some that we didn't. The expected information is that these implants, when placed in the subglandular position, maintain the desired anatomic shape with extra lower pole projection. This information is reassuring because the objective of using this specific type of implant is indeed the creation of lower pole fullness. The unexpected information is that these implants, widely called form stable, are in fact NOT form stable. Significant alterations in the implant form are noted when comparing the supine dimensions with the prone measurements. The question that many surgeons would now ask is, what happens to these implants in the upright position (especially because breasts are infrequently visualized in the prone position)? Unfortunately, the authors are unable to obtain this information because of current limitations in MRI systems. Irrespective of the unexpected finding, the surgeon can have reasonable confidence in telling patients that anatomic implants will maintain their lower pole projection inside the body, not just outside.

R. L. Ruberg, MD

A Prospective Study of 708 Form-Stable Silicone Gel Breast Implants

Grant Stevens W, Hirsch EM, Tenenbaum MJ, et al (Marina del Rey, CA; Northwestern Univ Feinberg School of Medicine, Chicago, IL; Washington Univ School of Medicine, St Louis, MO)
Aesth Surg J 30:693-701, 2010

Background.—Form-stable silicone gel breast implants represent the fifth generation of silicone gel augmentation devices. Additional crosslinking between the silicone molecules allows these implants to retain their shape, especially in the vertical position.

Objective.—The authors evaluate the efficacy of Silimed form-stable silicone gel breast implants.

Methods.—A total of 355 patients (708 implants) were enrolled prospectively over a 60-month period. Data were collected on patient demographics, implant factors, complications, and revisions. Chi-square analysis and Fisher's exact test were implemented to compare groups with respect to differences in complication and revision rates.

Results.—The overall tissue-related complication rate was 8.2% per patient, or 4.1% per breast. The overall implant-related cosmetic complication rate was 2.5% per patient, or 1.3% per implant. The overall implant-related complication rate, which was represented by the capsular contracture (CC) rate, was 1.4% per patient and 0.7% per implant. There were no complications in any of the reconstruction patients. There were no deep vein thromboses, pulmonary emboli, myocardial infarctions, or deaths among the patients in this study. In addition, there were no instances of flap necrosis, hematoma, or loss of implant integrity. The overall complication rate was 9.6% per patient, or 4.8% per implant. The overall tissue-related revision rate was 5.4% per patient, with the most common tissue-related reason for revision being unacceptable scarring. The overall implant-related cosmetic revision rate was 7.6% per patient, with the most common reason for revision in this category being size change. The overall implant-related revision rate was 1.1% per patient and was solely due to CC.

Conclusions.—This study demonstrates that form-stable silicone gel breast implants are safe and have a complication profile similar to other models of silicone breast implants, with a lower CC rate and a decreased incidence of wrinkling compared to fourth-generation silicone gel implants (as well as other published studies of fifth-generation implants).

▶ This article is valuable for a number of different reasons. First, it represents a study of a significant number of patients operated on in the United States; most previous studies of fifth generation (form-stable) silicone gel implants have been performed in foreign countries. Second, the authors are able to demonstrate a high rate of successful augmentation cases using periareolar incisions—including periareolar submuscular placement in a number of cases. Most early studies emphasized the need to use larger incisions to insert these relatively inflexible devices, thus ruling out periareolar incisions. These authors do report that patients with small-diameter areolas may not be able to have implant placement through the periareolar route (unless they agree to smaller implants). Finally, the capsular contracture rate with these implants was as good as, or even better than, the rate reported with any other type of implant. At the time of this writing, these devices are not available for general use in the United States. Based on the findings reported in this study, they may become very popular when released for use by all surgeons.

R. L. Ruberg, MD

Breastfeeding After Augmentation Mammaplasty with Saline Implants
Cruz NI, Korchin L (Univ of Puerto Rico, San Juan)
Ann Plast Surg 64:530-533, 2010

It has been reported that breastfeeding problems occur in women who have breast implants.

The breastfeeding success of women who had augmentation with saline implants and subsequently had a live birth (n = 107) was compared with that of women of similar age who had hypoplastic breasts and had children before their consultation (n = 105). A self-administered 11-item questionnaire was used to collect data on demographics and breastfeeding success. The information requested included age, weight, height, whether breastfeeding was attempted, if it was successful, and the need to supplement. Additional information requested from the study group included position of breast scar, implant volume, and whether loss of nipple sensation had occurred after the surgery (as judged by the patient).

The groups were not significantly different in age (22 ± 7 vs. 23 ± 5). There was, however, a significant difference ($P < 0.05$) in the breastfeeding success and need to supplement feedings. Successful breastfeeding occurred in 88% of the control and 63% of the study group. A need to supplement breastfeeding occurred in 27% of the control group but increased to 46% in the study group. No significant difference ($P > 0.05$) was found in the breastfeeding experience between periareolar and inframammary approaches. Loss of nipple sensation after augmentation mammaplasty was reported by 2% of both the periareolar and inframammary subgroups.

The success rate of breastfeeding decreases ~25% and the need to supplement breastfeeding increases 19% in young women with hypoplastic breasts after augmentation mammaplasty, irrespective of whether a periareolar or inframammary approach is used.

▶ This study does replicate others that have shown a decrease in breastfeeding in patients with small breasts after augmentation mammoplasty with saline implants. Similar results have been reported following implantation with silicone gel implants. It is somewhat surprising that the authors found no difference in the difficulty in breastfeeding between those who had inframammary incisions and those who had periareolar incisions, as opposed to the report of Hurst.[1] The problem with these studies are that none have really identified specific factors that may be causing the difficulty. Although the authors included a control group, said to be similar to the study group, we do not know that is true. For example, we do not know if the overall health of the patients, their socioeconomic conditions, the amount of glandular material in each patient's breast, or various other factors including psychological ones, as regards breastfeeding in general and breastfeeding as it might prove negative for the aesthetic result, really were equivalent in the 2 groups.

S. H. Miller, MD, MPH

Reference

1. Hurst NM. Lactation after augmentation mammaplasty. *Obstet Gynecol.* 1996; 87:30-34.

Conservative Augmentation with Periareolar Mastopexy Reduces Complications and Treats a Variety of Breast Types: A 5-Year Retrospective Review of 100 Consecutive Patients
Cannon CL III, Lindsey JT (Tulane Univ School of Medicine, New Orleans, LA)
Ann Plast Surg 64:516-521, 2010

Augmentation with mastopexy remains a challenge because reported complication and revision rates remain high. Previous publications are difficult to interpret because of inclusion of a broad array of mastopexy techniques and different implant styles and placements. This is a review of 100 consecutive augmentation/mastopexy patients performed by a single surgeon using a single procedure, implant style, and placement.

Between January 2003 and December 2008, 100 female patients underwent primary augmentation mammoplasty with periareolar mastopexy. All patients had either grade II or grade III ptosis, or tubular deformity. All implants were Allergan style 168 (270–390 mL saline prosthesis).

All patients (N = 100) were available for follow-up, an average 8.3 months postoperatively (1.5–21 months). Overall complication rate was 11%. Nonimplant-related complication rate was 6%—2 widened scars, 3 hypertrophic scars, and 1 partial nipple necrosis. Implant-related complication rate was 5%—2 deflations, 1 capsular contracture, 1 implant shifting, and 1 infection.

Augmentation mammoplasty with periareolar mastopexy treats a wide variety of breast types including tubular deformity and grade II and III ptosis. Planned nipple-areolar elevation should be 4 cm or less. Vertical and horizontal skin envelope redraping is tailored for each case.

▶ This article reports a series of 100 consecutive reasonably similar periareolar augmentation/mastopexy cases from which some tentative conclusions can be drawn. Instead of a conglomeration of varied cases by different surgeons, this series encompasses only cases using the same technique, by the same surgeon, using the same type of implant. The key word in this entire article is the description of the augmentation approach by the surgeons: conservative. As has been reported many times in the past, this procedure (periareolar mastopexy/augmentation) has been shown to have a high complication rate and a high lawsuit rate. These authors report a relatively low complication rate, which they attribute to their conservative approach. The limitations, which they apply to the selection process, are appropriately outlined in Table 3 in the original article. Some may argue that it is even safer to limit the patients even more than proposed in the article—for example, to even smaller implants. The authors are willing to show their complications and illustrate how they have addressed these. The representative examples of cases without complication show results, which are quite satisfactory.

R. L. Ruberg, MD

The Use of Human Acellular Dermal Matrix for the Correction of Secondary Deformities after Breast Augmentation: Results and Costs
Hartzell TL, Taghinia AH, Chang J, et al (Brigham and Women's Hosp, Boston, MA)
Plast Reconstr Surg 126:1711-1720, 2010

Background.—Secondary breast deformities following breast augmentation constitute some of the most challenging and difficult problems to correct. Although the application and efficacy of human acellular dermal matrix in breast reconstruction has been previously reported, there is little information in the literature relating to its indications, results, or cost in aesthetic breast surgery.

Methods.—This study retrospectively reviewed a single surgeon's experience in correcting secondary deformities with human acellular dermal matrix after breast augmentation from 2005 to 2009. A total of 23 patients (38 breasts) were included in the study.

Results.—There were 28 breasts with surface irregularities and 22 breasts with implant malposition (12 had both). On average, 1.13 sheets of human acellular dermal matrix were used per breast per operation. At the authors' institution, this material equates to a cost to the patient of $3536 to $4856 per breast (depending on sheet size and thickness). Twenty of 23 patients (87 percent) [32 of 38 breasts (84 percent)] had improvement in their breast deformity after breast revision surgery. Three patients (six breasts) needed another cosmetic breast operation before the end of the follow-up period: two because of persistent surface irregularities and one with a request for larger implants. One patient (3 percent) had an infection in one breast, requiring removal of the human acellular dermal matrix.

Conclusions.—Human acellular dermal matrix is a useful and safe adjunct for correction of contour deformities after breast augmentation. Its high cost, however, may be a deterrent to widespread use in self-pay patients.

▶ It is not surprising that acellular dermal matrix can play an important role in the correction of postaugmentation breast deformities, given the multiple reports of success in treating similar problems in postmastectomy patients. This article verifies the validity of the approach and documents some helpful techniques for addressing a variety of challenging deformities. The real question that most patients and surgeons face in these cases is not whether the techniques work, but how to cover the costs associated with the use of this rather expensive product. The authors provide us with a realistic cost (not just a catalog price) for use of the acellular dermal matrix. They do suggest several options for reducing the patient cost for these surgical revision procedures but don't directly tell us the exact approach they use in charging their own patients. In the preoperative discussion, the surgeon must not only introduce the idea of the increased cost of using this product but must also prepare the patient for a range of costs, because it is not always clear how many sheets of the product will be required until the surgeon directly visualizes the deformity in the operating room. Therefore, both the cases and the billing can be challenging.

R. L. Ruberg, MD

General

Clinical Analyses of Clustered Microcalcifications after Autologous Fat Injection for Breast Augmentation

Wang C-F, Zhou Z, Yan Y-J, et al (Meitan General Hosp, Beijing, People's Republic of China; Peking Union Med College Hosp, Beijing, People's Republic of China)
Plast Reconstr Surg 127:1669-1673, 2011

Background.—Autologous fat injection for breast augmentation has been disputed with regard to its complications for many years, especially regarding calcifications, most of which present with benign features. In previous studies, clustered microcalcifications were not observed after fat injection for breast augmentation, which are usually regarded as malignant calcifications.

Methods.—From July of 1999 to December of 2009, autologous fat injection for breast augmentation was performed for both breasts in 48 patients. Eight patients with clustered microcalcifications found by mammography after surgery were analyzed retrospectively. For the nonpalpable breast lesions in three patients, the clustered microcalcifications were resected with the help of needle localized breast biopsy. The palpable lump, including clustered microcalcifications, was resected 1 cm away from its border in the other patients. All of the specimens were submitted to pathologic examination.

Results.—The digitized mammographic films of eight of 48 patients (16.7 percent) showed clustered microcalcifications after autologous fat injection, which were highly suspected of being breast carcinoma microcalcifications, whereas all pathologic examinations indicated fat necroses.

Conclusions.—Clustered microcalcifications can be found after autologous fat injection for breast augmentation, which cannot be distinguished from malignancy. The mammographic confusion constitutes the problem rather than the success of the procedure itself, and the method should continue to be prohibited.

▶ In the face of growing enthusiasm for autologous fat injection of the breast, this article presents a distinctly negative message. However, many authors in many published studies reach the exact opposite conclusion about fat injection, namely, that it is a safe, effective, and indicated procedure for treatment for a variety of breast contour problems. Those who continue to advocate fat injection would cite multiple problems with studies of this issue, such as this one: There is no uniformity in techniques used for fat injection; there is no clear evidence that nonsurgical pretreatment expansion of the breast is or is not of value; there are many different techniques of mammography that might give differing conclusions, etc. So where does that leave the individual practitioner? The very cautious person would refrain from the use of fat injection until all the evidence is in, all the variables have been considered, and a consensus opinion is issued. But such a definitive conclusion may be years away. In today's world, it appears as though most surgeons are willing to proceed with fat injection, with the expectation that ultimately the negative conclusions in this particular article will be overturned by the weight of the evidence. Current practice therefore supports cautious continued use of fat injection for correction of breast deformities despite the negative voice of a few investigators.

R. L. Ruberg, MD

Radiographic Findings after Breast Augmentation by Autologous Fat Transfer
Veber M, Tourasse C, Toussoun G, et al (Univ of Lyon—Léon Bérard Cancer Ctr, France; Jean Mermoz Private Hosp, Lyon, France; Univ of Lyon, France)
Plast Reconstr Surg 127:1289-1299, 2011

Background.—Fat transfer to healthy breasts, that is, in women with no history of breast disease, particularly breast cancer, is becoming increasingly popular. The main issue remains whether the transfer of fat cells to the native breast hampers breast imaging. This pilot study aimed to assess the effectiveness of radiographic evaluation after breast lipomodeling and to propose objective elements for the detection of mammographic signs, and for postoperative evaluation of breast density and Breast Imaging Reporting and Data System (American College of Radiology) classification.

Methods.—The authors retrospectively reviewed the radiographic findings of patients undergoing breast lipomodeling between 2000 and 2008. A descriptive semiologic analysis was conducted. Then, the authors compared breast tissue density and Breast Imaging Reporting and Data System categorization in 20 patients with preoperative and postoperative images available for review.

Results.—The descriptive analysis identified 16 percent of mammograms with microcalcifications, 9 percent with macrocalcifications, 25 percent with clear well-focused images of cystic lesions, and 12 percent with tissue remodeling. The comparative study showed no statistically significant difference between breast density findings before and after fat injection, whether using the American College of Radiology classification or a personalized rating system. Similarly, no significant difference was observed using the American College of Radiology Breast Imaging Reporting and Data System categorization before and after fat grafting.

Conclusions.—Radiographic follow-up of breasts treated with fat grafting is not problematic and should not be a hindrance to the procedure. However, the authors' preliminary results should be confirmed in larger series, and the radiographic follow-up of women undergoing breast lipomodeling should be standardized to ensure reproducibility and improve patient safety.

▶ The increasing popularity of fat grafting to the breast for both cosmetic and reconstructive purposes makes this an important, although imperfect, study. The initial response to descriptions of fat grafting of the breast by organized plastic surgery was overwhelmingly negative, and the procedure was condemned. Multiple authors have since then confirmed the effectiveness of this approach for contour improvement in reconstructive cases, and then later for simple breast augmentation, without evidence of adverse effects. But the question as to what problems might be encountered when performing post-treatment mammograms has been repeatedly raised. Now there is growing evidence that there are no clearly adverse effects, and this article adds to that body of knowledge. But several cautions must be stated. The article's title refers to findings after breast augmentation, but only 2 of the 76 patients in this study truly had breast augmentation, that is, fat injection (without implant) in an otherwise normal breast. Secondly, the procedure definitely did result in radiographic changes; however, these changes simply were not considered to be of major consequence. Therefore, with a persistent degree of caution, we can state that fat injection for all types of breast contouring is PROBABLY a safe and acceptable procedure. The authors support this conclusion but clearly state that more confirmatory studies are needed.

R. L. Ruberg, MD

Phosphorylcholine-Coated Silicone Implants: Effect on Inflammatory Response and Fibrous Capsule Formation
Zeplin PH, Larena-Avellaneda A, Jordan M, et al (Univ Hosp, Wuerzburg, Germany; et al)
Ann Plast Surg 65:560-564, 2010

Introduction.—The formation of capsular fibrosis around silicone breast implants is a common complication in reconstructive and plastic surgery. Foreign body reaction-induced infections are quite common because of the hydrophobic surface properties of silicone and are, in addition, considered to be a causative factor of capsular fibrosis.

Methods.—In this experimental pilot study, 2 groups of 7 Sprague-Dawley rats were established to evaluate the periprosthetic collagen synthesis after implantation of coated silicone implants. In the first group, the textured minisilicone implants were implanted submuscularly. The second group received the biotechnologically, surface-modified phosphorylcholine (PC)-coated implants. After a 3-month period, all the rats were killed, and the capsules were examined in a histologic (hematoxylin-eosin and Masson-trichrom) and immunohistologic way (CD4, CD8, CD68, TGF-beta, fibroblasts, collagen type I, and collagen type III).

Results.—Significant differences were found to occur between the PC-coated and standard, textured implants with respect to the inflammatory reaction and collagen synthesis.

Conclusions.—The production of hydrophilic surfaces in silicone implants by way of PC-coating causes a decrease in the inflammatory reaction, and thus, a reduction of periprosthetic fibrosis. This could form the basis of a cost-effective, preventive, and therapeutic strategy with respect to the decrease in capsular fibrosis occurrence.

▶ The mechanism by which bacterial adhesion (the first step in biofilm formation) to solid surfaces is decreased by adsorbed plasma proteins is not well understood. Studies support the hypothesis that substrate hydrophobicity is a more important contributor to nonspecific adhesion than bacterial surface itself. Consequently, instead of using antimicrobial agents to reduce the number of bacteria in an implant milieu, the use of surfaces that repel bacteria or those with coating that modify an inflammatory reaction may prove to be a successful alternative. Modalities that may prevent early adhesion of microbes (formation of biofilm), excessive collagen deposition, and ultimately capsular contracture formation have been tested. Natural phosphorylcholine is a nonthrombogenic component of the outer layer of erythrocytes. Synthetic forms of phosphorylcholine are used as coating on drug-eluting stents. They demonstrate no adverse clinical effect on healing of the arterial wall. Application and testing of this phospholipid as a coating material preventing early steps of reactions leading to biofilm formation (bacterial adhesion) is an interesting choice because of its durability, nonreactivity with drugs, and ability to undergo sterilization using standard methods without effect on its structure or efficacy. Phosphorylcholine may reduce biofilm formation and procoagulant and inflammatory responses; therefore, it is an important candidate for further research on the control of capsular contracture.

M. Dobke, MD, PhD

Subclinical (Biofilm) Infection Causes Capsular Contracture in a Porcine Model following Augmentation Mammaplasty

Tamboto H, Vickery K, Deva AK (Univ of New South Wales, Sydney, Australia)
Plast Reconstr Surg 126:835-842, 2010

Background.—Capsular contracture remains the most common complication following augmentation mammaplasty. The infective hypothesis implicates subclinical infection with biofilm in its pathogenesis. The authors developed an in vivo model of subclinical infection and biofilm formation to further investigate this.

Methods.—Adult female pigs underwent augmentation mammaplasty using miniature gel-filled implants. *Staphylococcus epidermidis* was inoculated into some of the periprosthetics as compared with control pockets, which were not inoculated. Implants were left in situ for 13 weeks, after which clinical assessment with the Baker technique was performed. Implants and capsules were then removed and subjected to laboratory analysis to detect biofilm.

Results.—Fifty-one breast augmentations were performed in six pigs: 36 in submammary pockets inoculated with *S. epidermidis* and 15 in uninoculated pockets. Twenty-six of the 36 inoculated implants (72.2 percent) resulted in biofilm production. Pocket inoculation was strongly associated with biofilm formation ($p = 0.0095$). The presence of biofilm in the inoculated pockets was also significantly associated with the subsequent development of capsular contracture as compared with the uninoculated pockets ($p < 0.05$). Of the 15 uninoculated pockets, seven developed contracture. Five of these, however, demonstrated the presence of biofilm caused by native porcine *S. epidermidis*. Of the 31 biofilm-positive specimens, 25 (80.6 percent) developed capsular contracture. Using univariate analysis, biofilm formation was associated with a fourfold increased risk of developing contracture (odds ratio, 4.1667; 95 percent confidence interval, 1.1939 to 14.5413).

Conclusion.—Using this in vivo model, the authors have demonstrated a causal link between subclinical infection, biofilm formation, and capsular contracture.

▶ This experimental study provides strong evidence linking subclinical infection with biofilm presence and capsular contracture and reaffirms previous circumstantial evidence from clinical studies.[1] This well-designed study provides hard-to-dispute support to the theory that biofilm may precipitate processes leading to the formation of capsular contracture. However, it is important to note that because the biofilm itself is an immunologically and biochemically complex entity and microbes embedded into glycocalyx may change chemistry of biologically active products they secrete, the formation of capsular contracture should not be attributed to simple biofilm growth but rather to a still little-known host—implant surface interactions.[2] Further research to characterize these interactions is needed to establish a fund of knowledge necessary for design of specific interventions interrupting or preventing biofilm formation and ultimately reduction of the rate of capsular contracture.

M. Dobke, MD, PhD

References

1. Virden C, Dobke M, Stein P, Parsons L, Frank D. Subclinical infection of the silicone breast implant surface as a possible cause of capsular contracture. *Aesthetic Plast Surg.* 1992;16:173-179.
2. Dobke M, Svahn J, Vastine V, Landon B, Stein P, Parsons L. Characterization of microbial presence at the surface of silicone mammary implants. *Ann Plast Surg.* 1995;34:563-569.

Cancer and Reconstruction

Surgical and Financial Implications of Genetic Counseling and Requests for Concurrent Prophylactic Mastectomy
Murphy RX Jr, Namey T, Eid S, et al (The Lehigh Valley Health Network, Allentown, PA)
Ann Plast Surg 64:684-687, 2010

Risk assessment evaluation and breast cancer (*BRCA*) testing can occur in situations where a woman considers herself to be at increased risk for developing breast cancer or her physicians, either during routine evaluation or after diagnosis of unilateral breast cancer, consider her to be at risk for harboring a genetic predisposition to breast malignancy. This study examined the impact of risk assessment counseling on trends in breast surgery and cost of care.

A retrospective chart review was performed from January 1, 1999 to December 31, 2008 for women older than 18 years who underwent breast surgery for malignancy or prophylaxis, had at least 1-year follow-up, and underwent genetic counseling. From the total number of women treated at our institution who underwent unilateral or bilateral mastectomy, we identified 102 women who underwent genetic counseling and selected 199 patients who did not undergo counseling to create a 4:1 retrospective case–control study. Patients who underwent *BRCA* gene testing and/or counseling were compared with patients who did not (controls). The study was powered at 70%, and α was set at 0.05.

Counseled patients were >9 times more likely to undergo bilateral mastectomies (odds ratio = 9.18). They were younger (46.4 vs. 61.8) and incurred higher total costs ($10,810 vs. $7,266) ($P < 0.002$). The same trend was observed in each group. In counseled and control groups, younger women chose bilateral mastectomies (mean 44.4; 55.5), whereas older women chose unilateral procedures (mean 49.8; 63.02) ($P < 0.014$). Total cost for bilateral mastectomies was greater than unilateral mastectomies for both groups. Of 55 counseled patients undergoing mastectomies (85 breasts), 78 (92%) breasts were reconstructed, whereas 113 (49%) of 230 breasts were reconstructed in the control group.

There was a statistically significant association between counseling with *BRCA* testing and decision to undergo bilateral as opposed to unilateral mastectomies. Younger women were also more likely to choose bilateral mastectomies whether or not they underwent counseling. Furthermore, a greater proportion of counseled women who underwent reconstruction opted to have bilateral implants. At our institution, younger women tend to choose costlier options.

▶ Genetic testing to determine the presence of *BRCA1* and *BRCA2* genes assesses the risk for those who are positive to develop breast cancer, and appropriate counseling of the patients regarding their options for therapy is becoming increasingly important. Although the lifetime risk for women with *BRCA1* and *BRCA2* genes to develop breast cancer is roughly 5 times greater than those without these genes, the lifetime risk for these women to develop ovarian cancer is even greater, roughly 1.4% in the general population to 15% to 40% in those carrying these genes. One must ask during the process of counseling the patients in this study—recognizing the focus on prophylactic mastectomy—whether the issue of ovarian cancer was discussed and whether treatment options were offered. We must also be aware that most studies on consequences and the lifetime risk of having the *BRCA* genes have been formulated on large family populations with many members having the *BRCA* genes. Actual information on whether these risk factors are the same in the general population is unknown at this time. It is unclear to me whether all patients who were counseled underwent *BRCA* testing, and if they did not undergo BRCA testing, what was the reason for the counseling? How many women with negative *BRCA1* and *BRCA2* genes had mastectomy and why? Why did the younger women in this study choose to have bilateral mastectomy? These and many other questions remain to be answered. It is imperative that cancer centers in the United States organize studies to help provide us with more information.

S. H. Miller, MD, MPH

Association of Risk-Reducing Surgery in *BRCA1* or *BRCA2* Mutation Carriers With Cancer Risk and Mortality
Domchek SM, Friebel TM, Singer CF, et al (Univ of Pennsylvania School of Medicine, Philadelphia; Med Univ of Vienna, Austria; et al)
JAMA 304:967-975, 2010

Context.—Mastectomy and salpingo-oophorectomy are widely used by carriers of *BRCA1* or *BRCA2* mutations to reduce their risks of breast and ovarian cancer.

Objective.—To estimate risk and mortality reduction stratified by mutation and prior cancer status.

Design, Setting, and Participants.—Prospective, multicenter cohort study of 2482 women with *BRCA1* or *BRCA2* mutations ascertained between 1974 and 2008. The study was conducted at 22 clinical and research genetics centers in Europe and North America to assess the relationship of risk-reducing mastectomy or salpingo-oophorectomy with cancer outcomes. The women were followed up until the end of 2009.

Main Outcomes Measures.—Breast and ovarian cancer risk, cancer-specific mortality, and overall mortality.

Results.—No breast cancers were diagnosed in the 247 women with risk-reducing mastectomy compared with 98 women of 1372 diagnosed with breast cancer who did not have risk-reducing mastectomy. Compared with women who did not undergo risk-reducing salpingo-oophorectomy, women who underwent salpingo-oophorectomy had a lower risk of ovarian cancer, including those with prior breast cancer (6% vs 1%, respectively; hazard ratio [HR], 0.14; 95% confidence interval [CI], 0.04-0.59) and those without prior breast cancer (6% vs 2%; HR, 0.28 [95% CI, 0.12-0.69]), and a lower risk of first diagnosis of breast cancer in *BRCA1* mutation carriers (20% vs 14%; HR, 0.63 [95% CI, 0.41-0.96]) and *BRCA2* mutation carriers (23% vs 7%; HR, 0.36 [95% CI, 0.16-0.82]). Compared with women who did not undergo risk-reducing salpingo-oophorectomy, undergoing salpingo-oophorectomy was associated with lower all-cause mortality (10% vs 3%; HR, 0.40 [95% CI, 0.26-0.61]), breast cancer–specific mortality (6% vs 2%; HR, 0.44 [95% CI, 0.26-0.76]), and ovarian cancer–specific mortality (3% vs 0.4%; HR, 0.21 [95% CI, 0.06-0.80]).

Conclusions.—Among a cohort of women with *BRCA1* and *BRCA2* mutations, the use of risk-reducing mastectomy was associated with a lower risk of breast cancer; risk-reducing salpingo-oophorectomy was associated with a lower risk of ovarian cancer, first diagnosis of breast cancer, all-cause mortality, breast cancer—specific mortality, and ovarian cancer—specific mortality.

▶ This is a very important large, multi-institutional, international, observational study regarding risk of the development of breast and ovarian cancers in women with *BRCA1* and *BRCA2* mutations. The study clearly documents the benefits of prophylactic mastectomy and salpingo-oophorectomy on significantly reducing the risk of developing breast cancer in the former and the risk of developing ovarian cancer, including those with/without previous breast cancer. One of the unanswered questions remains: when is the most propitious time to perform the mastectomy and/or the salpingo-oophorectomy? All of those who chose not to undergo surgery and the group against whom the study group was compared were offered intensive screening. It is unclear if in the case of breast cancer screening in these high-risk patients, MRI mammograms are a better tool than routine mammograms. It is also unclear whether those who did not have the surgery were, in fact, compliant with the screening protocol.

S. H. Miller, MD, MPH

Trends in Contralateral Prophylactic Mastectomy for Unilateral Cancer: A Report From the National Cancer Data Base, 1998–2007
Yao K, Stewart AK, Winchester DJ, et al (Univ of Chicago, Evanston, IL; American College of Surgeons, Chicago, IL)
Ann Surg Oncol 17:2554-2562, 2010

Background.—Several studies have reported an increased rate of contralateral prophylactic mastectomy (CPM) in patients with unilateral breast cancer. This study reports on CPM trends from the American College of Surgeon's National Cancer Data Base (NCDB) diagnosed over a 10-year period.

Methods.—Data about women diagnosed with unilateral breast cancer between 1998 and 2007 undergoing CPM were extracted from the NCDB. Temporal trends were analyzed across patient demographic, tumor, and provider characteristics. Logistic regression models identified characteristics independently associated with use of CPM.

Results.—A total of 1,166,456 patients, of whom 23,218 patients underwent CPM, were reviewed; use increased from 0.4% in 1998 to 4.7% in 2007 of surgically treated patients. The greatest comparative increases in CPM was among white patients <40 years of age residing in high socioeconomic status areas with private or managed care insurance plans and treated at high-volume medical centers in the Midwest region of the country. A greater proportion of patients with in-situ disease undergo CPM compared to invasive disease. Independent factors associated with CPM include patient demographic and socioeconomic factors, tumor stage and histopathology, and provider characteristics.

Conclusions.—Although an increase in the proportion of surgically treated women undergoing CPM was universally observed across a broad range of patient, biological, and provider factors, the increase was more noticeably associated with patient-related factors rather than tumor or biological characteristics. Further studies are needed to determine why patients seem to choose CPM and whether a survival benefit can be associated with this choice of surgical management.

▶ The findings in this study, as important as they are, are a beginning and only that. It is not surprising that young, relatively well-off patients with adequate insurance coverage and relatively low-risk disease would opt for going all out to prevent death from breast cancer. Further, logic, both lay and professional, would seem to dictate that removal of all or most of the tissues susceptible to the malignancy should assure prolonged survival. Follow-up studies need to be done that can specifically address the motivation for contralateral prophylactic mastectomy (CPM) as it relates to issues such as family history and outcomes of those with breast cancer, genetic testing such as *BRCA1* and *BRCA2*, use of MRI, and the recommendations of the patient's physicians. Additional studies need to address the issue of why certain centers and not others perform far more CPMs without good evidence of improved outcomes. Finally, definitive data on the effects of such surgery on ultimate outcomes will be important for patient education and guidance.

S. H. Miller, MD, MPH

Reporting Clinical Outcomes of Breast Reconstruction: A Systematic Review

Potter S, Brigic A, Whiting PF, et al (Univ of Bristol, UK; Yeovil District Hosp NHS Foundation Trust, Somerset, UK; et al)
J Natl Cancer Inst 103:31-46, 2011

Background.—Breast reconstruction after mastectomy for cancer requires accurate evaluation to inform evidence-based participatory decision making, but the standards of outcome reporting after breast reconstruction have not previously been considered.

Methods.—We used extensive searches to identify articles reporting surgical outcomes of breast reconstruction. We extracted data using published criteria for complication reporting modified to reflect reconstructive practice. Study designs included randomized controlled trials, cohort studies, and case series. The Cochrane Risk of Bias tool was used to critically appraise all study designs. Other criteria used to assess the studies were selection and funding bias, statistical power calculations, and institutional review board approval. Wilcoxon signed rank tests were used to compare the breadth and frequency of study outcomes, and χ^2 tests were used to compare the number of studies in each group reporting each of the published criteria. All statistical tests were two-sided.

Results.—Surgical complications following breast reconstruction in 42 146 women were evaluated in 134 studies. These included 11 (8.2%) randomized trials, 74 (55.2%) cohort studies, and 49 (36.6%) case series. Fifty-three percent of studies demonstrated a disparity between methods and results in the numbers of complications reported. Complications were defined by 87 (64.9%) studies and graded by 78 (58.2%). Details such as the duration of follow-up and risk factors for adverse outcomes were omitted from 47 (35.1%) and 58 (43.3%) studies, respectively. Overall, the studies defined fewer than 20% of the complications they reported, and the definitions were largely inconsistent.

Conclusions.—The results of this systematic review suggest that outcome reporting in breast reconstruction is inconsistent and lacks methodological rigor. The development of a standardized core outcome set is recommended to improve outcome reporting in breast reconstruction.

▶ This is a very important article for all plastic surgeons and our national organizations to carefully read, ponder, and hopefully organize and standardize outcomes research efforts in this country. The authors evaluated 134 articles, published in English between 1995 and 2009, detailing information about complications in some 42 000 patients who underwent breast reconstruction. Not surprisingly, they concluded that the published reports of outcomes following breast reconstruction are largely anecdotal and of little help in educating ourselves, our trainees, and our patients. Because we have no nationally standardized outcomes defined and accepted by all, we will continue to fail to understand and more importantly correct our failures. Until we can truly define, standardize, and measure complications and patient expectations with focused survey instruments, such as BREAST-Q, rather than generic survey instruments, such as 36-Item Short Form Health Survey, we will continue to have significant numbers of patients whose expectations have not been met. Further information on this subject is available in a study conducted by the National Health Service.[1]

S. H. Miller, MD

Reference

1. The National Mastectomy and Breast Reconstruction Audit. A national audit of provision and outcomes of mastectomy and breast reconstruction surgery for women in England. Third Annual Report, http://www.ic.nhs.uk/services/national-clinical-audit-support-programme-ncasp/cancer/mastectomy-and-breast-reconstruction, April 25, 2011.

Reduction mammaplasty: An advantageous option for breast conserving surgery in large-breasted patients
Hernanz F, Regaño S, Vega A, et al (Univ of Cantabria, Santander, Spain)
Surg Oncol 19:e95-e102, 2010

Oncoplastic breast conserving surgery is a good approach for large-breasted women with breast cancer, as it increases the rate of breast conserving surgery, improves cosmetic results and prevents both cosmetic sequelae and the symptoms associated with macromastia. We reviewed ten publications in which 276 patients had been treated with bilateral reduction mammaplasty. All showed the same conclusion: women with breast cancer and macromastia candidates for breast conserving surgery could obtain clear oncological and cosmetic advantages and an improvement in quality of life if they were treated using bilateral reduction onco-therapeutic mammaplasty.

▶ The combination of lumpectomy and reduction mammaplasty has become an accepted form of breast conservation surgery for patients with appropriate tumors. This article reviews a number of different studies and summarizes the evidence that shows that this approach is oncologically sound. Some controversy exists as to whether this procedure should be done by a single breast surgeon with oncoplastic training, or a team that includes the surgical oncologist/breast surgeon and an independent plastic surgeon. Most plastic surgeons would, of course, recommend the latter approach in order to maximize both the oncologic effectiveness and the aesthetic outcome of the procedure. For example, experience in using a variety of different pedicles for breast reduction allows the plastic surgeon to facilitate the lumpectomy in a greater variety of locations in the breast. When the combined approach is used, the plastic surgeon ideally is present for the resection and the reduction in order to protect the pedicle and minimize the unnecessary removal of benign tissue, which can contribute to the best final aesthetic outcome.

R. L. Ruberg, MD

Breast Reduction in the Irradiated Breast: Evidence for the Role of Breast Reduction at the Time of Lumpectomy
Parrett BM, Schook C, Morris D (Harvard Med School, Boston, MA)
Breast J 16:498-502, 2010

Given the high incidence of breast cancer in our society, it is common to encounter patients with macromastia who desire breast reduction after breast-conserving therapy by lumpectomy and radiation. We hypothesize that radiation leads to a significant increase in postoperative complications after breast reduction. All patients with a history of unilateral breast lumpectomy and radiation who subsequently underwent bilateral breast reduction by a single surgeon from 2004 to 2008 were retrospectively reviewed. Outcomes including cellulitis, wound breakdown, seroma, and need for repeat operations were compared between the radiated and nonradiated breast. The Fisher's exact test was used for statistical analysis. Twelve patients (mean age, 57 years) underwent bilateral breast reduction a mean of 86 months after unilateral lumpectomy and radiation. The nonradiated breasts had no complications postoperatively. The radiated breasts had a significant increase in complications with a total of five breasts (42%, p < 0.04) having postoperative complications including cellulitis in two breasts, seroma requiring drainage in five breasts, two cases of fat necrosis, and one case of wound dehiscence. This resulted in two admissions for intravenous antibiotics and two repeat operative procedures. Additionally, three patients had significant breast asymmetry or contour deformities after reduction requiring operative revisions. Breast reduction after radiation leads to a significant increase in complications. Given this data, patients with macromastia undergoing breast conservation therapy for cancer should be considered for reduction at the time of lumpectomy and prior to radiation.

▶ Much has been written recently about the value of combining breast reduction with lumpectomy for breast cancer as part of the new approach called oncoplastic surgery. This article adds additional evidence for the benefit of this approach by showing the potential complications if the reduction is done after radiation and not as part of the original tumor extirpation. Nevertheless, the article should not be interpreted as condemning reduction mammaplasty in patients who have had previous lumpectomy and radiation. The authors do report a significant increase in complications in these patients, but one could still assume that these complications can be balanced by the benefits usually seen after breast reduction. The article suggests some steps to minimize complications in these patients. In my own experience, I have performed breast reduction after lumpectomy and radiation in a few patients (perhaps 3 patients) with only minimal problems. All of these were patients who did not consider breast reduction surgery until many years after their cancer treatment. However, the authors make a good point of introducing the discussion of breast reduction during the planning for lumpectomy in patients with symptomatic macromastia. I think that the evidence shows that the performance of the combined procedure (lumpectomy and reduction followed by radiation) will logically lead to the best result for these patients, with the minimum number of operative procedures.

R. L. Ruberg, MD

Current Practice Among Plastic Surgeons of Antibiotic Prophylaxis and Closed-Suction Drains in Breast Reconstruction: Experience, Evidence, and Implications for Postoperative Care
Phillips BT, Wang ED, Mirrer J, et al (Stony Brook Univ Med Ctr, NY; Stony Brook Univ School of Medicine, NY)
Ann Plast Surg 66:460-465, 2011

Background.—Despite their widespread use, there are no evidence-based guidelines on the management of closed-suction drains or antibiotics in postmastectomy breast reconstruction. The purpose of this study was to assess consensus and variation in postoperative care among plastic surgeons.

Methods.—The authors designed and administered a self-reported, anonymous survey to 4669 American Society of Plastic Surgeons and Canadian Society of Plastic Surgeons members in October 2009.

Results.—A total of 650 completed surveys were available for analysis. A majority (>81%) of respondents reported using closed-suction drains in breast reconstruction. Most surgeons (>93%) used a volume criteria for drain removal, most commonly when drain output was ≤30 mL over 24 hours (>86%). Preoperative antibiotic use was nearly universal (98%), usually consisting of intravenous cefazolin (97%). Postoperative care demonstrated less uniformity with outpatient antibiotics administered by 72% of respondents. Surgeons were divided on when to discontinue outpatient antibiotics: 46% preferred concomitant discontinuation with drains, whereas 52% preferred a specific postoperative day. No clear consensus was observed for the number (1 or 2) or type (Jackson-Pratt or Blake) of drains used. Respondents were further divided on the restriction of postoperative showering with drains and the use of acellular dermal matrix.

Conclusions.—These results demonstrate a consensus for drain use, drain removal, and preoperative antibiotic administration. There was no consensus for number or type of drain used, postoperative antibiotic use, shower restrictions, and use of acellular dermal matrix. Our results further emphasize the need for evidence-based postoperative-care guidelines specific to breast reconstruction.

▶ This study emphasizes the many problems associated with the use of survey studies. In the first place, a response rate of roughly 14% leads one with a great deal of discomfort in trying to generalize any of the results/consensus reached. More useful studies could be generated if several institutions agreed on protocols to (1) randomize the use and type of pre- and postoperative antibiotics versus nonuse (with postoperative infection measures as an outcome) and (2) randomize patients as to the duration of treatment with the antibiotics, based on specific days versus volume of drainage in those patients with drains (again with postoperative infection as an outcome) along with randomized arms for the study of patients with and without drains from the standpoint of the development of postoperative fluid collections and infection rates. Are there outcome differences whether or not antibiotics and drains are used? Once that is answered, are there differences in the timing and way they are used?

S. H. Miller, MD, MPH

Becker expander implants: Truly a long term single stage reconstruction?
Chew BK, Yip C, Malyon AD (Glasgow Royal Infirmary, UK)
J Plast Reconstr Aesthet Surg 63:1300-1304, 2010

Despite being more expensive than conventional tissue expanders, Becker expanders offer the advantage of single stage breast reconstruction. However, the large series in published literature which report good outcomes of Becker expanders in breast reconstruction have a mean follow up period of less than three years. This does not allow for definitive conclusions as to whether the Becker expander truly meets its design goal of a lasting single stage breast reconstruction.

This study is a retrospective case note review of all patients who underwent breast reconstruction using a Becker expander at our unit from 1993 to 1998, with a mean follow up of 12.5 years. Sixty-eight Becker-only breast reconstructions were carried out following oncological and risk-reducing mastectomies, and for congenital hypoplasias.

There was a high premature overall explantation rate with 68% of expanders removed by 5 years due to complications which included poor aesthetics, capsular contracture and infection. The mean time to explantation for these patients was only 23 months, and time to 50% overall expander removal ('half life') was just 30 months. On subgroup analysis, patients in the congenital hypoplasias group had a significantly better rate of expander retention with 67% remaining in situ at 10 years. In comparison, patients in the oncological and risk-reducing mastectomy groups had implant retention rates of 2% and 7% respectively.

The Becker expander does not appear to meet its design purpose of lasting single stage breast reconstruction in post-mastectomy cases. In contrast, it appears to have significantly better longevity when used for congenital hypoplasias.

▶ The Becker expander implant was designed to allow immediate reconstruction of the breast after mastectomy with a device that started out as a tissue expander but ended up as a silicone gel implant after valve removal. This device is not currently available for general use in the United States but other expander implants are (although they are not gel devices). I used many of these devices a number of years ago, and the results were acceptable. The problem is that since that time, other more aesthetically pleasing methods of reconstruction have become available. As a result, the potential value of an expander implant has been reduced significantly. This study provides us with evidence that many of the original Becker devices had to be removed (for a carefully analyzed list of reasons), often relatively early after the reconstructive procedure. Although currently available teardrop shaped expander implants might be an improvement on the round Becker shape, these are still likely to be subject to the same types of complications, most prominently aesthetic considerations, such as malposition and capsular contracture. The expander implant is still available for reconstructive purposes, but it should be used only with full understanding of its limitations.

R. L. Ruberg, MD

Evaluation of Outcomes in Breast Reconstructions Combining Lower Abdominal Free Flaps and Permanent Implants

Roehl KR, Baumann DP, Chevray PM, et al (Univ of Texas M D Anderson Cancer Ctr, Houston)

Plast Reconstr Surg 126:349-357, 2010

Background.—The purpose of this study was to evaluate outcomes in breast reconstruction combining lower abdominal flaps with implants and to compare the impact of timing of implant placement on complication and revision rates.

Methods.—A retrospective review of all patients who underwent free transverse rectus abdominis musculocutaneous, muscle sparing transverse rectus abdominis musculocutaneous, deep inferior epigastric perforator, or superficial inferior epigastric perforator flaps with implants at a single center over the past decade was performed. Patients were classified as having implant placement at the time of flap reconstruction or during a second procedure. The flap types, implant types/planes, flap and implant-related complications, and revision rates were compared between the groups.

Results.—Sixty-nine patients underwent 110 abdominal free flap breast reconstructions with an implant (immediate placement group, 35 patients; staged placement group, 34 patients). The mean follow-up periods were 32 months and 43 months for the immediate placement and staged placement groups, respectively. There was no statistically significant difference in flap type, implant type or plane, flap-related complications, or early implant-related complications between groups. The immediate placement group had a significantly higher rate of late implant-related complications: 25 percent (15 of 59) versus 4 percent (two of 51) in the staged placement group ($p = 0.007$). The implant revision rate was 63 percent (22 of 35) in the immediate placement group versus 26 percent (nine of 34) in the staged placement group ($p = 0.081$).

Conclusions.—The authors conclude that it is safe to combine implants with autologous lower abdominal free flaps for breast reconstruction. However, it may be preferable to perform this procedure in a staged fashion to minimize late complications and the need for future revisions because of complications or dissatisfaction with the aesthetic result.

▶ Even though this is a retrospective study, it still provides us with valuable information regarding the combination of free flap breast reconstruction with implant placement. Clearly the need for an implant along with an abdominal flap is limited. The authors indicate that this subset of breast reconstruction patients principally includes those with very limited abdominal tissue or those needing bilateral reconstructions of substantial size. At their institution, which performs a very large number of breast reconstructions, the cases included in this series represented only about 3% of the total number of reconstructions. Although the revision rate for immediate implant patients was almost two-thirds, a significant number of these patients (17%) simply underwent exchange of a saline to a silicone implant. Had these patients received a silicone implant immediately, it appears that the revision rate could have fallen to less than 50%. So perhaps it would be reasonable to perform the reconstruction plus immediate implantation in those patients who really would prefer to avoid a second operation, as long as they knew that there was a 50-50 chance that additional surgery would be needed. But the safest approach, based on the information provided by these authors, is to intentionally postpone the implant placement to a later date.

R. L. Ruberg, MD

Evaluation of Outcomes in Breast Reconstructions Combining Lower Abdominal Free Flaps and Permanent Implants

Roehl KR, Baumann DP, Chevray PM, et al (Univ of Texas M D Anderson Cancer Ctr, Houston)
Plast Reconstr Surg 126:349-357, 2010

Background.—The purpose of this study was to evaluate outcomes in breast reconstruction combining lower abdominal flaps with implants and to compare the impact of timing of implant placement on complication and revision rates.

Methods.—A retrospective review of all patients who underwent free transverse rectus abdominis musculocutaneous, muscle-sparing transverse rectus abdominis musculocutaneous, deep inferior epigastric perforator, or superficial inferior epigastric perforator flaps with implants at a single center over the past decade was performed. Patients were classified as having implant placement at the time of flap reconstruction or during a second procedure. The flap types, implant types/planes, flap and implant-related complications, and revision rates were compared between the groups.

Results.—Sixty-nine patients underwent 110 abdominal free flap breast reconstructions with an implant (immediate placement group, 35 patients; staged placement group, 34 patients). The mean follow-up periods were 32 months and 43 months for the immediate placement and staged placement groups, respectively. There was no statistically significant difference in flap type, implant type or plane, flap-related complications, or early implant-related complications between groups. The immediate placement group had a significantly higher rate of late implant-related complications: 25 percent (15 of 59) versus 4 percent (two of 51) in the staged placement group ($p = 0.007$). The implant revision rate was 63 percent (22 of 35) in the immediate placement group versus 26 percent (nine of 34) in the staged placement group ($p = 0.081$).

Conclusions.—The authors conclude that it is safe to combine implants with autologous lower abdominal free flaps for breast reconstruction. However, it may be preferable to perform this procedure in a staged

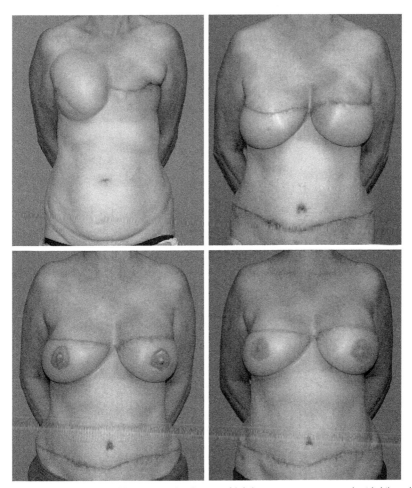

FIGURE 1.—A 67-year-old woman with a history of left breast cancer was treated with bilateral mastectomies and immediate reconstruction with tissue expanders. She was subsequently treated with irradiation of the left side of the chest and lost the tissue expander. She presented to one of the authors (P.M.C.) and underwent removal of the 580-cc right breast tissue expander and delayed bilateral breast reconstruction with bilateral 150-cc textured postoperatively adjustable saline implants and a free DIEP flap for the right breast, and a muscle-sparing free TRAM flap for the left breast. (*Above, left*) Preoperative view. (*Above, right*) Postoperative view 5 weeks after surgery. (*Below, left*) Postoperative view 1 week after nipple-areola micropigmentation, 2 months after bilateral reconstructed breast revision and nipple reconstruction, and 4 months after the initial surgery. (*Below, right*) Postoperative view 11 months after lower abdominal free flap and saline implant surgery. (Reprinted from Roehl KR, Baumann DP, Chevray PM, et al. Evaluation of outcomes in breast reconstructions combining lower abdominal free flaps and permanent implants. *Plast Reconstr Surg.* 2010;126:349-357.)

fashion to minimize late complications and the need for future revisions because of complications or dissatisfaction with the aesthetic result (Fig 1).

▶ An important question has been posed by the authors: does the timing of breast reconstruction, in a small subset of patients with limited abdominal tissue using a combination of a lower abdominal flap and an implant affect the aesthetic outcome and the need for surgical revisions? They conclude that in patients who undergo staged reconstruction, late implant-related complications and the need for secondary surgical procedures is decreased. Intuitively, the results were predictable. Immediate breast reconstructions, especially when redundant, amorphous, unshaped tissues have not had time to stabilize, are more likely to develop late aesthetic complications. There are several unanswered questions in my mind relating to the retrospective analysis and nonrandomized selection of patients. I am curious as to whether the number of perforators in each of the free flaps had any bearing on the outcomes. I would think that it is incumbent upon the authors, perhaps in combination with other centers, to look at this issue in more detail and in a prospective manner, to increase the size and equivalency of the groups studied, and finally, to evaluate and compare the outcomes using these flaps with the results obtainable from combining the latissimus dorsi flap and implants.

S. H. Miller, MD, MPH

Practice Patterns in Venous Thromboembolism Prophylaxis: A Survey of 606 Reconstructive Breast Surgeons
Pannucci CJ, Oppenheimer AJ, Wilkins EG (Univ of Michigan, Ann Arbor)
Ann Plast Surg 64:732-737, 2010

Current practice patterns for venous thrombembolism (VTE) prophylaxis in autogenous breast reconstruction are unknown. A web-based survey on VTE prophylaxis was distributed to all American Society of Plastic Surgery members in the United States with a clinical interest in autogenous tissue breast reconstruction (N − 3584). A total of 606 completed surveys were returned for a response rate of 16.9%. Overall compliance with established guidelines was low (25%). High volume surgeons (43% vs. 22%) and surgeons in academic practice (42% vs. 22%) were significantly more likely to report prophylaxis regimens consistent with American College of Chest Physicians guidelines (ACCP) recommendations. Subgroup analysis of 72 surgeons who specifically report conformance to ACCP guidelines demonstrated only 38% actually provided prophylaxis consistent with ACCP recommendations. VTE is a potentially fatal complication of autogenous breast reconstruction. Further research is necessary to create VTE prophylaxis guidelines specific to patients undergoing these procedures. The need for surgeon education on appropriate prophylaxis cannot be overemphasized.

▶ This is a critically important article primarily because of the lack of participation by plastic surgeons. The plastic surgery community has long recognized the importance of venous thrombosis prophylaxis in patients undergoing plastic surgical procedures, especially those with cancer. Additionally, the practice of plastic surgery calls for evidence-based guidelines and to validate its good work even in tangential areas of plastic surgery practice, such as appropriate pre- and postoperative care, including prophylaxis to prevent postoperative deep venous thrombosis and pulmonary embolism. Certainly the medical and surgical literature, including that from the world of plastic surgery, has been replete with articles documenting the need for prophylaxis and the appropriate protocols necessary to accomplish such prophylaxis.[1,2] It is disheartening for this important and relatively short survey to have had such a low response rate and a low overall compliance rate with generally accepted guidelines for venous thrombosis prophylaxis, and even more disheartening is the failure to actually provide prophylaxis in accordance with the widely accepted recommendations of the American College of Chest Physicians. I believe such surveys are critical to establish guidelines for acceptable plastic surgical practice, and the entire community of plastic surgeon needs to participate in them.

S. H. Miller, MD, MPH

References

1. Caprinia JA. Thrombosis risk assessment as a guide to quality patient care. *Dis Mon.* 2005;51:70-78.
2. Hatef DA, Kenkel JM, Nguyen MQ. Thromboembolic risk assessment and the efficacy of enoxaparin prophylaxis in excisional body contouring surgery. *Plast Reconstr Surg.* 2008;122:269-279.

Resource implications of bilateral autologous breast reconstruction — a single centre's seven year experience
Molina AR, Ponniah A, Simcock J, et al (Cambridge Univ Hosps NHS Trust, UK)
J Plast Reconstr Aesthet Surg 63:1588-1591, 2010

Introduction and Aims.– Since the recent introduction of "Payment by Results" as part of NHS financial reforms, it has been noted that there is an imbalance between allocated Healthcare Resource Group tariffs and actual resource use for certain procedures. This study was undertaken to assess the impression that bilateral breast reconstruction using autologous flaps is under-funded.

Material and Methods.—Patients who underwent bilateral flap breast reconstruction following mastectomy between 2000 and 2006 at Addenbrooke's University Hospital were identified. Resource cost analysis for each patient was based on the following parameters: number of operating consultants, theatre running costs, and length of hospital stay. The estimated hospital costs were then compared to the national tariff for the Healthcare Resource Group "Complex Breast Reconstruction using Flaps".

Key Results.—Over the 7-year period 24 patients underwent bilateral flap breast reconstruction (7 paired latissimus dorsi and 17 paired abdominal flaps). The mean operative time was 9.4 h (£4.5/min), the mean hospital stay was 10 days (£150/day) and ten patients required 2 consultants (£34/h) operating. The average total cost equated to £5 492.

Conclusion.—The allocated tariff of £4 053 is insufficient, even before the inclusion of hidden costs. Bilateral free flap breast reconstructions are grossly under-funded at present. With increasing financial pressures on NHS Trusts there may be a drive towards simpler operations, which receive proportionally greater remuneration.

▶ This is an interesting retrospective anecdotal study that certainly mirrors experiences in the United States with regard to underpayment for microsurgical procedures of all types. Specifically with regards to complex autologous breast reconstructions, failure to take into account patient comorbidities and how they effect costs is grossly unfair. Equally problematic is how to deal with the inequities, from the standpoint of the health care provider and the patient, associated with immediate versus delayed breast reconstruction. Perhaps it is necessary to consider a fair global fee covering similar treatments for the entire illness regardless of when they are provided, that is, complete or partial mastectomy and immediate or delayed complex flap reconstruction. One of the major drawbacks in these types of studies is to have enough data to be certain about whether the comparisons being made are truly about resource-based costs, prices charged to patients, or the entities paying the bill.

S. H. Miller, MD, MPH

Free Transverse Rectus Abdominis Myocutaneous Flap for Breast Reconstruction in Patients with Prior Abdominal Contouring Procedures
Jandali S, Nelson JA, Wu LC, et al (Univ of Pennsylvania Health System, Philadelphia)
J Reconstr Microsurg 26:607-614, 2010

With an increasing number of women undergoing abdominal liposuction and abdominoplasties, patients who have a history of an abdominal-contouring procedure are now presenting to plastic surgeons with breast cancer and are interested in autologous breast reconstruction. Based on the principle of vascular ingrowth and experience of seeing intact perforators arise from the rectus abdominis muscle in repeat abdominoplasty patients, it was hypothesized that these new perforators could adequately and safely supply the abdominal skin island as a flap in this patient population. A retrospective chart review was performed searching for cases of free transverse rectus abdominis myocutaneous (TRAM) or deep inferior epigastric perforator (DIEP) flap breast reconstruction in patients with a prior history of either abdominal liposuction, abdominoplasty, or both. Three successful cases of free TRAM flap breast reconstruction were performed in patients who had undergone previous full abdominoplasties. Additionally, three successful cases of free TRAM or DIEP flaps were performed in patients after abdominal liposuction. Major complications included one anterial thrombosis in which the flap was salvaged. This study demonstrates the feasibility and viability of free TRAM flaps after previous abdominoplasty and DIEP flaps following prior abdominal liposuction. This is an important advance in the potential uses of the free TRAM flap.

▶ Use of free vascularized abdominal tissue for breast reconstruction in patients who have undergone previous full abdominoplasty would appear to be contra-indicated because of transection of perforators during the previous operation. Similar procedures after abdominal liposuction alone would likely be less risky but still of concern. Based on the limited experience of these surgeons, free tissue transfer in both these circumstances can indeed be done with a reasonable chance of success. The authors considered but did not delay their flaps. They do recommend preoperative imaging of the vessels of the abdomen, although they note that small perforators that have regenerated after abdominoplasty may not be visible in such studies. Clearly, a great deal of caution and a comparable amount of patient counseling would be required before undertaking these procedures. But if the skill of the surgeon and the will of the patient are maximal, this procedure appears now to be justified.

R. L. Ruberg, MD

Comparison of Morbidity, Functional Outcome, and Satisfaction following Bilateral TRAM versus Bilateral DIEP Flap Breast Reconstruction
Chun YS, Sinha I, Turko A, et al (Brigham and Women's Hosp, Boston, MA; Beth Israel Deaconess Med Ctr, Boston, MA)
Plast Reconstr Surg 126:1133-1141, 2010

Background.—The potential for donor-site morbidity associated with bilateral pedicled transverse rectus abdominis myocutaneous (TRAM) flap breast reconstruction has led to the popularization of deep inferior epigastric artery perforator (DIEP) flap reconstruction. This study compares postoperative morbidity and satisfaction following bilateral pedicled TRAM and DIEP flap reconstruction.

Methods.—One hundred five women with bilateral pedicled TRAM flaps were compared with 58 women with bilateral DIEP flap reconstruction. Medical records were reviewed for complications and demographic data. Postoperative follow-up data were obtained through Short Form-36, Functional Assessment of Cancer Therapy-Breast, Michigan Breast Satisfaction, and Qualitative Assessment of Back Pain surveys.

Results.—The mean follow-up interval was 6.2 years in the bilateral TRAM group and 2.3 years in the bilateral DIEP group ($p < 0.001$). Demographic data were otherwise similar. Abdominal hernias occurred in three TRAM patients (2.9 percent) and in no DIEP patients, whereas abdominal bulges occurred in three TRAM patients (2.9 percent) and four DIEP patients (6.9 percent); these differences were not statistically significant. Fat necrosis occurred less frequently in the TRAM group ($p = 0.04$). Postoperative survey results revealed no significant difference in patient satisfaction, incidence of back pain, or physical function. The

TRAM group scored higher in the Medical Outcome Study Short Form-36 subjective energy category ($p = 0.01$) and mean Functional Assessment of Cancer Therapy-Breast score ($p = 0.01$).

Conclusions.—This study suggests no significant differences in donor-site morbidity, survey-based functional outcome, or patient satisfaction between bilateral TRAM and DIEP flap breast reconstruction. Although perforator flaps represent an important technological advancement, bilateral pedicled TRAM flap reconstruction still represents a good option for autologous breast reconstruction.

▶ This is an important beginning to evaluating the risks and benefits of 2 very popular and useful techniques for breast reconstruction using autologous tissue. We always need to be mindful as plastic and reconstructive surgeons that preference for one type of elective procedure or another should be based on its safety, morbidity, and patient outcome. It should also be evaluated appropriately and scientifically, rather than entirely on the choice of the surgeon. Studies measuring abdominal wall strength following pedicled transverse rectus abdominis myocutaneous breast reconstruction as opposed to deep inferior epigastric artery perforator (DIEP) flaps state that the former results in greater degree of weakness, but few actually determined that the weaknesses were of clinical significance.[1] This study is important, but its limitations include its small number of patients and average length of follow-up, its retrospective nature and having 2 different surgeons in 2 different institutions each performing only 1 type of surgery, and pedicled versus DIEP flap and each necessitating different methods for abdominal wall closure. The authors did make use of several tools to evaluate functional outcome and found no differences, but no attempt was made to actually measure abdominal wall strength and correlate that with the functional outcomes achieved. Finally, no attempt was made to compare costs at the 2 institutions.

S. H. Miller, MD, MPH

Reference

1. Atisha D, Alderman AK. A systematic review of abdominal wall function following abdominal flaps for postmastectomy breast reconstruction. *Ann Plast Surg.* 2009;63:222-230.

A single center comparison of one versus two venous anastomoses in 564 consecutive DIEP flaps: investigating the effect on venous congestion and flap survival
Enajat M, Rozen WM, Whitaker IS, et al (Uppsala Clinic Hosp, Sweden; The Univ of Melbourne, Parkville, Victoria, Australia; Morriston Hosp, Swansea, UK)
Microsurgery 30:185-191, 2010

Background.—Venous complications have been reported as the more frequently encountered vascular complications seen in the transfer of deep inferior epigastric artery (DIEA) perforator (DIEP) flaps, with a variety of techniques described for augmenting the venous drainage of these flaps to minimize venous congestion. The benefits of such techniques have not been shown to be of clinical benefit on a large scale due to the small number of cases in published series.

Methods.—A retrospective study of 564 consecutive DIEP flaps at a single institution was undertaken, comparing the prospective use of one venous anastomosis (273 cases) to two anastomoses (291 cases). The secondary donor vein comprised a second DIEA venae commitante in 7.9% of cases and a superficial inferior epigastric vein (SIEV) in 92.1%. Clinical outcomes were assessed, in particular rates of venous congestion.

Results.—The use of two venous anastomoses resulted in a significant reduction in the number of cases of venous congestion to zero (0 vs. 7, $P = 0.006$). All other outcomes were similar between groups. Notably, the use of a secondary vein did not result in any significant increase in operative time (385 minutes vs. 383 minutes, $P = 0.57$).

Conclusions.—The use of a secondary vein in the drainage of a DIEP flap can significantly reduce the incidence of venous congestion, with no detriment to complication rates. Consideration of incorporating both the superficial and deep venous systems is an approach that may further improve the venous drainage of the flap.

▶ With the increasing adoption of deep inferior epigastric perforator (DIEP) flaps, there has been the growing sense that the incidence of venous congestion is higher than that in the era of the free vertical rectus abdominis musculo-cutaneous (VRAM). Venous congestion can lead to fat necrosis, partial or complete flap loss. This large series (more than 500 flaps) from a single institution proposes that additional measures may be required to counter this trend. Specifically, they propose that for DIEP flaps, venous anastomosis to both the deep (vena commitans of the deep inferior epigastric artery) and superficial (superficial inferior epigastric vein [SIEV]) systems is required to decrease the incidence of venous congestion. In 273 cases with a single-vein anastomosis, there were 7 cases of venous congestion, compared with 0 cases in which 2 veins were anastomosed ($P = .006$). Interestingly, most of the second veins were SIEVs that were anastomosed to the cephalic veins through an anterior axillary incision. These were performed using clips or coupling devices and did not add any additional operative time. Although this was a retrospective study, it suggests that the increase in venous congestion can be prevented using a relatively simple approach. What is needed now is a preoperative way to predict which patients are at high risk of venous congestion so that this can be a planned part of the operative procedure rather than something that requires intraoperative decision making.

G. C. Gurtner, MD

Fibrin sealant decreases postoperative drainage in immediate breast reconstruction by deep inferior epigastric perforator flap after mastectomy with axillary dissection

Hivelin M, Heusse JL, Matar N, et al (Henri Mondor Hosp, Creteil, France; Hôpital Sud-Rennes-Rennes Univ, France)
Microsurgery 31:18-25, 2011

Background.—Serosanguinous drainage after breast reconstruction by deep inferior epigastric perforator flap (DIEP) can limit patient's discharge. We introduced fibrin sealant in immediate breast reconstruction by DIEP flap to reduce drainage after mastectomy with axillary dissection.

Materials and Methods.—We performed an open study on 30 consecutive female aged from 28 to 63 years old. All underwent immediate breast reconstructions by DIEP flaps after mastectomy and axillary dissection for cancer. Patients were divided in group 1 ($N = 15$) without fibrin sealant and group 2 ($N = 15$) where the flap, thoracic, and axillary areas were sprayed with 5 mL of liquid fibrin sealant before drains insertion. There was no difference in the patient's BMI, height, weight or age between both the groups. Blake suction drains were placed under the flap and in the axillary area.

Results.—No adverse effects were reported, after a 20-month median follow-up. Drainage volumes or durations were not correlated to the patient's BMI, nor the height, weight or age. Thoracic drainage duration was longer than abdominal drainage in both the groups. Average drained volumes from the thoracic area were lower (427 vs. 552 mL; $P = 0.015$) and thoracic drains were removed earlier (5.47 vs. 6.33 days $P = 0.022$), in group 2 than in group 1. The length of stay was also reduced after the use of fibrin sealant (5.53 vs. 6.33 days; $P = 0.032$).

Conclusion.—This study introduce the interest of fibrin sealant to significantly decrease the postoperative drainage volume and duration in the thoracic area after immediate breast reconstruction by DIEP flap.

▶ This is an interesting study from France recording the use of Tissucol, a fibrin sealant manufactured by Baxter, in some patients who underwent mastectomy, axillary dissection, and immediate deep inferior epigastric perforator flap breast reconstruction. The authors report that in the 15 patients who had the sealant applied, a statistically significant reduction in postoperative thoracic drainage and length of hospital stay was achieved, when compared with the 15 patients who did not have the sealant applied. To be fair, the study group and the control groups were handled by a single surgeon, but at 2 distinctly different periods so that all patients who did not receive sealant were operated in 2007 to 2008, and those who did receive sealant were operated on in 2008 to 2009. Furthermore, while reduction in drainage and length of stay were statistically different, I am not sure that they really were clinically significant. No attempt was made to compare the use of sealant against wound quilting, and the presumption was made that sending people home with drains was not desirable because of the risk of infection. The authors do take into account the cost of the Tissucol versus an extra day in a surgery unit to suggest that the use of this sealant is cost effective. The study needs to be broadened and enlarged, keeping in mind the proposed outcome that really demonstrates a clinically significant, as well as financial cost, advantage to the use of quilting or even sending patients home with drains.

S. H. Miller, MD, MPH

Clinical experience with the lateral septocutaneous superior gluteal artery perforator flap for autologous breast reconstruction
Rad AN, Flores JI, Prucz RB, et al (The Johns Hopkins Univ, Baltimore, MD)
Microsurgery 30:339-347, 2010

Background.—Superior gluteal artery perforator (SGAP) flaps are a useful adjunct for autologous microvascular breast reconstruction. However, limitations of short pedicle length, complex anatomy, and donor site deformity make it an unpopular choice. Our goals were to define the anatomic characteristics of SGAPs in cadavers, and report preliminary clinical and radiographic results of using the lateral septocutaneous perforating branches of the superior gluteal artery (LSGAP) as the basis for a modified gluteal flap.

Methods.—We performed 12 cadaveric dissections and retrospectively reviewed 12 consecutive breast reconstruction patients with gluteal flaps (19 flaps: 9 LSGAP, 10 traditional SGAP) over a 12-month period. The LSGAP flap was converted to traditional SGAP in 53% of flaps because of dominance of a traditional intramuscular perforator. Preoperative 3D computed tomography angiography (CTA) and cadaveric dissections were used to define anatomy. Anatomic, demographic, radiographic, perioperative, and outcomes data were analyzed. Mean follow-up was 4 ± 3.4 months (range 4 weeks to 10 months).

Results.—Compared with the pedicle in the SGAP flap, the mean pedicle length in the LSGAP flap was 1.54 times longer by CTA, 2.05 times longer by cadaver dissection, and 2.36 times longer by intraoperative bilateral measurement. These differences were statistically significant ($P < 0.001$). Clinically, 100% of the flaps survived.

Conclusions.—LSGAP flap reconstruction is advantageous, when feasible, because of the septocutaneous pedicle dissection and gain in pedicle length that make microsurgical anastomoses easier without compromising gluteus function (Fig 4).

▶ This is an interesting early study of the potential of a lateral septocutaneous perforator flap (LSGAP) for breast reconstruction rather than a standard superior gluteal artery perforator flap (SGAP) when the patient does not have adequate abdominal wall tissue for breast reconstruction. The standard SGAP flap, while useful in the armamentarium of reconstructive breast surgeons is less popular because of the complexity of harvesting the flap and the major deformity created in the donor site. Although the advantages of the LGSAP

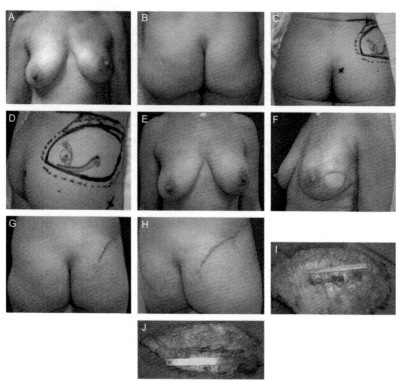

FIGURE 4.—(A) This is a 47-year-old female with invasive left ductal carcinoma who received a nipple-sparing mastectomy. She had preoperative breast asymmetry with grade I ptosis on the right. (B) The abdominal donor site was inadequate, therefore LSGAP was planned. Note lower lateral buttock "saddle bag" deformity. (C and D) Flap outline. Dotted lines represent beveled edge of deep gluteal fat. The most medial tip of the flap captures the central intramuscular perforators, which support the traditional SGAP flap. (E and F) Postoperative result following nipple-sparing mastectomy and flap with restoration of volume and improved symmetry. (G and H) Donor site spares central buttock mound. Lower lateral "saddle bag" has been improved in contour with a scar still hidden within the "bikini line." (I) Traditional SGAP pedicle length is 5.5 cm in this case example, whereas (J) LSGAP pedicle length measures 13 cm in a different patient, a ratio of lengths of 2.36. [Color figure can be viewed in the online issue, which is available at www.interscience.wiley.com.] (Reprinted from Rad AN, Flores JI, Prucz RB, et al. Clinical experience with the lateral septocutaneous superior gluteal artery perforator flap for autologous breast reconstruction. *Microsurgery.* 2010;30:339-347, with permission from Wiley-Liss, Inc.)

seem quite evident, such as longer pedicle length, less prone to compromise gluteus function and much less prone to deformity of the buttock, the lateral septal perforator vessels were inadequate for use in more than 50% of the dissections forcing use of the traditional central SGAP vessels. This modification does seem to have potential, but further study is necessary to fully understand its benefits and limitations.

S. H. Miller, MD, MPH

Is a Second Free Flap Still an Option in a Failed Free Flap Breast Reconstruction?

Hamdi M, Andrades P, Thiessen F, et al (Gent Univ Hosp, Belgium)
Plast Reconstr Surg 126:375-384, 2010

Background.—Salvage of a failed autologous breast reconstruction is a complex and challenging problem. The purpose of this study was to analyze the indications, methods, and outcomes of tertiary surgery in patients with a failed autologous breast reconstruction.

Methods.—A retrospective chart review was performed for all patients who underwent breast reconstruction with autologous tissue performed by the senior author (M.H.) between 2002 and 2009. Special emphasis was made to evaluate the first reconstruction performed, causes of failure, indications for tertiary reconstruction, and outcomes. A preoperative hematologic workout was performed. For patients who were classified within the highest group of thromboembolism, specific prophylactic measurements were taken for the tertiary surgery.

Results.—Of 688 patients who underwent autologous breast reconstruction, a total of 14 patients required tertiary breast reconstruction. Hypercoagulability was found in three patients resulting from disorders such as lupus anticoagulant positivity and antiphospholipid syndrome. Six patients (43 percent) underwent a combination of local skin flaps and/or implant reconstructions. Eight patients (57 percent) underwent nine microvascular breast reconstructions: five superior gluteal artery perforator flaps, three transverse myocutaneous gracilis flaps, and one deep inferior epigastric artery perforator flap. Two of nine flaps (22 percent) required quaternary reconstructions because of a failure of the second free flap. Additional corrections such as revision lipofilling, scar revision, contralateral breast shaping, implant change, and capsulotomies were performed in 92.7 percent of the patients, with a mean follow-up of 37 months (range, 6 months to 7 years).

Conclusions.—Tertiary surgery after autologous breast reconstruction failure has limited options and further reoperations are often needed. Careful patient history and selective blood tests may reveal hidden coagulation disorders. When a second free flap is planned, primary and secondary antithrombotic therapy should be considered.

▶ This article provides evidence that a second free flap after failed free flap breast reconstruction can be an appropriate and justified procedure provided that a number of important criteria are met: (1) a careful analysis of the reasons for the initial flap failure is carried out; (2) reasonable alternatives are considered; and (3) every possible extra precaution (including consideration of antithrombotic therapy) is taken. If the original free flap was chosen because it would provide the optimal result for reconstruction in a particular patient, then doing something other than a second free flap (eg, a latissimus dorsi flap plus implant) would likely yield a less-than-optimal result after the original flap failed. It clearly is important to determine that the patient is willing to undergo another complicated, time-consuming, and expensive salvage procedure. But if the patient is willing and the appropriate steps have been taken, the surgeon is justified in proceeding with a second free flap.

R. L. Ruberg, MD

Postoperative Monitoring of Free Flaps in Autologous Breast Reconstruction: A Multicenter Comparison of 398 Flaps Using Clinical Monitoring, Microdialysis, and the Implantable Doppler Probe
Whitaker IS, Rozen WM, Chubb D, et al (Uppsala Univ Hosp, Sweden; Univ of Melbourne, Victoria, Australia; et al)
J Reconstr Microsurg 26:409-416, 2010

Many techniques for flap monitoring following free tissue transfer have been described; however, there is little evidence that any of these techniques allow for greater rates of flap salvage over clinical monitoring alone. We sought to compare three established monitoring techniques across three experienced microsurgical centers in a comparable cohort of patients. A retrospective, matched cohort study of 398 consecutive free flaps in 347 patients undergoing autologous breast reconstruction was undertaken across three institutions during the same 3-year period, with a single form of postoperative monitoring used at each institution: clinical monitoring alone, the Cook-Swartz implantable Doppler probe, or microdialysis. Both objective and subjective measures of efficacy were assessed. Clinical monitoring alone, the implantable Doppler probe, and microdialysis showed statistically similar rates of flap salvage. False-negative rates were also statistically similar (only seen in the clinically monitored group). However, there was a statistically significant increase in false-positive alarms causing needless take-backs to theater in the microdialysis and implantable Doppler arms, $p < 0.001$. This study did not find any technique superior to clinical monitoring alone. New monitoring technologies should be compared objectively with clinical monitoring as the current standard in postoperative flap monitoring.

▶ This is an interesting retrospective matched study from Australia detailing an experience in 3 different centers monitoring free flaps used for breast reconstruction. The authors conclude that in their study, clinical monitoring was as effective and efficient as monitoring with a Doppler probe system, Cook-Schwartz, and/or microdialysis when assessing final salvage rate and false-negative rates but that the 2 types of monitoring devices produced increased numbers of false positives. This is in contradiction to the study reported by Rozen et al.[1] In truth, though, only 1 of 111 patients being monitored by the Doppler probe system had a false positive, and ultimately the overall survival of these flaps is very high thus providing a very small cohort of flap salvage cases to study. In light of the disparity of experience in the 3 centers, one must wonder why the type of monitoring was not randomized among the 3. It is also of interest that in the only group with documented false negatives, the clinical monitoring group, 2 flaps had significant necrosis, and one wonders why they were not returned to the operating room before they developed necrosis. The development of accurate cost-effective monitoring of flap modalities is essential in buried free flaps and tissue transfers.

S. H. Miller, MD, MPH

Reference

1. Rozen WM, Chubb D, Whitaker IS, Acosta R. The efficacy of postoperative monitoring: a single surgeon comparison of clinical monitoring and the implantable Doppler Probe in 547 consecutive free flaps. *Microsurgery.* 2010;30:105-110.

Effects of Vasopressor Administration on the Outcomes of Microsurgical Breast Reconstruction

Chen C, Nguyen M-D, Bar-Meir E, et al (Dept of Surgery, Boston, MA; et al)
Ann Plast Surg 65:28-31, 2010

The use of vasopressors during microsurgery is still debated. General anesthesia often induces hypotension, but microsurgeons are reluctant to use intraoperative vasopressors with the potential risks of vasoconstriction. A retrospective review was performed on 187 consecutive patients undergoing 258 deep inferior epigastric perforator flaps, free transverse rectus abdominis myocutaneous flap, and muscle-sparing free transverse rectus abdominis myocutaneous flap operations. A total of 102 patients (140 flaps) received intraoperative ephedrine and/or phenylephrine and 85 patients (118 flaps) did not. The administration of vasopressors did not affect the rates of reoperation, complete flap loss, partial flap loss, or fat necrosis. Patients recciving vasopressors had no differences in operative time, number of perforators, or number of rows of perforators harvested. There was no statistically significant association between dosage, timing, and complications. Although we do not recommend routine vasopressor use during microsurgery, administration does not seem to increase complications in microsurgical breast reconstruction.

▶ Development of a hypotensive state often accompanies the administration of a general anesthetic. Many surgeons, including microsurgeons, concerned about the effects of vasoconstriction, are very reluctant to use vasopressors to overcome hypotension during the course of a general anesthetic. These authors have provided us with a retrospective case study comparing 2 groups of patients, those who received vasopressors and those who did not, undergoing a variety of free flap breast reconstructions. They conclude that in this study no increase in complications were apparent. Although their findings might provide a measure of comfort to others using abdominal free flaps for breast reconstruction, there are far too many uncontrolled variables in this study for its ready acceptance and generalization to all areas of microsurgery. Two different vasopressors, ephedrine and phenylephrine, were used and each has a different primary mechanism of action. Additionally, the dosages of the vasopressors varied for different patients. It is unclear whether the 2 groups were truly alike in all variables other than the use of vasopressors. Finally, could these results be replicated in flaps harvested from and inserted into different anatomic locations?

The major problem with the animal studies reported is that the design in all of the studies varied as to the experimental animal used, the type of flap studied, pedicle versus free flap, and the types of vasopressors used and their routes of administration. It would seem to me that an experimental protocol could and should be developed to address the question, Are vasopressors deleterious in microsurgery?

S. H. Miller, MD

Effects of Vasopressor Administration on the Outcomes of Microsurgical Breast Reconstruction

Chen C, Nguyen M-D, Bar-Meir E, et al (Dept of Surgery, Boston, MA; et al)
Ann Plast Surg 65:28-31, 2010

The use of vasopressors during microsurgery is still debated. General anesthesia often induces hypotension, but microsurgeons are reluctant to use intraoperative vasopressors with the potential risks of vasoconstriction. A retrospective review was performed on 187 consecutive patients undergoing 258 deep inferior epigastric perforator flaps, free transverse rectus abdominis myocutaneous flap, and muscle-sparing free transverse rectus abdominis myocutaneous flap operations. A total of 102 patients (140 flaps) received intraoperative ephedrine and/or phenylephrine and 85 patients (118 flaps) did not. The administration of vasopressors did not affect the rates of reoperation, complete flap loss, partial flap loss, or fat necrosis. Patients receiving vasopressors had no differences in operative time, number of perforators, or number of rows of perforators harvested. There was no statistically significant association between dosage, timing, and complications. Although we do not recommend routine vasopressor use during microsurgery, administration does not seem to increase complications in microsurgical breast reconstruction.

▶ This is a nicely done study that suffers only from a lack of numbers. The conclusion that vasopressor administration does not affect outcome is comforting. On the other hand, we should not be too comforted so that the indication for vasopressor administration is changed. My belief is that there is still no substitute for volume. I would also wonder if there is a difference between end-to-end and end-to-side anastamoses with vasopressor use.

D. J. Smith, Jr, MD

Cold ischemia in microvascular breast reconstruction

Lee DT, Lee G (Stanford Univ, Palo Alto, CA)
Microsurgery 30:361-367, 2010

Introduction.—A major drawback to microvascular free flap breast reconstruction is the length of operation—up to 9 hours or more for bilateral reconstruction. This takes a significant mental and physical toll on the surgical team, producing fatigue that may compromise surgical outcome. To facilitate the operation we have incorporated a period of cold ischemia of the flaps such that members of the surgical team can alternate a brief respite during the operation.

Methods.—We retrospectively reviewed our series of microvascular free flap breast reconstructions performed over a four-year period in which cold ischemia of the flaps were induced.

Results.—Seventy patients underwent free flap breast reconstruction with 104 flaps. Mean cold ischemia time for all flaps was 2 hours 36 min. Average rest time per surgeon per case was 35 min. Complications included two total flap losses (1.9%), one partial flap loss (1.0%), one anastomotic thrombosis (1.0%), two hematomas (1.9%), three fat necrosis (2.9%), and two delayed healing (1.9%). Statistical analysis revealed that the probability of complications is inversely related to cold ischemia time ($P = 0.0163$).

Conclusion.—Cold ischemia facilitates breast reconstruction by allowing the surgical team to alternate breaks during the operation. This helps reduce surgeon fatigue and is well tolerated by the flap. Thus, we believe that the use of cold ischemia is safe and advantageous in microvascular breast reconstruction.

▶ The planned use of cold ischemia as part of the free flap procedure is interesting. Because the outcome of any procedure cannot be predicted, it stands to reason that the authors are recommending this for all procedures. The level of detail is impressive: protecting the vascular pedicle from the ice, turning every 15 minutes, and manipulation of the ice slush machine. More important, and to some degree lost in the article, is the importance of overall planning. These authors have given a great deal of thought to working as a team to improve outcome. My guess is that the cold ischemia is only one of several improvements made in their free flap surgery.

D. J. Smith, Jr, MD

Aesthetic outcome and oncological safety of nipple—areola complex replantation after mastectomy and immediate breast reconstruction

Wirth R, Banic A, Erni D (Univ of Bern, Switzerland)
J Plast Reconstr Aesthet Surg 63:1490-1494, 2010

Immediate breast reconstruction (IBR) has become an established procedure for women necessitating mastectomy. Traditionally, the nipple—areola complex (NAC) is resected during this procedure. The NAC, in turn, is a principal factor determining aesthetic outcome after breast reconstruction, and due to its particular texture and shape, a natural-looking NAC can barely be reconstructed with other tissues. The aim of this study was to assess the oncological safety as well as morbidity and aesthetic outcome after replantation of the NAC some days after IBR.

Retrospective analysis of 85 patients receiving 88 mastectomies and IBR between 1998 and 2007 was conducted. NAC ($n = 29$) or the nipple alone ($n = 23$) were replanted 7 days (median, range 2—10 days) after IBR in 49 patients, provided the subareolar tissue was histologically negative for tumour infiltration. Local recurrence rate was assessed after 49 months (median, range 6—120 months). Aesthetic outcome was evaluated by clinical assessment during routine follow-up at least 12 months after the last intervention.

Malignant involvement of the subareolar tissue was found in eight cases (9.1%). Patients qualifying for NAC replantation were in stage 0 in 29%, stage I in 15%, stage IIa in 31%, stage IIb in 17% and stage III in 8%. Total or partial necrosis occurred in 69% and 26% if the entire NAC or only the nipple were replanted, respectively ($P < 0.01$). Depigmentation was seen in 52% and corrective surgery was done in 11 out of 52 NAC or nipple replantations. Local recurrence and isolated regional lymph node metastasis were observed in one single case each. Another 5.8% of the patients showed distant metastases.

We conclude that the replantation of the NAC in IBR is oncologically safe, provided the subareolar tissue is free of tumour. However, the long-term aesthetic outcome of NAC replantation is not satisfying, which advocates replanting the nipple alone (Fig 1).

▶ This is a large, retrospective, uncontrolled study of the safety and aesthetic outcome after replantation of the nipple-areolar complex (NAC) and/or nipple following immediate breast reconstruction. The authors address the issue of oncologic safety by only replanting the NAC or nipple after careful review of permanent sections of the tissue beneath the NAC/nipple as opposed to the use of frozen sections because the latter have been associated with a high false-negative rate. While promoting safety, this protocol required them to store the NAC and/or nipples and delay replantation for between 2 to 10 days. While stating that this delay in replantation had little effect on the end result, a relatively high incidence of complete or partial necrosis and depigmentation, the number of patients studied were quite small and I am unsure that the duration of storage had no effect on the aesthetic outcome. Overall, the

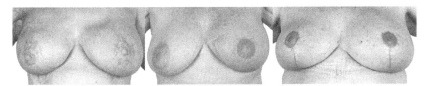

FIGURE 1.—View of replanted NAC's in three different patients 12 months postoperatively, showing poor (left), moderate (middle) and good (right) results. 56 years old patient after bilateral SSM and TRAM reconstruction (left). 65 years old patient after unilateral SSM and TRAM reconstruction (middle). 47 year old patient after SSM and TRAM reconstruction on the left side and adaptive reduction mammoplasty on the right side (right). (Reprinted from Wirth R, Banic A, Erni D. Aesthetic outcome and oncological safety of nipple–areola complex replantation after mastectomy and immediate breast reconstruction. *J Plast Reconstr Aesthet Surg*. 2010;63:1490-1494, with permission from British Association of Plastic, Reconstructive and Aesthetic Surgeons.)

authors concluded that in spite of the high failure/complication rates, the procedure, when it worked provided better results than could be obtained with other methods of NAC reconstruction and when it fails little has been lost. This opinion requires further study and documentation.

S. H. Miller, MD, MPH

Surgical Correction and Reconstruction of the Nipple-Areola Complex: Current Review of Techniques
Boccola MA, Savage J, Rozen WM, et al (Univ of Melbourne, Victoria, Australia)
J Reconstr Microsurg 26:589-600, 2010

Nipple malformations are common congenital or acquired conditions that can have tremendous cosmetic, psychological, breast-feeding, sexual, and hygienic ramifications. Ideal reconstruction of the nipple-areola complex (NAC) requires symmetry in position, size, shape, texture, pigmentation, and permanent projection, and although many technical descriptions of NAC reconstruction exist in the medical literature, there are insufficient data presented to accurately compare outcomes. The current article comprises a thorough review of the literature, exploring the techniques described for NAC reconstruction, comparing reported outcomes and complications, and providing an evidence-based approach to NAC reconstruction. The findings of the review suggest that evidence regarding surgical correction of nipple deformity and complete NAC reconstruction is lacking, and loss of nipple projection over time is a pervasive problem common to all flap techniques. A combination of a single pedicle local flap with tattooing for complete NAC reconstruction is currently the most supported method; however, data concerning which type of reconstruction is best suited to immediate versus delayed and type of breast mound remain to be examined.

▶ This is an excellent very comprehensive review article dealing with the correction and the reconstruction of the nipple-areola complex (NAC). As such, it provides the reader, in 1 location, with the literature on the subject as published in the English language. The authors provide information on the correction of inverted and hypertrophic nipples and NACs removed during the course of treatment of breast carcinoma. They correctly point out the paucity of information regarding the best method for nipple-areola reconstruction, especially when the reconstruction is performed immediately rather than when delayed. Ideally, if one had no oncological concerns about the native NAC and a partial mastectomy was to be performed, the best results would likely be achieved using the patient's own NAC. If that is not possible, the 2 main difficulties with reconstruction of the NAC, regardless of the method used, remain loss of projection of the nipple and failure to provide a good color match, on a long-term basis, of the reconstructed areola.

S. H. Miller, MD, MPH

Application of Screening Principles to the Reconstructed Breast
Zakhireh J, Fowble B, Esserman LJ (Univ of California, San Francisco)
J Clin Oncol 28:173-180, 2010

A significant number of women choose mastectomy for the treatment of early and locally advanced breast cancer. Advances in reconstruction techniques and greater awareness of options have led to an increased use of immediate breast reconstruction, which has resulted in uncertainty for the management of surveillance for local recurrence. In this article, we review mastectomy and reconstruction trends and how these techniques affect the frequency and location of local recurrence. The data on surveillance imaging of the reconstructed breast are extremely limited. However, by assessing the potential role for imaging in this setting and applying the principles of screening, we have identified that there is a potential theoretic advantage of surveillance imaging in a very small subset of women: those with autologous tissue reconstructions and moderate to high risk of recurrence. A prospective registry study of surveillance imaging in this target population would be the appropriate way to determine its benefit and its impact on survival outcomes. In this review article, we will detail the reasons that should allow clinicians to forego routine surveillance imaging in the majority of women who undergo mastectomy and reconstruction (Table 1).

▶ This study is of importance to all general surgeons performing mastectomies and all plastic surgeons performing breast reconstructions after prophylactic and/or therapeutic mastectomy. The question addressed is after reconstruction, what type of postoperative surveillance (physical examination, mammography, and magnetic resonance imaging) is best and when should it be performed to detect locoregional recurrences, which, as a consequence of early detection and treatment, can positively impact patient survival? Unfortunately, no studies are currently available that establish clinical guidelines. The authors conclude that physical examination is sufficient for implant reconstructions when the

TABLE 1.—Prognostic Risk Factors That Influence Locoregional Recurrence* After Mastectomy

Characteristic	Favorable	Intermediate	Poor
Patient characteristics	Age > 35 years	Age < 50 years; premenopausal	Age ≤ 35 years
Clinical staging	T1-2	T3	T4; T3 with any positive lymph nodes
Tumor characteristics	Low to intermediate grade	High grade	Positive margins
	LVI absent	LVI present	
	ER/PR positive	Extracapsular extension	
		Multicentricity	
Lymph node status	Negative lymph nodes	1-3 positive lymph nodes	> 4 positive lymph nodes
Response to neoadjuvant chemotherapy	Yp T1-2, N0	Yp T1-2, N1-3, age > 35 years	Yp T3 with any positive lymph nodes
	Initial stage I-II with complete pathologic response after neoadjuvant chemotherapy	Initial stage IIIA with complete response to chemotherapy	Initial stage IIIB with complete response to neoadjuvant chemotherapy
		Stage II with residual disease in nodes or breast	Stage III with residual disease in nodes or breast

NOTE. Data adapted.[17,18,29,30,70-74]
Abbreviations: LVI, lymphovascular invasion; ER, estrogen receptor; PR, progesterone receptor; Yp, after neoadjuvant chemotherapy.
Editor's Note: Please refer to original journal article for full references.
*Estimated locoregional recurrence risk for a 5-year period: low risk, < 10%; intermediate risk, 10% to 20%; high risk, > 20%.

implant is placed behind the pectoralis muscle but in fact offer little evidence for this statement. Generally speaking, they have suggested that routine radiologic surveillance is best done with mammography in moderate- to high-risk patients (Figs 1 and 2 in the original article) who have undergone autologous breast reconstruction, but they clearly documented the lack of specific evidence to support this stance. I agree with their suggestion that we need a prospective registry study to determine how best to follow up with breast cancer patients who have been reconstructed, when to use imaging, what type of imaging, and in which patients will it prove most beneficial.

S. H. Miller, MD, MPH

Determining the Oncological Risk of Autologous Lipoaspirate Grafting for Post-Mastectomy Breast Reconstruction
Rigotti G, Marchi A, Stringhini P, et al (Azienda Ospedaliera di Verona, P. le Stefani, Italy; et al)
Aesth Plast Surg 34:475-480, 2010

This study compares the incidence of local and regional recurrence of breast cancer between two contiguous time windows in a homogeneous population of 137 patients who underwent fat tissue transplant after modified radical mastectomy. Median follow-up time was 7.6 years and the follow-up period was divided into two contiguous time windows, the first starting at the date of the radical mastectomy and ending at the first lipoaspirate grafting session and the second beginning at the time of the first lipoaspirate grafting session and ending at the end of the total follow-up time. Although this study did not employ an independent control group, the incidence of local recurrence of breast cancer was found to be comparable between the two periods and in line with data from similar patient populations enrolled in large multicenter clinical trials and who did not undergo postsurgical fat tissue grafting. Statistical comparison of disease-free survival curves revealed no significant differences in relapse rate between the two patient subgroups before fat grafting and after fat grafting. Although further confirmation is needed from multicenter randomized clinical trials, our results support the hypothesis that autologous lipoaspirate transplant combines striking regenerative properties with no or marginal effects on the probability of post-mastectomy locoregional recurrence of breast cancer.

▶ This report provides further support for the safety of autologous fat grafts as part of breast reconstruction. While we await supporting studies with longer follow-up intervals, we can feel more comfortable in offering this additional technique to our breast cancer patients.

K. A. Gutowski, MD

Early Results Using Ultrasound-Assisted Liposuction as a Treatment for Fat Necrosis in Breast Reconstruction

Hassa A, Curtis MS, Colakoglu S, et al (Univ of Western Ontario, London, Ontario, Canada; Beth Israel Deaconess Med Ctr, Boston, MA)
Plast Reconstr Surg 126:762-768, 2010

Background.—Fat necrosis is a common complication from autologous breast reconstruction that can compromise the aesthetic outcome and can be confused with recurrent breast cancer. Removal of fat necrosis through direct excision can be difficult with lesions in the periphery and may result in contour deformities. The article describes a case series of patients with fat necrosis treated with ultrasound-assisted liposuction.

Methods.—A retrospective database was created consisting of consecutive patients treated with ultrasound-assisted liposuction at a single academic institution. Patient demographics and complications were identified, including initial size of fat necrosis, number of ultrasound-assisted liposuction treatments, and final size of fat necrosis. Surgical technique was standardized over the entire series.

Results.—There were 54 breast reconstructions with fat necrosis treated with ultrasound-assisted liposuction. The average initial size of fat necrosis was 2.72 cm. Twenty-seven lesions (50.0 percent) were treated once, 20 (37.0 percent) were treated twice, and seven (13.0 percent) were treated three times. The final size of fat necrosis was 0.44 cm ($p < 0.0001$), with an average time to follow-up of 17.8 months. Complete resolution (<0.5 cm) was seen in 44 lesions (81.5 percent). Only one complication, a thermal burn, was seen from ultrasound-assisted liposuction, and this resolved with conservative management.

Conclusions.—This case series describes the successful use of ultrasound-assisted liposuction for treatment of fat necrosis after autologous breast reconstruction. The authors find this technique to be safe, effective, and reproducible, as the majority of fat necrosis areas resolved with one or two treatments (Figs 2 and 5).

▶ This preliminary retrospective study of the use of ultrasound-assisted liposuction for fat necrosis following breast reconstruction is interesting and potentially useful in the right group of patients but raises several unanswered questions. The incidence of fat necrosis is subject to wide interpretation depending on the type of flap used for reconstruction, the technique(s) used to diagnose necrosis, and how long after the reconstruction the diagnosis was made. The authors state that fat necrosis should be treated because of the following 3 issues: (1) aesthetics, but of course small areas of fat necrosis, less than 2 cm, may not be apparent at all to the patient, or others, so that the indications for treatment based on size and aesthetic appearance need to be further studied; (2) most patients with fat necrosis do not have pain or discomfort, so that indication needs to be more

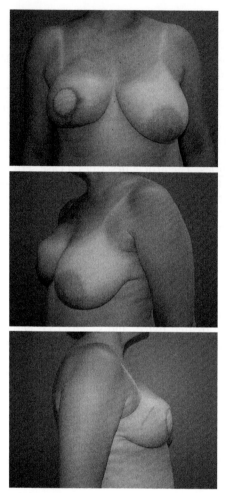

FIGURE 2.—Superior pole fat necrosis (4 cm) seen at 3 months after mastectomy and DIEP flap reconstruction. (*Above*) Anterior view. (*Center*) Oblique view (the area of fat necrosis at the superior pole of the far breast). (*Below*) Lateral view. (Reprinted from Hassa A, Curtis MS, Colakoglu S, et al. Early results using ultrasound-assisted liposuction as a treatment for fat necrosis in breast reconstruction. *Plast Reconstr Surg*. 2010;126:762-768.)

clearly delineated; and (3) cancer recurrence is quite small and needs to be ruled in or out long before liposuction is undertaken especially because the technique has not been demonstrated to be able to identify tumor cells in the aspirate. Finally, the issue of cost-benefit analysis of the technique needs to be addressed.

S. H. Miller, MD, MPH

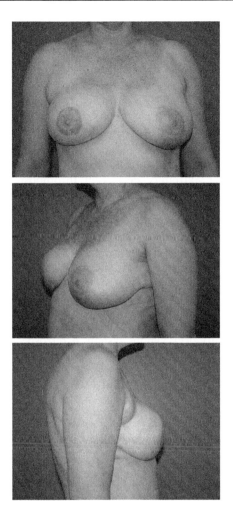

FIGURE 5.—Same patient as shown in Figure 2, 30 months after a single ultrasound-assisted liposuction treatment to the area of fat necrosis. Note complete resolution of the superior pole contour irregularity. On examination, there was complete softening of the lesion, with no firmness. (*Above*) Anterior view. (*Center*) Oblique view. (*Below*) Lateral view. (Reprinted from Hassa A, Curtis MS, Colakoglu S, et al. Early results using ultrasound-assisted liposuction as a treatment for fat necrosis in breast reconstruction. *Plast Reconstr Surg.* 2010;126:762-768.)

Venous Thromboembolism following Microsurgical Breast Reconstruction: An Objective Analysis in 225 Consecutive Patients Using Low-Molecular-Weight Heparin Prophylaxis

Lemaine V, McCarthy C, Kaplan K, et al (Memorial Sloan-Kettering Cancer Ctr, NY)

Plast Reconstr Surg 127:1399-1406, 2011

Background.—Free flap breast reconstruction involves major risk factors for postsurgical venous thromboembolism. The main study objectives were (1) to estimate objectively the incidence of symptomatic and asymptomatic lower extremity deep vein thrombosis in patients who received postoperative thromboprophylaxis after free flap breast reconstruction, (2) to evaluate the safety of low-molecular-weight heparin postoperatively, and (3) to assess the incidence of symptomatic pulmonary embolism or sudden death.

Methods.—A cohort study of 225 consecutive patients who underwent abdominally based free flap breast reconstruction at a single cancer center was conducted. The postoperative thromboprophylaxis regimen was based on the American College of Chest Physicians guidelines. A study group of 118 patients systematically underwent bilateral lower extremity duplex ultrasound before hospital discharge to assess objectively the status of the lower extremity deep venous system. A retrospective cohort of 107 women who were not systematically screened for deep vein thrombosis was used for comparison.

Results.—The incidence of postoperative deep vein thrombosis confirmed by duplex ultrasound was 3.4 percent in the study group, all events being clinically silent. Bleeding complications in the entire patient sample were estimated at 5.3 percent. Partial flap loss and total flap loss rates were 2.7 and 1.9 percent, respectively. No venous thromboembolism event was diagnosed in the control group.

Conclusions.—This report shows that the objective incidence of deep vein thrombosis was 3.4 percent within 5 postoperative days in this patient population. The authors' findings support the use of triple thromboprophylaxis and demonstrate that low-molecular-weight heparin is a safe and effective method for prevention of venous thromboembolism in this population.

▶ This is the first epidemiological study to objectively assess the incidence of deep vein thrombosis in women receiving thromboprophylaxis following microsurgical breast reconstruction. The results demonstrate that this method of prophylaxis is highly effective in preventing venous thromboembolism events in the vast majority of women undergoing microvascular breast reconstruction. This provides early confirmation of this treatment modality. Although there are several shortcomings, that is, sample size, overall it confirms the importance of this methodology. The onus is quickly shifting to acceptance of this methodology.

D. J. Smith, Jr, MD

7 Scars and Wound Healing

Scars

Scar Prevention Using Laser-Assisted Skin Healing (LASH) in Plastic Surgery

Capon A, Iarmarcovai G, Gonnelli D, et al (Service de Chirurgie Plastique et Réparatrice, CHRU, Lille, France; Service de Chirurgie Plastique et Réparatrice, APHM, Marseille, France; et al)

Aesth Plast Surg 34:438-446, 2010

Background.—The use of lasers has been proposed for scar revision. A recent pilot clinical study demonstrated that lasers could also be used immediately after surgery to reduce the appearance of scars. The LASH (Laser-Assisted Skin Healing) technique induces a temperature elevation in the skin which modifies the wound-healing process. We report a prospective comparative clinical trial aimed at evaluating an 810-nm diode-laser system to accelerate and improve the healing process in surgical scars immediately after skin closure.

Methods.—Twenty-nine women and 1 man (mean age = 41.4 years; Fitzpatrick skin types I-IV) were included to evaluate the safety and performance of the laser system. The laser dose (or fluence in J/cm^2) was selected as a function of phototype and skin thickness. Each surgical incision (e.g., abdominoplasty) was divided into two parts. An 8-cm segment was treated with the laser immediately after skin closure. A separate 8-cm segment was left untreated as a control. Clinical evaluations (overall appearance ratings, comparative scar scale) of all scars were conducted at 10 days, 3 months, and 12 months by both surgeon and patients. Profilometry analysis from silicone replicas of the skin was done at 12 months. Wilcoxon signed-rank test analyses were performed.

Results.—Twenty-two patients were treated using a high dose (80–130 J/cm^2) and 8 patients with a low dose (<80 J/cm^2). At 12 months in the high-dose group, both surgeon and patients reported an improvement rate of the laser-treated segment over the control area of 72.73 and 59.10%, respectively. For these patients, profilometry results showed a decrease in scar height of 38.1% ($p = 0.027$) at 12 months for the laser-treated segment versus control. Three patients treated with higher doses (>115 J/cm^2) experienced superficial burns on the laser-treated segment, which resolved in about 5–7 days. For the eight patients treated at low dosage (<80 J/cm^2), there was no significant difference in the treated segment versus the control segment. No side effects were observed.

Conclusion.—This prospective comparative trial demonstrates that an 810-nm diode laser treatment, performed immediately after surgery, can improve the appearance of a surgical scar. The dose plays a great role in scar improvement and must be well controlled. There is interest in LASH for hypertrophic scar revision. LASH can be used to prevent and reduce scars in plastic surgery.

▶ This approach of dealing with unfavorable postoperative scars by pretreating with laser therapy at the time of skin closure is innovative and shows a statistical improvement in scar appearance compared with no treatment. However, while the scar ratings did show a better scar appearance on the high-dose laser treatment areas, it was difficult for this editor to see a visual difference based on the actual 12-month postoperative patient photographs presented in this article. From a practical perspective, it may not be realistic to offer this additional treatment for surgeries performed at hospitals or surgery centers where a laser is not routinely available. Perhaps a better approach would be to apply the laser treatment at the time of the first postoperative visit to the surgeon's office.

K. A. Gutowski, MD

Wound Healing

Biologic dressings
Junkins-Hopkins JM (Johns Hopkins Med Insts, Baltimore, MD)
J Am Acad Dermatol 64:e5-e7, 2011

Background.—Various human and skin substitutes are available for use as biologic dressings. The choice of product relies on multiple factors, such as type, size, and depth of the wound; comorbid conditions; and patient preferences. The advantages and disadvantages of various biologic dressings were outlined.

Products.—Epicel is an epidermal autograft cultured from healthy human skin and has a 1-day half-life. It is most useful as a lifesaving intervention in burn patients, but also successful for pyoderma gangrenosum and epidermolysis bullosa.

Dermal and composite biologic dressings include Apligraf, which contains living allogeneic cells. The epidermal component is neonatal foreskin keratinocytes seeded on a dermal component of neonatal foreskin fibroblasts in a matrix of bovine type I collagen. When stored at 68° to 73° F, a 0.75-cm disk has a 10-day shelf life. This temporary wound cover is secured to the sterile, debrided, and edema-free wound bed using sutures or dressing and changed weekly. Apligraf's performance is significantly better than compression in healing large, deep venous ulcers present for more than a year. Osteomyelitis and amputation rates are lower with Apligraf, and scars may be more pliable and less vascular than healing with secondary intention.

Orocel is a biologic cellular matrix of neonatal foreskin epidermal keratinocytes and dermal fibroblasts cultured onto a preformed porous sponge. It is cryopreserved rather than fresh like Apligraf.

Among the synthetic dermal substitutes are Dermagraft, which comprises neonatal fibroblasts cultured on a scaffold of polyglactin 910. This frozen product stimulates the ingrowth of fibrovascular tissue and epithelialization and has a shelf life of 6 months. Its primary use is in healing complex surgical wounds with secondary closure.

Integra is a bilaminar skin equivalent composed of a porous matrix of cross-linked bovine collagen and shark-derived glycosaminoglycan. A semipermeable silicone layer is attached to serve as an epidermis. Integra prevents water loss, provides a flexible wound covering, and serves as a scaffold that promotes neovascularization and new dermal growth. It is usually used for partial and full-thickness wounds; pressure, diabetic, and chronic vascular and venous ulcers; and surgical wounds. This single-use product must be applied on a flat, uniform wound that has been completely and surgically debrided. Online training is required to obtain a certification number for purchase and the application procedure is not convenient. Integra is readily available, can cover large surfaces, and has a shelf life of 2 years at room temperature. It inhibits scar formation and wound contraction, making it especially useful for keloid repair.

The acellular dermal matrix device Alloderm is derived from human cadaveric skin screened for transmissible agents and stripped of cells that may induce rejection. It encourages revascularization and provides a template for dermal regeneration. Its shelf life is 2 years, and it is ideal for wounds with large soft tissue defects.

Biobrane is a temporary synthetic dressing consisting of a nylon mesh bonded to a silicone membrane. It aids in water loss control and reepithelialization, especially in fresh wounds at low risk for infection.

Porcine xenografts come from swine small intestinal submucosa or skin grafts that have been harvested, soaked in antibiotic and bleach, and irradiated to ensure sterility. These nonliving biologic dressings are usually frozen and have a shelf life of 2 years. Sutures or dressings secure them to a clean wound base. Grafts are assessed for necrosis or infection after about 7 days, when they may be replaced, removed, permanently grafted in, left to granulate in, or allowed to desiccate or fall off in 2 to 3 weeks. These temporary dressings relieve pain, protect vital structures, permit partial closure and granulation before final repair, and facilitate reepithelialization in surgical sites that may have poor healing. As temporary dressings, porcine grafts help predict final graft viability. They are easy to apply, readily available, and inexpensive.

Conclusions.—Many factors enter into the choice of biologic dressing material. Bioengineered devices may offer an advantage over standard wound therapy. Human cell-n-derived wound care products used for venous and diabetic ulcers may be cost effective in selected patients because treatment time is shorter, there are fewer complications, and fewer patients need admission to care facilities, offsetting the initial product cost. Use of these devices requires careful patient selection, knowledge of each product's characteristics and imitations, and further research into their cost effectiveness.

▶ Many of our referrals are from dermatologists. It is reasonable to be aware of their literature and approach to treating wounds. This concise presentation reviews biologic dressings and has a representative bibliography.

R. E. Salisbury, MD

Dermal substitutes do well on dura: Comparison of split skin grafting +/−artificial dermis for reconstruction of full-thickness calvarial defects
Wain RAJ, Shah SHA, Senarath-Yapa K, et al (Royal Preston Hosp, Lancashire, UK)
J Plast Reconstr Aesth Surg 63:e826-e828, 2010

Large, full-thickness calvarial defects present a series of significant reconstructive challenges involving a range of techniques, including local and free flaps. Occasionally these conventional methods may not be possible due to technical, or patient, factors. Artificial dermis is already widely used in burns surgery and is increasing in oncological reconstruction. We believe that artificial dermis coupled with split-thickness skin grafting provides an excellent option for closure of these defects when other techniques are not appropriate.

▶ This excellent case report clearly states that this technique is only suggested when more conventional methods for reconstruction are not available. The authors' good results mirror those of burn centers for the past 10 years.

R. E. Salisbury, MD

Evidence-based recommendations for the use of Negative Pressure Wound Therapy in traumatic wounds and reconstructive surgery: Steps towards an international consensus
Runkel N, (International Expert Panel on Negative Pressure Wound Therapy [NPWT-EP]) (Univ of Freiburg, Germany; et al)
Injury 42:S1-S12, 2011

Negative pressure wound therapy (NPWT) has become widely adopted over the last 15 years and over 1000 peer reviewed publications are available describing its use. Despite this, there remains uncertainty regarding several aspects of usage. In order to respond to this gap a global expert panel was convened to develop evidence-based recommendations describing the use of NPWT. In this paper the results of the study of evidence in traumatic wounds (including soft tissue defects, open fractures and burns) and reconstructive procedures (including flaps and grafts) are reported.

Evidence-based recommendations were obtained by a systematic review of the literature, grading of evidence, drafting of the recommendations by a global expert panel, followed by a formal consultative consensus development program in which 422 independent healthcare professionals were able to agree or disagree with the recommendations. The criteria for agreement were set at 80 approval. Evidence and recommendations were graded according to the SIGN (Scottish Intercollegiate Guidelines Network) classification system.

Twelve recommendations were developed in total; 4 for soft tissue trauma and open fracture injuries, 1 for burn injuries, 3 for flaps and 4 for skin grafts. The present evidence base is strongest for the use of NPWT on skin grafts and weakest as a primary treatment for burns. In the consultative process, 11/12 of the proposed recommendations reached the 80 agreement threshold.

The development of evidence-based recommendations for NPWT with direct validation from a large group of practicing clinicians offers a broader basis for consensus than work by an expert panel alone.

▶ The value of this article is not so much in the specific therapeutic recommendations as it is in the introduction of the concept of the importance of evidence-based recommendations for a specific therapeutic modality (negative pressure wound therapy [NPWT]). In today's world of contested funding for medical procedures and therapies, the use of evidence-based principles will likely go a long way toward securing payment (reimbursement) for procedures that are clearly documented to be effective. Having said that, one has to admit that this article provides only limited evidence that NPWT is absolutely effective and indicated, and only for 1 of the 12 applications of NPWT considered in the article, namely, use of NPWT for skin graft procedures. Using a scale of recommendations from A (must use) to D (possible benefit), most of the applications scored a B recommendation (should, but not must, use) or lower. An example of a B level recommendation in the article would be that "NPWT SHOULD be considered when primary closure is not possible after or in between debridements as a bridge to definitive closure." The reader may wish to review the results for all 12 of the applications to find further justification for a proposed usage of NPWT. In the future, one would hope that we will have many more articles reporting evidence-based recommendations for multiple aspects of plastic surgical practice.

R. L. Ruberg, MD

Extensive allergic reaction to a new wound closure device (Prineo™)
Dunst KM, Auboeck J, Zahel B, et al (General Hosp Linz, Krankenhausstrasse, Austria)
Allergy 65:798-799, 2010

Background.—New wound closure devices are being developed to permit rapid and safe skin closure. Cyanoacrylates have been especially useful as sutureless skin closure agents and facilitate rapid and easy wound closure. A two-component wound closure system (Prineo) consists of a self-adhering mesh and a liquid adhesive (octyl-2-cyanoacrylate). Allergic reactions to the adhesive alone have been reported, but a possible reaction to the combination product has now emerged.

> *Case Report.*—Woman, 44, with breast hyperplasia underwent breast reduction surgery. Subcutaneous wound closure was achieved with interrupted 3-0 glycollide/lactide copolymer absorbable sutures, with a distance of 1 cm in the deep dermis. The skin edges were approximated, then the Prineo skin closure system was applied, following manufacturer's instructions. Light bandages were used. At a routine checkup on the tenth day after surgery the patient complained of severe itching. When the self-adhering dressing was removed, there was an extensive skin reaction in the area where the Prineo system had been used. The system was removed completely and topical corticosteroid skin ointment was applied. After wound healing, the patient came for treatment of persistent skin discoloration and for diagnostic assessment. Allergy testing performed using epicutaneous patching 2 months after the initial adverse event revealed a moderate positive allergic reaction to both components of the Prineo system. Azelaic acid ointment 20% was applied for the hyperpigmentation. Four months later the site had a satisfactory scar with mild residual hyperpigmentation.

Conclusions.—The wound closure system Prineo combines the effectiveness of octyl-2-cyanoacrylate and a self-adhering mesh to achieve safe and reliable closure of long skin incisions. An adverse reaction was reported, showing that there is a potential for bothersome and possibly hazardous cutaneous responses to this system. This product is quite new and permits quick, smooth skin closures, which will make it attractive for use in surgical situations. The surgeon must be aware of the potential for severe skin reactions and inform the patient about the possibility.

▶ This is an important case report describing an allergic reaction to the new Prineo wound closure device. This device consists of a standard cyanoacrylate adhesive and a self-adhering mesh component. The case report describes a healthy patient undergoing a standard breast reduction who had the Prineo device attached to the wise pattern incisions to close them. The patient did well but developed severe pruritus and a skin reaction beneath the Prineo device, which was removed. Subsequent allergy testing revealed hypersensitivity to both the cyanoacrylate and mesh components of the device. Although hypersensitivity to cyanoacrylates has been reported, this is the first report of an allergy to the self-adhering mesh. Certainly, this is likely to be a rare event, but this patient had troublesome hyperpigmentation that took several months to resolve even with active treatment. Thus, caution is probably warranted in cosmetically sensitive areas, such as the face, arms, and legs. We will certainly get a better understanding of the true incidence with increasing adoption of the device worldwide.

G. C. Gurtner, MD

Comparison of 10 Hemostatic Dressings in a Groin Transection Model in Swine

Arnaud F, Parreño-Sadalan D, Tomori T, et al (Naval Med Res Ctr, Silver Spring, MD; Uniformed Services Univ of Health Science, Bethesda, MD; et al)
J Trauma 67:848-855, 2009

Background.—Major improvements have been made in the development of novel dressings with hemostatic properties to control heavy bleeding in noncompressible areas. To test the relative efficacy of different formulations in bleeding control, recently manufactured products need to be compared using a severe injury model.

Methods.—Ten hemostatic dressings and the standard gauze bandage were tested in anesthetized Yorkshire pigs hemorrhaged by full transection of the femoral vasculature at the level of the groin. Application of these dressings with a 5-minute compression period (at ~ 200 mm Hg) was followed with a subsequent infusion of colloid for a period of 30 minutes. Primary outcomes were survival and amount and incidence of bleeding after dressing application. Vital signs and wound temperature were continuously recorded throughout the 3-hour experimental observation.

Results.—These findings indicated that four dressings were effective in improving bleeding control and superior to the standard gauze bandage. This also correlated with increased survival rates. Absorbent property, flexibility, and the hemostatic agent itself were identified as the critical factors in controlling bleeding on a noncompressible transected vascular and tissue injury.

Conclusions.—Celox, QuikClot ACS⁺, WoundStat, and X-Sponge ranked superior in terms of low incidence of rebleeding, volume of blood loss, maintenance of mean arterial pressure >40 mm Hg, and survival.

▶ There are an incredible number of seemingly identical products that are commercially available as hemostatic aids or agents. All come with similar claims regarding their ability to stop bleeding and improve survival in the case of major hemorrhage. The authors of this study have done the surgical community in general a huge service by examining 10 different commercially available wound hemostatic agents, including mineral (zeolite, kaolin) and chitin (shrimp shell) based in granular, sponge, or gauze form. These were used in a rigorously controlled femoral artery and vein transection model in pigs to assess blood loss, toxicity, and mortality. All the dressings performed better than standard gauze dressings, which was the control. Given the large number of experimental groups, there was no statistically significant difference between 10 different agents. However, the best-performing dressings were in powder or granular form rather than rigid or block form. A combination of absorbency and activation of the clotting system seemed optimal. As these agents migrate from trauma application to more elective procedures, this article will provide a valuable source of information to compare the different products.

G. C. Gurtner, MD

Hyperbaric Oxygen: Its Mechanisms and Efficacy
Thom SR (Univ of Pennsylvania Med Ctr, Philadelphia)
Plast Reconstr Surg 127:131S-141S, 2011

Background.—This article outlines therapeutic mechanisms of hyperbaric oxygen therapy and reviews data on its efficacy for clinical problems seen by plastic and reconstructive surgeons.

Methods.—The information in this review was obtained from the peer-reviewed medical literature.

Results.—Principal mechanisms of hyperbaric oxygen are based on intracellular generation of reactive species of oxygen and nitrogen. Reactive species are recognized to play a central role in cell signal transduction cascades, and the discussion will focus on these pathways. Systematic reviews and randomized clinical trials support clinical use of hyperbaric oxygen for refractory diabetic wound-healing and radiation injuries; treatment of compromised flaps and grafts and ischemia-reperfusion disorders is supported by animal studies and a small number of clinical trials, but further studies are warranted.

Conclusions.—Clinical and mechanistic data support use of hyperbaric oxygen for a variety of disorders. Further work is needed to clarify clinical utility for some disorders and to hone patient selection criteria to improve cost efficacy.

▶ Many of us are unfamiliar with the use of hyperbaric oxygen therapy in clinical plastic surgery practice. In part, this is because hyperbaric treatment is often conducted in stand-alone, for-profit outpatient centers, giving the therapy a fringe appearance. Many of us have also taken care of difficult wounds that have been treated for months in hyperbaric facilities, often at great expense to the patient. This article provides an excellent overview of the clinical and scientific evidence for the use of hyperbaric therapy in a variety of clinical scenarios. Surprisingly, the evidence for the use of hyperbaric oxygen is best for the treatment of diabetic wounds, where randomized controlled studies have shown that hyperbaric oxygen both accelerates healing and decreases amputation rates. There are even some data suggesting that hyperbaric therapy is cost-effective in certain settings if patients are followed long enough. The data are less clear-cut for radiation injury, reperfusion injury, and the salvage of compromised flaps and grafts. Hopefully, this overview will help plastic surgeons gain a better understanding of when this modality might be useful for the difficult problems they see every day.

G. C. Gurtner, MD

Randomized clinical trial of Chinese herbal medications to reduce wound complications after mastectomy for breast carcinoma
Chen J, Lv Q, Yu M, et al (Sichuan Univ, China; et al)
Br J Surg 97:1798-1804, 2010

Background.—Ischaemia and necrosis of skin flaps is a common complication after mastectomy. This study evaluated the influence of anisodamine and *Salvia miltiorrhiza* on wound complications after mastectomy for breast cancer.

Methods.—Ninety patients undergoing mastectomy for breast carcinoma were divided into three groups. Group 1 received routine wound care, group 2 received intravenous *Salvia miltiorrhiza* after surgery for 3 days and group 3 similarly received intravenous anisodamine. Skin flaps were observed on postoperative days 4 and 8; areas of wound ischaemia and necrosis were graded and adverse events recorded.

Results.—There was no difference in demographic characteristics between the groups. At 4 days after surgery the rate of ischaemia and necrosis in groups 2 and 3 was significantly reduced compared with that in control group 1 (median wound score 6·80 *versus* 23·38, $P = 0·002$, and 3·76 *versus* 23·38, $P < 0·001$, respectively). This improvement in groups 2 and 3 continued to postoperative day 8 (both $P < 0·001$), but wound scores at this stage were better in group 3 than in group 2 (1·82 *versus* 6·92 respectively; $P = 0·022$). The volume of wound drainage was lower in group 3 than in group 1 ($P = 0·004$). The incidence of adverse effects was highest in group 3, and two patients in this group discontinued treatment. No significant complications were noted in group 2.

Conclusion.—Anisodamine and *S. miltiorrhiza* were both effective in reducing skin flap ischaemia and necrosis after mastectomy, although anisodamine was associated with a higher rate of adverse effects (Fig 1).

▶ This is a very interesting prospective randomized and carefully controlled study of the effects of 2 Chinese herbal medications on skin flap ischemia and necrosis following mastectomies, the majority of which were simple. All the operations were performed by the same surgeon in a manner clearly described. The results were evaluated by 3 doctors (identity and relationship to the operating team unknown) and a computer-assisted colorimetric analysis and were then averaged to assign each wound an ischemia-necrosis score. Both medications were administered intravenously for 3 days postoperatively, and both reduced

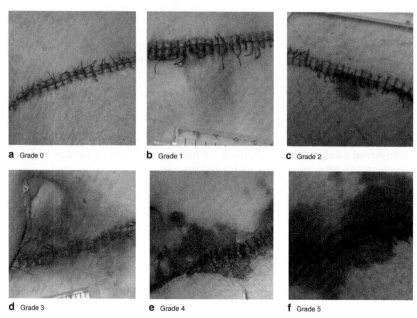

a Grade 0   **b** Grade 1   **c** Grade 2

d Grade 3   **e** Grade 4   **f** Grade 5

FIGURE 1.—Representative images showing different grades of ischaemia and necrosis. a Grade 0, normal (no ischaemia); b–f grades 1–5, increasing degree of ischaemia and necrosis. (Reprinted from Chen J, Lv Q, Yu M, et al. Randomized clinical trial of Chinese herbal medications to reduce wound complications after mastectomy for breast carcinoma. *Br J Surg.* 2010;97:1798-1804, Copyright © 2010, British Journal of Surgery Society Ltd. Reproduced with permission. Permission is granted by John Wiley & Sons Ltd on behalf of the BJSS Ltd.)

the incidence of ischemia and necrosis compared with the controls. The anisodamine, a synthetic version of a natural substance, seemed to be more effective than *Salvia*, a naturally occurring herb, but also more toxic in the sense of causing side effects. Several questions arise regarding the materials used as to their purity, their effective chemical composition, as well as dose-response curves for maximum effect. Additional studies, by other authors using similar protocols, need to be done in larger series of patients and perhaps even broadening the population studied to include other types of flaps.

S. H. Miller, MD, MPH

Adipose-Derived Stem Cells for Wound Healing Applications
Cherubino M, Rubin JP, Miljkovic N, et al (Univ of Pittsburgh, PA)
Ann Plast Surg 66:210-215, 2011

Nonhealing wounds remain a significant challenge for plastic surgeons. More than 600,000 people suffer from venous ulcers and 1.5 to 3 million people are being treated for pressure sores every year in the United States. The use of tissue engineering techniques such as stem-cell therapy and gene therapy to improve wound healing is a promising strategy. Adipose tissue represents a source of cells that may be able to enhance wound healing. Adipose-derived stem cells (ASCs) are adult stem cells that are easily harvested and of great interest for plastic surgeons. Specifically, ASCs secrete angiogenic growth factors that can induce tissue regeneration. This review describes innovative research strategies using ASCs therapies for treatment of chronic, nonhealing wounds.

▶ Wound healing remains an unmet need for millions of patients worldwide. Stem cells have been proposed to be a potential solution for this problem. For plastic surgeons, the appeal of fat-derived stem cells that could potentially be harvested through a liposuctionlike procedure is very appealing. However, significant problems remain. Despite the widespread interest and enthusiasm, the largest clinical series remains Rigotti's experience of 20 patients that was published 4 years ago. Why is this? For a potentially game changing technology, the pace of technology development has been uncomfortably slow. The reasons for this are varied, but as a specialty, the time is now for us to take a leadership position in the use of these types of approaches in patients. This article proposes a reasonable framework with which to move forward as plastic surgeons. It is important that we remain leaders in this field that is clearly within our area of expertise.

G. C. Gurtner, MD

Cell Therapy in Tendon Disorders: What Is the Current Evidence?

Obaid H, Connell D (Doncaster Royal Infirmary, UK; Royal Natl Orthopaedic Hosp, Stanmore, Middlesex, UK)
Am J Sports Med 38:2123-2132, 2010

Background.—Various types of tissue-derived cells are being experimented with for the treatment of tendinopathy, tendon repair, and use in tissue engineering.

Purpose.—The aim of this systematic review is to explore the current evidence with a view to evaluate the potential of this therapeutic intervention.

Study Design.—Systematic review.

Methods.—A review of the literature was conducted using PubMed. Search criteria included keywords "tendinopathy," "tendinitis," "tendinosis," "epicondylitis," "stem cell," and "cell therapy." Articles not written in English language were excluded.

Results.—A total number of 379 articles were identified and a critical appraisal of the relevant articles was undertaken, which encompassed human and animal research. The review included articles related to various tissue-derived cells such as tendon progenitors, adipose tissue, synovium, muscle, bone marrow, and skin. The utility of cell therapy in tissue engineering and rotator cuff repair was also assessed.

Conclusion.—With the limitation of the available evidence, the literature suggests that cell therapy is applicable and may be effective for the treatment of tendinopathy. However, further research into the precise biological mechanisms, long-term implications, and cost-effectiveness is needed.

▶ This is a really thorough well-referenced overview of the status of cell therapy in tendon disorders. If you are looking for immediate clinical applicability, this article is not for you. If you are looking to stay current and aware of what is on the horizon, this is a perfect overview.

D. J. Smith, Jr, MD

8 Grafts, Flaps, and Microsurgery

Grafts

Management of split thickness skin graft donor sites: A prospective clinical trial for comparison of five different dressing materials

Demirtas Y, Yagmur C, Soylemez F, et al (Ondokuz Mayis Univ Med School, Kurupelit, Samsun, Turkey)

Burns 36:999-1005, 2010

Introduction.—Split-thickness skin grafting (STSG) is a frequently used reconstructive technique but is associated with a large variation regarding the management of the donor site. The aim of this study is to compare five different dressings for management of the STSG donor site in a prospective trial.

Patients and Methods.—100 consecutive patients, in whom reconstruction with STSG was performed, were included into the study. The grafts are harvested in a standard manner and the donor sites were dressed with one of the following materials: Aquacel® Ag, Bactigras® with Melolin®, Comfeel® Plus Transparent, Opsite® Flexigrid and Adaptic®. The materials are compared regarding to the time required for complete epithelialization, pain sensed by the patients, incidence of infection, scar formation, ease of application and the cost.

Results.—The earliest complete epithelialization was observed for Aquacel® Ag and the latest for Bactigras® with Melolin®. Comfeel® Plus Transparent was the most painless dressing and Bactigras® with Melolin® was the most painful. The incidence of infection was highest for Bactigras® with Melolin®. Opsite® Flexigrid was the most economical dressing and Aquacel® Ag was the most expensive one.

Conclusion.—The aim is to provide the earliest complete epithelialization with minimal patient discomfort and lower cost in management of the STSG donor sites. None of the tested materials were ideal regarding these criteria, but Comfeel® Plus Transparent, as the least painful and one of the most economical materials, may be offered as the dressing of choice among the tested materials.

▶ This is an interesting prospective study to determine which of several different dressing materials placed on split-thickness graft donor sites was the best in terms of rapidity of 90% epithelialization, pain, infection rates, cost, and scar formation. Five different common materials were numbered and placed on the wounds in consecutive order, with only 1 dressing per patient. In reality, only 4 were tested, since one of the materials, Adaptic, was not always available. Perhaps even more important than the specific conclusions—that is, that Comfeel Plus Transparent was the least painful and one of the most economical materials and thus recommended—was the reaffirmation of the general principles for donor site care; donor sites should be protected by occlusive dressings that can easily be applied, remain adherent, and ideally allow visualization of the healing site. The authors were unable to determine differences in infection rate because of the small numbers of wounds studied. Furthermore, some of the statistical differences observed may be of limited practical use. For example, the 90% healing rate ranged from 8.1(.9) to 10.5(2.4), but whether or not healing of the donor site was stable without subsequent breakdown, as is not uncommon in donor site wounds, and the ultimate amount of scar formation in the healed wound was different for the dressing tested is unknown. Longer follow-up to address the questions of rates of infection and course and quality of healing need to be performed.

S. H. Miller, MD, MPH

Basic fibroblast growth factor is beneficial for postoperative color uniformity in split-thickness skin grafting
Akita S, Akino K, Yakabe A, et al (Nagasaki Univ, Japan)
Wound Repair Regen 18:560-566, 2010

Color changes of visible and exposed body surfaces, such as the face and extremities, after burn injury or surgery, such as skin grafting, flap, or sclerotherapy for vascular malformations, are sometimes a concern. The consequences reduce the satisfaction of both patients and physicians. An easy and reproducible method has not yet been established for an objective analysis of color changes; therefore, we tested a hand-held color analyzer (NF-333; Nippon Denshoku Co. Ltd) with data transport to a computer database and analysis software for posttreatment skin color change. The parameters included L, a, and b, which measure clarity, red, and yellow, respectively. Two groups were prospectively divided with 20 (11 females and nine males) patients per group. One group received skin grafting plus basic fibroblast growth factor (bFGF) spray daily and the other group received only skin grafting. The patients were randomized by the date of their first visit to our hospital. Patients were treated with bFGF on odd days, while patients who came on even days were included in the non-bFGF-treated

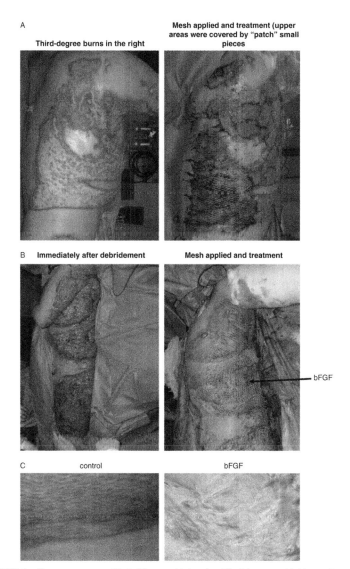

A — Third-degree burns in the right

Mesh applied and treatment (upper areas were covered by "patch" small pieces)

B — Immediately after debridement

Mesh applied and treatment

— bFGF

C — control

bFGF

FIGURE 3.—Burn torso cases. (A) A 55- year-old female with right torso thirddegree burns treated with only 0.01 in. mesh skin grafting from the lateral thigh. The right panel shows the mesh skin grafting after the complete eschar debridement over the fat tissue. (B) A 56-year-old female with left torso third-degree burns treated with basic fibroblast growth factor (bFGF) treatment and 0.01 in. split-thickness mesh skin grafting from the lateral thigh. The third-degree burn areas were debrided to the fat layer and bFGF treatment with coverage by 0.01 in. split-thickness mesh skin grafting. The bFGF spraying over the mesh skin grafting continued to complete wound healing. (C) Eighteen-months postoperatively, the close-up views of the grafted wound color match. The control skin color compared with the intact skin in the lower half showed more reddish and darker in the left, while the color of the bFGF-treated group matched well with the intact skin and showed clear in the left lower quadrant of the view. (Reprinted from Akita S, Akino K, Yakabe A, et al. Basic fibroblast growth factor is beneficial for postoperative color uniformity in split-thickness skin grafting. *Wound Repair Regen.* 2010;18:560-566, with permission from the Wound Healing Society.)

group. The donor site for skin grafting was the lateral thighs and the thickness was similar in both groups. The results were compared at 1-year posttreatment follow-up. Clinical and objective assessments of the scars were performed 1 to 1½ years after complete healing. Color change differentials in comparison with the surrounding skin were lower with bFGF treatment in all parameters ($p < 0.01$), along with clinical assessment with the Vancouver Scar Scale; therefore, the treatment contribute to a better color match with skin grafting postoperatively (Fig 3).

▶ This is an interesting addition to several previous reports on the benefits of treating skin grafts with basic fibroblast growth factor (bFGF). Previously, the authors have shown accelerated wound healing and a better quality of scar with the early administration of bFGF.[1] In this prospective, randomized study, the authors have demonstrated that grafted wounds treated with bFGF spray daily resulted in wounds, evaluated at 1 year, whose color more closely matched the surrounding skin, demonstrated by a Japan-manufactured color analyzer, than those wounds grafted but not treated with bFGF spray. Furthermore, they confirmed their earlier studies that demonstrated the benefits on overall healing of grafted sites treated with bFGF and were able to correlate the beneficial changes in healing of the grafts with the color changes documented by the color analyzer. Further studies by other centers to confirm these findings certainly seem warranted.

S. H. Miller, MD, MPH

Reference

1. Akita S, Akino K, Imaizumi T, et al. The quality of pediatric burn scars is improved by early administration of basic fibroblast growth factor. *J Burn Care Res.* 2006; 27:333-338.

Acute and Chronic Complications of Intracortical Iliac Crest Bone Grafting Versus the Traditional Corticocancellous Technique for Spinal Fusion Surgery
Lementowski PW, Lucas P, Taddonio RF (Long Island Jewish Dept of Orthopedics, Great Neck, NY; New York Med College, Valhalla)
Orthopedics 240-247, 2010 [Epub ahead of print]

Although autologous bone graft from the iliac crest is the gold standard for most spinal fusion applications, it is known to cause significant graft-site morbidity. Unlike the traditional corticocancellous allograft, the intracortical method leaves the iliac crest in continuity and decreases the surgical incision and overall area of dissection. We hypothesized this modified technique would decrease pain and complication rate. We first performed an extensive literature review to ascertain which questions, variables, and results were found to be statistically significant regarding the postoperative course and complication rates in patients who underwent iliac crest bone grafting. We then created an Iliac Crest Bone Graft survey that was mailed to 293 patients who had undergone intracortical iliac crest bone graft at our institution to assess postoperative pain and complications.

One hundred one (34.5%) surveys were returned. Differences in chronic pain between the surgical types (cervical, lumbosacral, traumatic, and scoliosis) using the intracortical technique showed a trend toward statistical significance ($F=2.42$, $P<.071$); this trend was mostly due to no chronic pain reported in the cervical and traumatic groups. Patients experiencing chronic pain at their graft site using the intracortical technique had a statistically significant difference in pain between the same incision versus a separate incision ($F=5.05$, $P<.027$), with a separate incision having lower reported pain. After meta-analyses were performed with articles obtained in the literature search using the traditional corticocancellous technique and compared to our results, the only variable that obtained statistical significance was decreased chronic pain at 2 years with the intracortical method in our study ($P<.001$).

▶ Another article from the orthopedic literature that will be of interest to hand and craniofacial surgeons who do bone grafts. This study performed both a meta-analysis of the literature and a retrospective study on nearly 300 patients who underwent iliac crest bone grafting by a single surgeon. The intent was to examine the complication rates between a corticocancellous harvesting technique (taking strips of bone in the posterior iliac crest with osteotomes) and the more familiar technique of creating a trap door in the iliac crest to harvest cancellous medullary bone. The study did not demonstrate any difference in pain, postoperative cosmesis, or complications between the two techniques. What was striking was the amount of postoperative pain at relatively late time points. In both groups, the incidence of chronic pain (ie, pain lasting more than 6 months) was 20%, chronic numbness was 30%, and nearly a quarter of the patients reported impairment in activities of daily living. Although these high complication rates may be representative of the back pain patient population studied, it serves to underscore that iliac crest bone graft harvest is a morbid procedure and should not be undertaken lightly. The use of high-cost bone graft substitute may be warranted in light of these surprising findings.

G. C. Gurtner, MD

Compaction Bone Grafting in Tibial Plateau Fracture Fixation

Veitch SW, Stroud RM, Toms AD (Royal Devon and Exeter Hosp, UK)
J Trauma 68:980-983, 2010

Background.—Displaced tibial plateau fractures are traditionally treated with internal fixation using autologous bone grafting to provide structural support. In comminuted and osteoporotic fractures, there can be insufficient autograft available for this. Fresh-frozen bone allograft is readily available in sufficient quantity to fill all voids, is relatively inexpensive, and avoids donor site morbidity.

Methods.—We describe our technique and the early clinical and radiologic results of compaction morselized bone grafting (CMBG) for displaced tibial plateau fractures using fresh-frozen allograft.

Results.—This technique has been performed since July 2006 on eight patients. One patient died of an unrelated cause 3 months after surgery and one patient failed to attend follow-up clinic. Clinical and radiologic follow-up was performed on the remaining six patients at an average 15 months (range, 12—19) after surgery. One patient underwent a manipulation under anesthesia at 3 months for knee stiffness. One patient developed a painless valgus deformity and underwent a corrective osteotomy at 15 months. The height of the tibial plateau on radiographs has been maintained to an excellent grade (less than 2 mm depression) in all but one patient.

Conclusion.—CMBG using fresh-frozen allograft in depressed tibial plateau fractures provides structural support sufficient to maintain the height of the tibial plateau, is associated with few complications in complex patients with large bone loss, and has theoretical advantages of graft incorporation and remodeling.

▶ Although this is an article from the orthopedic literature, it will be of considerable interest to plastic surgeons in the hand and craniofacial arenas. In both of these fields, there are numerous clinical scenarios where bone loss has occurred and bone grafting is required. Autologous iliac crest bone grafting is the gold standard in these situations, but in many cases, there is an inadequate amount of graft obtained. This has led to the proliferation of bone graft substitutes and bone graft extenders, few of which have much clinical evidence and all of which add considerable expense. These materials include hydroxyapatite blocks, powders, and calcium phosphate cements. The authors of this study practice in the resource-limited Canadian health care system and have developed and validated a low-cost alternative in a very challenging application. In depressed tibial plateau fractures, cadaveric femoral heads were obtained from a tissue bank and crushed into 5-mm chips and compacted into depressed tibial plateau fractures with good long-term results in 5 of 6 patients. Although the exact details of tissue processing were not provided, commercially available allografts are available in the United States and would probably be a cost-effective substitute for commercially available products.

G. C. Gurtner, MD

Clinical Flaps

The pudendal thigh flap for vaginal reconstruction: Optimising flap survival

Tham NLY, Pan W-R, Rozen WM, et al (Univ of Melbourne, Parkville, Victoria, Australia; et al)
J Plast Reconstr Aesthetic Surg 63:826-831, 2010

Background.—The pudendal thigh fasciocutaneous (PTF) flap is a useful flap in perineal reconstruction, that is reliable when small but is traditionally unreliable when large flaps are raised. Large flaps in particular, are associated with an increased incidence of apical necrosis. Thorough descriptions of the vascular anatomy of this flap have been lacking from the literature, with the current study evaluating this anatomy, aiming to provide the anatomical basis for vascular problems and for techniques to maximise its survival.

Methods.—Five unembalmed human cadaveric pelvis specimens were studied. Lead oxide injectant enabled radiographic and dissection analysis of the arterial anatomy of the integument of the perineum.

Results.—A consistent pattern of vascular supply was found in all specimens. 1: the blood supply to the pelvic floor was supplied sequentially by the posterior labial/scrotal arteries, cutaneous branches from the anterior branch of the obturator artery, and branches from the external pudendal arteries. 2: these vessels ran close to the midline, medial to the PTF flap. 3: the posterior labial/scrotal arteries were deep to the Colles' fascia and the branches from the obturator artery and external pudendal arteries were located superficial to the Colles' fascia.

Conclusion.—This study has demonstrated that the PTF flap is a three vascular territory flap and that the pedicle is situated close to the midline. This may explain why regions of the PTF flap may have a potentially precarious blood supply, and suggests that the PTF flap should be designed more medially. Given the third territory of supply to the apex of the flap, a delay procedure may help to avoid flap necrosis.

▶ The pudendal thigh fasciocutaneous (PTF) flap, sometimes called the Singapore flap, frequently is the best choice for reconstruction of defects in the perineal area and remains a useful option for partial or total vaginal reconstruction. Other musculocutaneous flaps (eg, vertical rectus abdominis or gracilis flaps) offer healthy, durable, and perhaps more reliable tissue for vaginal reconstruction but may have disadvantages in certain cases because of donor-site issues or excessive bulk. By more clearly defining the vascular supply of the PTF flap, the authors are able to recommend appropriate design alterations in the flap and provide a convincing rationale for delaying this flap before transfer, especially if a larger flap is needed as in total vaginal reconstruction. The description of the appropriate sites for thinning the flap (as illustrated in Fig 5 in the original article) is particularly useful.

R. L. Ruberg, MD

Reversed Gracilis Pedicle Flap for Coverage of a Total Knee Prosthesis
Tiengo C, Macchi V, Vigato E, et al (Univ of Padova, Italy)
J Bone Joint Surg Am 92:1640-1646, 2010

Background.—Poor wound-healing and skin necrosis are potentially devastating complications after total knee arthroplasty. Primary soft-tissue coverage with a medial or lateral gastrocnemius transposition flap is typically the first choice for reconstruction. The aim of this study was to evaluate the use of a distally based secondary-pedicle flap of the gracilis muscle for reconstruction of a soft-tissue defect.

Methods.—The characteristics of the distally based (secondary) pedicles of the gracilis muscle were studied with use of dissection (ten cadavers) and computed tomographic angiograms (fifty patients). On the basis of the anatomical features, an extended reversed gracilis flap based on the secondary pedicles was used in three patients with severe soft-tissue complications of total knee arthroplasty.

Results.—The mean number of secondary pedicles was 1.8 (range, one to four). The pedicles originated from the superficial femoral or popliteal artery. The most proximal pedicle was often the largest (mean caliber, 2.0 mm), and its point of entry into the gracilis muscle was an average (and standard deviation) of 21 ± 3.6 cm (range, 16 to 28 cm) from the ischiopubic branch. A significant positive association ($p = 0.001$; $r^2 = 0.49$) was found between the caliber of the proximal secondary pedicle and the number of other secondary pedicles. In all three patients, the adequate caliber of the secondary pedicles (as shown on preoperative computed tomographic angiograms) and good muscle vascularization confirmed the utility of the gracilis as a distally based pedicle flap.

Conclusions.—For the treatment of large soft-tissue defects of the patella or the proximal part of the knee, or for soft-tissue reconstruction over an exposed total knee prosthesis, the reversed gracilis pedicle flap

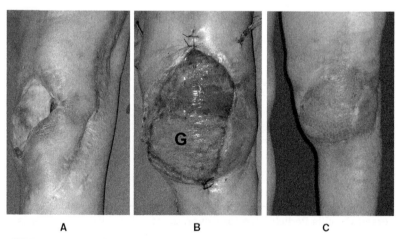

A   **B**   **C**

FIGURE 4.—Case 1. A forty-one-year-old man developed a large necrotic area of skin over the anterior surface of the knee seven days after delayed reimplantation of a knee prosthesis and a polyethylene terephthalate tendon implant. A: Surgical debridement completely exposed the prosthetic tendon and prosthetic implants. B: The distal portion of the defect was covered with a gastrocnemius pedicle flap and the gracilis (G) muscle flap was used to reconstruct the proximal half of the defect. C: Four months later, there was complete soft-tissue healing without evidence of infection. (Reprinted from Tiengo C, Macchi V, Vigato E, et al. Reversed gracilis pedicle flap for coverage of a total knee prosthesis. *J Bone Joint Surg Am.* 2010;92:1640-1646, with permission from The Journal of Bone and Joint Surgery, Incorporated.)

may be an alternative to, or may be integrated with, a lateral or medial gastrocnemius flap (Fig 4).

▶ This is an interesting, anatomical, radiographic, and clinical description of the use of reversed distally based secondary pedicled gracilis muscle flap for partial coverage of the superior aspect of the knee region, alone or in combination with a gastrocnemius flap. The key to their success was the use of computerized tomographic angiograms to document the presence of adequate secondary vessels and clamping of the primary pedicle to document actual adequacy of the blood flow through the secondary pedicles before finally committing to the use of the gracilis as a distally based flap. Needless to say, should these vessels not prove adequate, one could always convert the flap to a free flap. This variation should prove useful to reconstructive surgeons dealing with complex knee wounds, especially with the increasing numbers of knee replacements being performed in the United States.

S. H. Miller, MD, MPH

Microsurgery

Strategies to ensure success of microvascular free tissue transfer
Gardiner MD, Nanchahal J (Imperial College Healthcare NHS Trust, UK)
J Plast Reconstr Aesthet Surg 63:e665-e673, 2010

Free tissue transfer has revolutionised tissue reconstruction. Surgical technique is just one of many perioperative factors that determine the eventual outcome of the procedure. Many of these factors can be modified to ensure success. A search of the MEDLINE database using search terms related to perioperative management of free tissue transfer was performed. Further articles were identified by performing related-article searches in MEDLINE. The various perioperative factors that have been demon strated to affect clinical outcome are discussed along with the current evidence for their optimisation. We present an algorithm for the management of patients undergoing free tissue transfer.

▶ This article reviews preoperative, immediate postoperative, intraoperative, and postoperative modalities and monitoring of free tissue transfers. The authors searched the MEDLINE database and other articles to present an algorithm for the management of these patients. This is not an in-depth analysis. This is not a critical review. It is a quick read, nicely put together overview of the subject. It is also well referenced, so if you desire in-depth information, it is immediately available.

D. J. Smith, Jr, MD

Comparative Study of Different Combinations of Microvascular Anastomosis Types in a Rat Vasospasm Model: Versatility of End-to-Side Venous Anastomosis in Free Tissue Transfer for Extremity Reconstruction

Miyamoto S, Takushima A, Okazaki M, et al (Kyorin Univ School of Medicine, Tokyo, Japan)
J Trauma 66:831-834, 2009

Background.—There have been many studies comparing the patency rates of end-to-end and end-to-side microvascular anastomoses in both arteries and veins. Most of them failed to demonstrate a significant difference. The purpose of this study was to compare three different combinations of microvascular anastomoses in a rat vasospasm model, and determine which type of anastomosis is the most tolerant to vasospasm.

Methods.—Ninety Wistar rats were divided into three groups (n = 30 for each). In each group, a free pectoral skin flap was elevated and microsurgically transferred to the anterior cervical region. In group 1, end-to-end anastomoses were performed on both arteries and veins, in group 2 end-to-side anastomoses were performed on arteries and end-to-end anastomoses were performed on veins, and in group 3 end-to-end anastomoses were performed on arteries and end-to-side anastomoses were performed on veins. After revascularization, vasospasm was induced with topical epinephrine. Flap survival was assessed on day 3, and the success rates of the three groups were compared.

Results.—The flap success rate was 73.3% (22 of 30) in group 1, 66.7% (20 of 30) in group 2, and 96.7% (29 of 30) in group 3. The differences between groups 1 and 3 and between groups 2 and 3 were statistically significant. Overall, venous thrombosis was much more frequent than arterial thrombosis.

Conclusions.—In a rat epinephrine-induced vasospasm model, venous thrombosis was much more frequent than arterial thrombosis. The type of arterial anastomosis did not affect the success rate, but end-to-side venous anastomosis had a higher success rate than end-to-end venous anastomosis.

▶ This simple yet well-designed study provides useful information regarding the effectiveness of different types of anastomoses in microvascular free tissue transfer. The imposition of the vasospasm after the surgical procedure allows the anastomoses to be tested under more challenging conditions, perhaps comparable with those encountered in the clinical setting on many occasions. Certainly, the performance of an end-to-side venous anastomosis might not be possible in every clinical case, but an effort to use this approach appears justified based on the data supplied by these investigators. Of course, one must be cautious in applying rat data to human conditions. But the performance of a truly comparable randomized study on human beings would be next to impossible. So the data should be accepted as a useful (but not absolute) indicator of the value of the end-to-side venous anastomosis.

R. L. Ruberg, MD

A Minimally Invasive Technique for Burying Free Flaps and Grafts
Hartzell TL, Pribaz JJ (Brigham and Women's Hosp, Boston, MA)
J Reconstr Microsurg 27:79-82, 2011

The placement of large-volume flaps and grafts into a subcutaneous pocket often requires extensive incisions for accurate placement. We describe a technique that allows for the precise, atraumatic placement of these tissues through minimal incisions. No unusual or expensive surgical instrumentation is required, and the technique is easy to learn. We have found the technique especially useful in the augmentation of severe facial atrophy.

▶ This article is a gem. It contains 2 very clever ways of essentially blindly placing a needle deep within a subcutaneous pocket. For those of us who use free flaps or dermal fat grafts to restore volume in the breast or face (as for hemifacial microsomia), this is a very common occurrence. Suturing either of these deep within the subcutaneous pocket is essential for proper placement and the prevention of flap rolling in the perioperative period. Most of us use externally placed bolster suture tied over a xeroform pledget, although the authors of this article recommend DuoDERM or other hydrocolloid. The initial pass (from the external surface into the cavity) is performed by driving the needle into a Frazier-tip suction cannula with the suction on. The suture is then secured to the flap or graft and then the needle is grasped with 2 needle holders, one to drive the suture and the other to guard the tip, preventing snags as it is placed deep within the cavity and back out to the external surface. For any of us who have struggled to do this under direct vision, these pearls are worth their weight in gold, and I look forward to using them in my own practice in the near future.

G. C. Gurtner, MD

Postoperative monitoring of lower limb free flaps with the Cook-Swartz implantable Doppler probe: A clinical trial
Rozen WM, Enajat M, Whitaker IS, et al (Univ of Melbourne, Victoria, Australia; Uppsala Clinical Hosp, Sweden; Morriston Hosp, Swansea, UK)
Microsurgery 30:354-360, 2010

Background.—Free flaps to the lower limb have inherently high venous pressures, potentially impairing flap viability, which may lead to limb amputation if flap failure ensues. Adequate monitoring of flap perfusion is thus essential, with timely detection of flap compromise able to potentiate flap salvage. While clinical monitoring has been popularized, recent use of the implantable Doppler probe has been used with success in other free flap settings.

Methods.—A comparative study of 40 consecutive patients undergoing microvascular free flap reconstruction of lower limb defects was undertaken, with postoperative monitoring achieved with either clinical monitoring alone or the use of the Cook-Swartz implantable Doppler probe.

Results.—The use of the implantable Doppler probe was associated with salvage of 2/2 compromised flaps compared to salvage of 2/5 compromised flaps in the group undergoing clinical monitoring alone (salvage rate 100% vs. 40%, $P = 0.28$). While not statistically significant, this was a strong trend toward an improved flap salvage rate with the use of the implantable Doppler probe. There were no false positives or negatives in either group. One flap loss in the clinically monitored group resulted in limb amputation (the only amputation in the cohort).

Conclusion.—A trend toward early detection and salvage of flaps with anastomotic insufficiency was seen with the use of the Cook—Swartz implantable Doppler probe. These findings suggest a possible benefit of this technique as a stand-alone or adjunctive tool in the clinical monitoring of free flaps, with further investigation warranted into the broader application of these devices.

▶ This study makes the case, albeit without clear statistical significance, that the implantable Doppler probe allows a higher success rate in lower extremity free tissue transfers. Much has been written recently about the reliability of purely clinical monitoring in achieving a high rate of success with a whole variety of free flaps. In all likelihood, the critical factor in any of these studies is the competence and the experience of the individuals doing the clinical evaluation. The more experienced the evaluator, the less likely is there to be any additional benefit from the use of an evaluation device. So the information in this study can probably best be applied to institutions and to individuals with a lower level of experience in the monitoring of free flaps. In such circumstances, the supplementation of clinical evaluation with an implantable Doppler is likely to be of significant benefit.

R. L. Ruberg, MD

Perioperative Antibiotics in the Setting of Microvascular Free Tissue Transfer: Current Practices
Reiffel AJ, Kamdar MR, Kadouch DJM, et al (New York Presbyterian Hosp; et al)
J Reconstr Microsurg 26:401-407, 2010

Microvascular free tissue transfer is a ubiquitous and routine method of restoring anatomic defects. There is a paucity of data regarding the role of perioperative antibiotics in free tissue transfer. We designed a survey to explore usage patterns among microvascular surgeons and thereby define a standard of care. A 24-question survey regarding the perioperative antibiotic use in microvascular head and neck, breast, and lower extremity reconstruction was sent to all those members of the American Society for Reconstructive Microsurgery who had registered e-mail addresses

($n = 450$). Ninety-nine members responded. A first-generation cephalo-sporin is the most frequent choice of perioperative antibiotics across most categories: 93.5% for breast, 59.2% for head and neck, 91.1% for nontraumatic lower extremity, and 84.9% for traumatic noninfected lower extremity reconstruction. In penicillin-allergic patients, clindamycin is the most common choice. For traumatic lower extremity reconstruction in the presence of soft tissue infection or osteomyelitis, culture and sensi-tivity results determine the selection of perioperative antibiotics in 74%. A first-generation cephalosporin is the standard of care for perioperative antibiotic use in microvascular breast, head and neck, nontraumatic lower extremity, and traumatic noninfected lower extremity reconstruc-tion. No consensus exists regarding the appropriate duration of coverage. These data may serve as a guide until a large controlled prospective trial is performed and a standard of care is established.

▶ A review of clinical plastic surgery literature on prophylactic antibiotic administration reveals a dearth of carefully controlled, prospective, randomized trials. This study attempts to demonstrate the current use/trials of antibiotics in the setting of free tissue transfer through a nationwide survey. The title itself draws interest and attention given the paucity of information in the setting of free tissue transfer but does not provide support with evidence-based medicine. The authors do not provide validation of their survey tool. They do not provide the geographic distribution of surgeons or what percentage of surgeons they represent. Yet they claim to establish standard of care. I am very concerned with this. I believe the authors have a consensus of the surgeons who responded, not a standard of care. In fact, they state "These data may serve as a guide until a large controlled prospective trial is performed and a standard of care is established." Once again, this is consensus, not standard of care.

D. J. Smith, Jr, MD

Correction of hemifacial atrophy using free anterolateral thigh adipofascial flap

Teng L, Jin X, Wu G, et al (Plastic Surgery Hosp of Peking Union Med College, Beijing, PR China)

J Plast Reconstr Aesthet Surg 63:1110-1116, 2010

Treatment of hemifacial atrophy presents a challenge for reconstructive surgeons. Previous studies have described numerous methods for the correc-tion of facial asymmetry. We present our experience with treatment of hemi-facial atrophy using a microsurgical anterolateral thigh adipofascial flap procedure and other adjunctive measures. This method is similar to that used for the free anterolateral thigh flap, but only the deep fascia of the ante-rolateral thigh and subcutaneous fatty tissue above the fascia were harvested. This flap procedure was used in 32 patients with moderate or severe hemifa-cial atrophy. In the first stage, the anterolateral thigh adipofascial flap procedure was used in all the patients, of whom eight accepted a porous polyethylene implant along with the anterolateral thigh adipofascial flap to reconstruct the skeleton. In the second stage, ancillary procedures including porous polyethylene implantation, liposuction debulking, fat injection and flap re-suspension were performed to refine the outcome in 28 patients. The anterolateral thigh adipofascial flap is advantageous in that it can provide a reliable vascular pedicle with relatively thin, pliable soft tissue and direct primary closure of the donor site.

▶ The authors of this article show several impressive cases of facial contour restoration in patients with severe hemifacial atrophy. In the past, a number of different free tissue transfer techniques have been used in the management of this challenging deformity. More recently, fat injection alone has been applied in these cases, avoiding the need for more complex reconstructive techniques. The authors describe a new approach using a modification of the anterolateral thigh flap, with quite satisfactory results. Fat injection alone might still be the current first choice for relatively minor or even moderate degrees of deformity. However, in cases of severe deformity, major contour restoration can be achieved in a single stage with this flap, as opposed to multiple stages of fat grafting, which likely are required to achieve the same contour. Another important aspect of this article is the fine tuning of the initial result, which uses multiple modalities: synthetic hard-tissue implantation, liposuction, and lipoinjection. The authors show that whatever approach is used, multiple stages are required to achieve an optimal result.

R. L. Ruberg, MD

Fatty tissue atrophy of free flap used for head and neck reconstruction

Fujioka M, Masuda K, Imamura Y (Natl Hosp Organization Nagasaki Med Ctr, Ohmura, Japan)
Microsurgery 31:32-35, 2011

Background.—Many investigators have reported that microsurgical transplanted muscle shows a reduction in volume; however, changes in the size of transplanted fatty tissue have not been studied. The purpose of this study was to describe the degree of fatty tissue atrophy of microsurgical flaps.

Methods.—Nineteen patients who underwent head and neck reconstruction using free flaps between 2003 and 2008 were available for this study. They were divided into an irradiated (8 patients) and nonirradiated (11 patients) group. The free flaps used for reconstruction were rectus abdominal musculocutaneous, anterolateral thigh fasciocutaneous, and forearm flaps. This retrospective study utilized radiographs of magnetic resonance imaging or computed tomography, which were taken two to three and after six months postoperatively. The fatty tissue thickness of free flaps in each magnetic resonance imaging or computed tomography slice was measured. The transplanted fatty tissue thickness of the flap after more than six months was compared with the change in the normal fat thickness of the same slice, to avoid any bias caused by a change in diet due to the general postoperative condition.

Results.—The thickness of transplanted fatty tissue tends to decrease over period of 6–10 months after surgery. In the nonirradiated group, the mean postoperative fatty tissue thickness change in the free flaps was decreased by 15.9% (range, 0.3–31.4%). In the irradiated group, this change in the free flaps was decreased by 20.9% (range, 2.3–39.4%).

Conclusions.—Fatty tissue in free flaps shows atrophy over a period of six to nine months after surgery, and irradiation is more likely to result in severer fatty tissue atrophy.

▶ This is the first study with data documenting the atrophy of fatty tissue transferred as a free flap, so additional studies may be needed to confirm this finding. However, the information probably can be applied at this time. With 15% reduction in fatty volume expected, it would make sense to slightly overcorrect any contour reconstruction when using a flap that is largely fatty tissue. And if the predicted atrophy does not occur, in most cases, liposuction could easily be used to compensate for the failure of the expected atrophy. The data are specifically with reference to head and neck reconstruction, but it seems logical to extrapolate this finding to free flaps in other areas of the body (eg, breast) as well. The difference between 15% and 20% reductions is small enough that planning differently for radiated and nonradiated cases probably doesn't make sense.

R. L. Ruberg, MD

Aesthetic and Oncologic Outcome after Microsurgical Reconstruction of Complex Scalp and Forehead Defects after Malignant Tumor Resection: An Algorithm for Treatment

van Driel AA, Mureau MAM, Goldstein DP, et al (Erasmus Med Ctr, Rotterdam, The Netherlands; Univ Health Network, Toronto, Ontario, Canada; Univ of Washington Med Ctr, Seattle)
Plast Reconstr Surg 126:460-470, 2010

Background.—Limited follow-up data on aesthetic outcome and survival after microsurgical reconstruction of complex scalp and forehead defects are available. These data are important to improve reconstruction quality and patient counseling. The purpose of this study was to evaluate surgical, aesthetic, and oncologic outcome of free flap scalp and forehead reconstructions in the patient population of two academic centers.

Methods.—Retrospective data analysis of patients with a microsurgical reconstruction of the scalp or forehead between January of 1999 and June of 2008 was performed. Aesthetic outcome was assessed on a five-point Likert scale for flap color match, contour, and overall aesthetic result.

Results.—The group consisted of 84 patients with a mean follow-up time of 27 months (range, 1 to 95 months). Mean defect size was 134 cm^2 (range, 20 to 340 cm^2), with 46 percent full-thickness bone defects and 16 percent dura defects. The most commonly used free flaps were latissimus dorsi ($n = 34$) and anterolateral thigh ($n = 24$). Total flap failure occurred in five patients (6 percent). Disease-free survival and overall survival rates at 5 years were 57 and 65 percent, respectively. Additional operations for aesthetic reasons were performed in 19 patients (23 percent). Panel scores showed a significant lower satisfaction with reconstruction of defects that were located over the frontal scalp compared with other locations ($p = 0.004$).

Conclusions.—Microsurgical reconstruction in complex scalp and forehead defects is a safe procedure. From the authors' experience, they suggest an algorithm for reconstruction of these complex reconstructive defects that will most likely result in the best aesthetic result.

▶ This is a well-written, well-analyzed, retrospective review of 2 centers' experience with scalp and forehead reconstruction. The focus is on aesthetic and oncologic outcome, but there is much more. The detailed analysis of complications etc shows the importance of centers doing large numbers of cases. For example, failure rate is relatively comparable with other series but complications are significantly lower. The coup de gras is the algorithm. Don't be intimidated by its apparent complexity. It is nicely divided into the 3 anatomic areas necessary to replace. This is an article to put in your reference file.

D. J. Smith, Jr, MD

Iliac Crest Free Flap for Maxillary Reconstruction

Bianchi B, Ferri A, Ferrari S, et al (Univ and Hosp of Parma, Italy)
J Oral Maxillofac Surg 68:2706-2713, 2010

Purpose.—Reconstructing defects after maxillary resections presents a challenge for the reconstructive surgeon because of the critical role played by the maxillary skeleton in facial function and esthetics. Obturation, local or locoregional flaps, and soft tissue free flaps are good options for maxillary reconstruction; however, the lack of bone reconstruction often leads to ptosis of the facial tissues, particularly of the nasal base and columella, under the effects of gravity and makes it impossible to place osseous implants for dental rehabilitation. We present our experience with the iliac crest free flap for maxillary reconstruction, focusing on the advantages of this technique and particularly on flap positioning, which is dependent on defect site and size. Finally, 2 representative cases will be presented.

Patients and Methods.—Between January 1, 1996, and January 1, 2008, 14 patients were treated for maxillary reconstruction with an iliac crest free flap. In 6 patients, the floor of the orbit was included in the resection.

In 5 patients, we performed reconstructions using bone grafts harvested from the iliac crest, whereas in the remaining patient a titanium mesh was used.

Results.—All flaps were harvested and transposed. Minor complications included wound dehiscence in 2 cases, ectropion in 2, and nasal airway obstruction in 1. No major complications or donor site morbidity occurred. No oronasal communication or swallowing impairments developed in any patient. Seven patients completed oral rehabilitation with dental implant placement; the remaining 7 refused the treatment because of financial problems, and 4 patients were rehabilitated with a mobile prosthesis.

Conclusions.—The iliac crest free flap is an optimal method for maxillary defect reconstruction. The main advantages of the flap are the large amount of bone provided, its height, and the possibility of including the internal oblique muscle. Flap insetting is the key part of the procedure, and whether to use vertical or horizontal placement of the flap is the main consideration. Finally, the low rate of donor site morbidity reported in our patients, as in the recent literature, makes this flap even more safe and reliable.

▶ This article presents information that helps the reconstructive microsurgeon to choose between 3 currently recommended free flaps for bony reconstruction of maxillary defects: the scapular, fibular, and iliac crest flaps. The authors make the case for the iliac crest flap in selected cases because of the superior amount of bone available for transfer, particularly in larger defects. The addition of the internal oblique muscle to the flap greatly facilitates coverage of the transferred bone and minimizes the need for additional soft tissue manipulations. The authors have overcome one of the earlier problems with this flap, a short pedicle, by interposing an anterolateral thigh arteriovenous pedicle. The orientation of the bone needs to be tailored to the type of defect, and the article provides useful information as to how to optimize the orientation in different cases.

R. L. Ruberg, MD

The free vascularized fibular graft for bridging large skeletal defects of the upper extremity
Soucacos PN, Korompilias AV, Vekris MD, et al (Univ of Athens, Greece; Univ of Ioannina, Greece)
Microsurgery 31:190-197, 2011

Large skeletal defects of the upper extremity pose a serious clinical problem with potentially deleterious effects on both function and viability of the limb. Recent advances in the microsurgical techniques involved in free vascularized bone transfers for complex limb injuries have dramatically improved limb salvage and musculoskeletal reconstruction. This study evaluates the clinical and radiographic results of 18 patients who underwent reconstruction of large defects of the long bones of the upper extremity with free vascularized fibular bone grafts. Mean patient age was 27 years (7—43 years) and mean follow-up was 4 years (1—10 years). The results confirm the value of vascularized fibular grafts for bridging large bone defects in the upper extremity.

▶ This article provides important confirmation of the value of vascularized bone grafts (as opposed to more traditional types of reconstruction) for skeletal defects of significant size in the upper extremity. In this series, the defects averaged about 10 cm. The study showed satisfactory bony union at 37 of the 40 junction sites for the grafts that were studied. The authors rated their results as good or excellent in 94.4% of cases. An important part of the study was the evidence that free vascularized fibular grafts were applicable not only in simple cases with surgical or traumatic defects; the vascularized grafts were also effective in complex cases such as those involving previous reconstruction with resultant osteomyelitis or radiation necrosis. The bottom line appears to be that the larger the defect and the more complex the problem, the more VASCULARIZED bone, as opposed to other approaches, is needed for extremity reconstruction.

R. L. Ruberg, MD

Long-term outcome after free autogenous muscle transplantation for anal incontinence in children with anorectal malformations

Danielson J, Karlbom U, Graf W, et al (Akademiska Sjukhuset, Uppsala; et al)
J Pediatr Surg 45:2036-2040, 2010

Purpose.—Patients with high anorectal anomalies are often incontinent after reconstruction, particularly with the older forms of surgical treatment, that is, anorectal pull-through or Stephen's operations. In 1974, a new treatment for anal incontinence in children was introduced at the Akademiska Hospital: free autogenous muscle transplantation (FAMT) to the perirectal area. All the patients receiving FAMT were totally incontinent before the procedure and had no rectal sensitivity. The aim of this study was to evaluate the long-term functional outcome of this procedure.

Methods.—Twenty-two patients (17 males) operated on with FAMT below the age of 15 years were identified through records. One of the patients had died, and 2 were not available for follow-up. The remaining 19 were sent a validated bowel function questionnaire, and 15 (78.9%) of 19 patients responded (12 males). These 15 patients were compared with 15 patients with the same sex, age, and a similar malformation from our patient database.

Results.—At follow-up, after an average of 30 years postoperatively, 2 of 15 patients with FAMT had a stoma compared with 3 of 15 in the control group. The Miller incontinence score had a mean of 6.2 (median, 6; range, 0-15) in the FAMT group and 3.7 (median, 4; range, 0-12) in the control group. All patients in both groups could sense stool, and 11 of 13 patients in the FAMT group could distinguish between feces and flatus.

Conclusions.—The patients with FAMT had a slightly inferior anorectal function compared with the controls. Considering they were all totally incontinent before FAMT, we conclude that FAMT has an acceptable effect 30 years postoperatively. Therefore, we find that FAMT could be an alternative for anorectal malformation patients who are totally incontinent.

▶ While not many of us are involved with anorectal incontinence, this article is an interesting read. The ability to reevaluate a group of patients 30 years after a procedure is highly unusual. The use of free autogenous muscle transplantation (FAMT) was controversial. The high scores of the FAMT 30 years later are impressive, especially when compared with the control group. This really makes us think about the mechanism of FAMT.

D. J. Smith, Jr, MD

The inferior mesenteric vessels as recipients when performing free tissue transfer for pelvic defects following abdomino-perineal resection. A novel technique and review of intra-peritoneal recipient vessel options for microvascular transfer
Petrie NC, Chan JKK, Chave H, et al (Salisbury District Hosp, UK; Stoke Mandeville Hosp, Aylesbury, UK)
J Plast Reconstr Aesthet Surg 63:2133-2140, 2010

Successful microvascular transfer of tissue is dependent upon suitable vessels not only of the donor tissue but also at the recipient site. Congenital deformities, previous surgery, infection or irradiation at the recipient site may render vessels less suitable for this purpose. Under such circumstances it becomes desirable to identify suitable recipient vessels remote to the compromised area. In cases where external beam radiotherapy has been delivered, the superficial surface area damaged can be rather extensive precluding the use of even the longest of flap pedicles — a problem potentially addressed by searching for recipient vessels deep to the tissue planes affected. We report one such case where the inferior mesenteric vessels were used as recipient vessels for the microvascular transfer of a free Latissimus Dorsi musculocutaneous flap to reconstruct an extensive perineal defect following abdomino-perineal resection where the vessels would otherwise serve no purpose. Whilst a limited number of intra-peritoneal vessels have previously been reported as recipient vessels for free flap surgery there has not been, to our knowledge, any report of utilising the inferior mesenteric artery (Inf Mes A). Whilst based on a single case report, this article examines the literature describing microvascular transfer of tissue to compromised recipient sites and it reviews previously reported recipient vessel options available when reconstructing the perineum, abdominal wall or trunk with particular emphasis on intra-peritoneal options.

▶ This article represents only a single case report, yet it effectively introduces a new option for recipient vessels in an unusual reconstructive situation. The authors have found a limited number of reports (fewer than 10 cases) in which intra-abdominal vessels were used for free flap transfers. In this particular case, the performance of the abdominal-perineal resection freed the inferior mesenteric artery and vein for use as recipient vessels. Clearly, the combination of circumstances under which this approach might be used—previous external radiation therapy, prior vascular bypass procedures—would be unusual, but, when faced with this challenging circumstance, the authors successfully performed a novel procedure with a very satisfactory result.

R. L. Ruberg, MD

Reconstruction of an External Hemipelvectomy Defect with a Two-stage Fillet of Leg-Free Flap

Boehmler JH, Francis SH, Grawe RK, et al (The Ohio State Univ Med Ctr, Columbus)
J Reconstr Microsurg 26:271-276, 2010

The defect created by external hemipelvectomy for bone and soft tissue tumor resection is a challenge to reconstruct because of the exposure of bone, neurovascular structures, and peritoneal contents, particularly in the setting of previous radiotherapy. In a nonsalvageable limb with extensive tumor involvement and radiation damage, a free fillet of leg flap can be used to provide the necessary large volume of tissue for reconstruction without donor site morbidity. Because of the lengthy operative time for the hemipelvectomy procedure, the fillet of leg flap may be subject to long ischemia time and a subsequently compromised outcome. A two-stage fillet of leg flap for a hemipelvectomy defect was performed with two goals: to decrease ischemia time and to allow the necessary resuscitation of the patient between operative stages. Stage one was dissection of a lower fillet of leg flap, transfer and anastomosis to the contralateral femoral vessels, and temporary inset in the groin. The patient and flap were observed in the intensive care unit for several days. The patient returned to the operating room 3 days later for staged external hemipelvectomy and inset of the viable fillet of leg flap. Throughout follow-up, the reconstructive results and functional outcome were excellent.

▶ Although this represents just a single-case report, the article effectively demonstrates several important principles of reconstructive surgery. First of all, the authors are able to make effective use of a body part that would otherwise have been discarded. Also, instead of creating a new donor defect that had to be closed, the fillet-of-leg approach allowed the authors to in effect just dispose of the donor site. Then, by dividing the procedure (which had previously been done in a single lengthy operation) into 2 logical stages, the authors greatly reduced the flap ischemia time and also substantially reduced the operative time for each stage (likely reducing the chances of complications). So in this case, 2 separate shorter operations were likely to achieve a better and more reliable result than 1 very lengthy one. The postoperative photographs show what appears to be an adequate aesthetic and functional result in a very challenging case.

R. L. Ruberg, MD

Role of Microsurgery in Lower Extremity Reconstruction

Engel H, Lin C-H, Wei F-C (Chang Gung Univ, Taipei, Taiwan)
Plast Reconstr Surg 127:228S-238S, 2011

Developments in reconstructive microsurgery have heralded a new phase of limb-saving procedures. Although pedicled local fasciocutaneous or muscle flaps continue their useful role, microsurgical free tissue transfer is usually required for larger defects and also for areas without locoregional options. As this treatment modality has become more established, innovation and technical refinements have resulted in an evolution of flap surgery, including perforator and free-style free flaps, that has been applied to lower limb surgery. Effective outcome measures, bioelectronic prostheses, and composite tissue allotransplantation are the three major trends leading into a new era of lower limb reconstruction. This article outlines the role of microsurgical free tissue transfer for lower limb salvage and reconstruction.

▶ The authors present a complete but not in depth view of lower extremity reconstruction, particularly the role of microsurgery. For those doing lower extremity reconstruction day in and day out, this will probably not be helpful. For all others, this will give a quick, complete overview with excellent references. The view into the future is helpful and intriguing.

D. J. Smith, Jr, MD

Versatility of Chimeric Flap based on Thoracodorsal Vessels Incorporating Vascularized Scapular Bone and Latissimus Dorsi Myocutaneous Flap in Reconstructing Lower-extremity Bone Defects due to Osteomyelitis

Tachi M, Toriyabe S, Imai Y, et al (Tohoku Univ, Sendai, Japan; et al)
J Reconstr Microsurg 26:417-424, 2010

To treat lower-extremity osteomyelitis secondary to trauma, bone and soft tissue can be grafted at the same time using microsurgical techniques. We investigate the use of chimeric flaps based on thoracodorsal vessels incorporating vascularized scapular bone and latissimus dorsi myocutaneous flap to reconstruct bone and soft-tissue defects of the lower leg due to osteomyelitis. Ten patients with lower-extremity bone and soft-tissue defects due to osteomyelitis were treated. Vascularized scapular bones were raised on the angular branch of the thoracodorsal artery. Latissimus dorsi myocutaneous flaps were elevated simultaneously to reconstruct the soft tissue defects. All patients tolerated the procedure well. One patient developed an early venous thrombosis, which was successfully treated by thrombectomy. Mean follow-up time was 7 years and 8 months. Bone union without refracture was observed in all patients. The mean time required for bone union after surgery was 13.5 weeks. Donor-site morbidity was minimal. Chimeric flaps based on thoracodorsal vessels incorporating vascularized scapular bone and latissimus dorsi myocutaneous are safe and effective in the repair of lower-extremity bone and soft-tissue defects caused by osteomyelitis.

▶ This study is an interesting retrospective anecdotal report detailing the authors' experience with a free vascularized compound (chimeric) latissimus dorsi-scapular bone flap to treat osteomyelitis of the lower extremity. Ten patients were treated and all had complete union postoperatively, as opposed to reports of only 60% to 82% bone union in patients treated with free vascularized fibula flaps, presumably because the scapula has more cancellous bone than does the fibula.[1] Also, the authors state that donor site morbidity after this flap is far less than with the fibular flap. It is interesting that 6 of their patients had methicillin-resistant *Staphylococcus aureus* infection preoperatively and 3 did postoperatively, but the latter did not prevent healing, albeit somewhat delayed. Caveats to consider—use of scapular bone as a graft does not work well in circumferential defects because of a high incidence of postoperative fracture, and great care must be exercised to clear the recipient site of bacterial contamination and necrotic/sclerotic bone.

S. H. Miller, MD, MPH

Reference

1. Sano K, Hallock GG, Ozeki S, et al. Devastating massive knee reconstruction using the cornucopian chimera flap from the subscapular axis: two case reports. *J Reconstr Microsurg.* 2006;22:25-32.

Microsurgery for lymphedema: clinical research and long-term results
Campisi C, Bellini C, Campisi C, et al (Univ of Genoa, Italy; Inst G.Gaslini, Genoa, Italy)
Microsurgery 30:256-260, 2010

Objectives.—To report the wide clinical experience and the research studies in the microsurgical treatment of peripheral lymphedema.

Methods.—More than 1800 patients with peripheral lymphedema have been treated with microsurgical techniques. Derivative lymphatic micro-vascular procedures recognize today its most exemplary application in multiple lymphatic-venous anastomoses (LVA). In case of associated venous disease reconstructive lymphatic microsurgery techniques have been developed. Objective assessment was undertaken by water volumetry and lymphoscintigraphy.

Results.—Subjective improvement was noted in 87% of patients. Objectively, volume changes showed a significant improvement in 83%, with an average reduction of 67% of the excess volume. Of those patients followed-up, 85% have been able to discontinue the use of conservative measures, with an average follow-up of more than 10 years and average reduction in excess volume of 69%. There was a 87% reduction in the incidence of cellulitis after microsurgery.

Conclusions.—Microsurgical LVA have a place in the treatment of peripheral lymphedema, and should be the therapy of choice in patients who are not sufficiently responsive to nonsurgical treatment.

▶ This article is a little confounding to me. It has been some time since I have read or seen much in the literature about the microsurgical management of lymphedema. Now this. More than 1800 patients treated, 87% with subjective improvement, objective improvement in 83% with an average reduction of 67% of the excess volume, and 85% able to discontinue conservative measures. To be sure this speaks to the importance of a center of excellence. I am not aware of such concentrations with the United States, which implies we have not been able to reproduce these results.

D. J. Smith, Jr, MD

Miscellaneous

Professional Burnout Among Microvascular and Reconstructive Free-Flap Head and Neck Surgeons in the United States

Contag SP, Golub JS, Teknos TN, et al (Emory Voice Ctr, Atlanta, GA; Univ of Washington, Seattle; The Ohio State Univ Comprehensive Cancer Ctr, Columbus; et al)
Arch Otolaryngol Head Neck Surg 136:950-956, 2010

Objectives.—To determine the prevalence of professional burnout among microvascular free-flap (MVFF) head and neck surgeons and to identify modifiable risk factors with the intent to reduce MVFF surgeon burnout.

Design.—A cross-sectional, observational study.

Setting.—A questionnaire mailed to MVFF surgeons in the United States.

Participants.—A total of 60 MVFF surgeons.

Main Outcomes Measures.—Professional burnout was quantified using the Maslach Burnout Inventory—Human Services Study questionnaire, which defines burnout as the triad of high emotional exhaustion (EE), high depersonalization (DP), and low personal accomplishment. Additional data included demographic information and subjective assessment of professional stressors, satisfaction, self-efficacy, and support systems using Likert score scales. Potential risk factors for burnout were determined via significant association ($P < .05$) by Fisher exact tests and analyses of variance.

Results.—Of the 141 mailed surveys, 72 were returned, for a response rate of 51%, and 60 of the respondents were practicing MVFF surgeons. Two percent of the responding MVFF surgeons experienced high burnout (n = 1); 73%, moderate burnout (n = 44); and 25%, low burnout (n = 15). Compared with other otolaryngology academic faculty and department chairs, MVFF surgeons had similar or lower levels of burnout. On average, MVFF surgeons had low to moderate EE and DP scores. High EE was associated with excess workload, inadequate administration time, work invading family life, inability to care for personal health, poor perception of control over professional life, and frequency of irritable behavior toward loved ones ($P < .001$). On average, MVFF surgeons experienced high personal accomplishment.

Conclusions.—Most MVFF surgeons experience moderate professional burnout secondary to moderate EE and DP. This may be a problem of proper balance between professional obligations and personal life goals. Most MVFF surgeons, nonetheless, experience a high level of personal accomplishment in their profession.

▶ There has been a great deal of focus on the issue of burnout recently, especially in academic medical centers. This study of otolaryngologists performing significant volumes of microvascular procedures was done largely in an academic setting (87% of the respondents worked in an academic setting, and an additional 10% were in a modified academic environment). It was not surprising to find significant indicators of burnout in this high-powered group of surgeons performing complex procedures on a regular basis; what was surprising was that, for the most part, the problem existed to the same extent in other academic faculty members (ie, those not performing microsurgery) as well. However, perhaps the explanation for this comparable (and not higher) level of burnout may be that those performing this type of surgery simply don't keep doing this throughout their entire careers. Apparently, the average length of time that otolaryngologists practice this more intense form of surgery is only 7 years (T. N. Teknos, personal communication). So instead of waiting for more extreme burnout, these surgeons just stop doing microsurgical reconstruction. One might expect that the experiences of plastic surgeons doing similar procedures in areas throughout the body would be the same.

R. L. Ruberg, MD

Physicians' Perceptions, Preparedness for Reporting, and Experiences Related to Impaired and Incompetent Colleagues

DesRoches CM, Rao SR, Fromson JA, et al (Massachusetts General Hosp, Boston)

JAMA 304:187-193, 2010

Context.—Peer monitoring and reporting are the primary mechanisms for identifying physicians who are impaired or otherwise incompetent to practice, but data suggest that the rate of such reporting is lower than it should be.

Objective.—To understand physicians' beliefs, preparedness, and actual experiences related to colleagues who are impaired or incompetent to practice medicine.

Design, Setting, and Participants.—Nationally representative survey of 2938 eligible physicians practicing in the United States in 2009 in anesthesiology, cardiology, family practice, general surgery, internal medicine, pediatrics, and psychiatry. Overall, 1891 physicians (64.4%) responded.

Main Outcome Measures.—Beliefs about and preparedness for reporting and experiences with colleagues who practice medicine while impaired or who are incompetent in their medical practice.

Results.—Sixty-four percent (n = 1120) of surveyed physicians agreed with the professional commitment to report physicians who are significantly impaired or otherwise incompetent to practice. Nonetheless, only 69% (n = 1208) of physicians reported being prepared to effectively deal with impaired colleagues in their medical practice, and 64% (n = 1126) reported being so prepared to deal with incompetent colleagues. Seventeen percent (n = 309) of physicians had direct personal knowledge of a physician colleague who was incompetent to practice medicine in their hospital, group, or practice. Of those with this knowledge, 67% (n = 204) reported this colleague to the relevant authority. Underrepresented minorities and graduates of non-US medical schools were less likely than their counterparts to report, and physicians working in hospitals or medical schools were most likely to report. The most frequently cited reason for taking no action was the belief that someone else was taking care of the problem (19% [n = 58]), followed by the belief that nothing would happen as a result of the report (15% [n = 46]) and fear of retribution (12% [n = 36]).

Conclusion.—Overall, physicians support the professional commitment to report all instances of impaired or incompetent colleagues in their medical practice to a relevant authority; however, when faced with these situations, many do not report.

▶ This is an extremely important article for all physicians to read, to ponder, and to reflect upon. Universally, many people still believe that medicine is a classic profession with rights and responsibilities derived from a social contract between society and the profession established more than a century ago. Inherent in that contract was the concept that the profession should be autonomous and self-regulating and is best able to establish the standards and values that govern professional behavior and practice. This study clearly documents what many of us have believed: from the professional side at least, the social contract is broken. Unquestionably, most physicians maintain high ethical and professional standards, but the concern is with those who do not. Who is responsible for the detection and amelioration/remediation of those practitioners whose clinical practices are habitually or egregiously below the standards of care? It is disheartening to discover that more than one-third of the physicians surveyed were not certain of their obligation to report a colleague who is impaired or incompetent, one-third felt unprepared to deal with such colleagues, and a significant number of those who observed impaired or incompetent behavior in colleagues did not report such behavior. One is left with the impression that in today's practice environment, physicians themselves do not really support or feel comfortable with the obligation for self-regulation. Barriers to increased participation in self-regulation that need to be overcome before it is likely to improve are guarantees of anonymity for the reporting physician and for the complaints to be handled efficiently and justly. In addition, it is evident that professionalism is not just the responsibility of an individual physician to report incompetence but a responsibility for the entire professional community. For example, certifying and licensing boards are becoming more involved in the assessment of professionalism through their respective Maintenance of Certification and Maintenance of Licensure evaluations. To inform the decisions made by these bodies, it will be necessary for others in the community, medical societies, hospital staffs, and large medical organizations to participate in providing information about individual physician performance in the 6 core competencies, including professionalism, espoused by the Accreditation Council for Graduate Medical Education and the American Board of Medical Specialties.[1]

S. H. Miller, MD, MPH

Reference

1. American Board of Medical Specialties. About ABMS Maintenance of Certification, http://www.abms.org/Maintenance_of_Certification.

Article Index

Chapter 1: Congenital

Chapter 2: Neoplastic, Inflammatory and Degenerative Conditions

Chapter 3: Trauma

Chapter 4: Hand and Upper Extremity

Chapter 5: Aesthetic

Chapter 6: Breast

Chapter 7: Scars and Wound Healing

Chapter 8: Grafts, Flaps, and Microsurgery

Author Index

Printed and bound by CPI Group (UK) Ltd, Croydon, CR0 4YY

08/05/2025

01864678-0004